DATE DUE

DE 25 '94	MY 8 '97	JA 30 03
MR 17 '95	OC 9 '97	JE 9 03
MY 12 '95	DE 1 '97	AP 27 '04
JE 1 '95	DE 19 97	
OC 20 '95	AP 30 '98	JY 28 04
DE 8 '95	NO 30 '98	NO 18 '04
DE 22 '95	MY 01 '99	AP 29 05
AP 15 '96	MY 13 '99	DE 13 05
MY 10 '96	MY 27 '99	NO 26
RENEW	OC 21 '99	DE 19 07
MY 30 '96	NO 29 '99	OC 29
	AP 24 00	
MY 30 '96	MY 15 00	
DE 3 '96	AG 3 00	
DE 20 '96	DE 11 00	
	MY 15 01	
MR 25 '97	JE 11 01	

Deathright

DEATHRIGHT

Culture, Medicine, Politics, and the Right to Die

James M. Hoefler
with Brian E. Kamoie

Westview Press
Boulder • San Francisco • Oxford

Copyright © 1994 by James M. Hoefler

Published in 1994 in the United States of America by Westview Press, Inc., 5500 Central Avenue, Boulder, Colorado 80301-2877, and in the United Kingdom by Westview Press, 36 Lonsdale Road, Summertown, Oxford OX2 7EW

Library of Congress Cataloging-in-Publication Data
Hoefler, James M.
  Deathright : culture, medicine, politics, and the right to die /
James M. Hoefler, with Brian E. Kamoie
    p.   cm.
  Includes bibliographical references and index.
  ISBN 0-8133-1701-0 — ISBN 0-8133-1702-9 (pbk.)
  1. Right to die—Social aspects—United States.   2. Right to die—
Law and legislation—United States.   I. Kamoie, Brian E.
II. Title.
R726.H56   1994
174'.24—dc20
                                                                                      93-40907
                                                                                      CIP

Printed and bound in the United States of America

∞ The paper used in this publication meets the requirements
   of the American National Standard for Permanence of Paper
   for Printed Library Materials Z39.48-1984.

10   9   8   7   6   5   4   3   2   1

To Susan, Jill, and Jenny

Contents

9 Policy Activism, Restraint, Mediation, and the Right to Die

Tables and Figures

Tables

Figures

Preface

Policy Forces and Policymaking

Public policy is a curious thing, yet one might be excused for thinking otherwise since the policy process seems to be—and often is described as—the simple result of a straightforward transformation of public interest to government activity. Constituents—members of the community served by government—raise issues and express preferences through elections and interest-group activity. In response, these constituents get policy: a strategic and rational attempt to advance the public interest through government action. Nothing could be simpler. And nothing could be further from the truth about how public policy develops, especially when it comes to making policy in the right-to-die area.

We can understand right-to-die policy better if we think about the "policy forces" of restraint, activism, and mediation: pressures and stresses that push, pull, and shape policy into one form or another. Using this approach, one can understand the outcome of right-to-die policy at any given time, in any given place, as a product of a struggle—a mediated resultant that emerges when the forces of activism overwhelm the forces of restraint, forcing mediators to act.

Restraint

Consider first the policy forces of restraint. The fact that some issues are never raised as a matter of policy consideration is one of the big stories in any policy analysis, and the right to die is no exception. The forces of restraint often keep issues from percolating up to the attention of policymakers. And, just as importantly, once that percolation starts, these same forces of restraint can limit the scope and slow the speed of policy developments.

Policy change comes slowly in the United States, when it comes at all, because the forces of restraint are generally both inherent and formidable. Systemic forces of restraint have increasingly become sources of irritation for Americans. The separation of powers, bicameralism, single-member legislative districts, weak political parties, and federalism—all potential forces of restraint—are often at the root of complaints about bureaucratic inefficiency, gridlock, the "do-nothing Congress," and presidents who cannot seem to keep their promises. Additionally, a ruggedly individualistic political culture that tends to cast government in a skeptical light combines with an abiding faith in the hidden hand of free-market capitalism in adding to the policy inertia already built into the U.S. system.

In right-to-die cases, political culture and the constitutional system, though still important, serve only a supporting role as forces of restraint, and social and psychological predispositions in modern American society—predispositions that are manifest as a denial of mortality—take center stage. Restraint has begun to loosen its grip in recent years, however, as the forces of policy activism enable—and in some cases, force—policy-making mediators to overcome "do-nothing" inertia. Activism empowers policymakers to do more than muddle along with the status quo. It gives public servants the tools, the nerve, and the mandate to make changes in policy. The forces of activism, when they exist, work to overcome policy inertia so that at least *something*—though nothing in particular—gets done.

Activism

War, economic crises of all kinds, advancing technology, the machinations of policy entrepreneurs, traditional interest-group pressures, electoral mandates, and the magnifying (some might say distorting) effect the media have are just some of the primary factors that can serve as forces of policy activism. These forces—alone or in various combinations—stimulate the policy process by creating a climate that is friendly toward mediation. These activism forces are important not so much for shaping policy outcomes but for raising issues in the first place, in spite of the forces of restraint.

Dramatic advances in medical technology have combined with the emergence of the "rights culture" in America to create a climate that is conducive to right-to-die policymaking, despite the considerable forces of restraint that exist. To be sure, the forces of restraint have not gone away; they are simply being overwhelmed by the inexorable forces of right-to-die activism that have welled up in the past two decades or so.

Mediation

Ultimately, when restraint can no longer check the forces of activism entirely, a third sort of policy pressure enters the picture: the force of mediation. Mediation pressures shape the energy of activism, tempered by the forces of restraint, into a tangible policy response. Legislators make policy, so they are important mediation players. Presidents, governors, and mayors make policy as well; they, too, are potentially important actors in the mediation process. Judges also make policy, as do government bureaucrats and private-sector professionals. Academics and technical experts are part of the mediation process as well, although they play more of a supportive role.

Not all of these actors are equally important in mediating policy responses for every issue on the governmental agenda. The balance among them shifts with policy and with time. In the case of the right to die, the state courts have played a leading role in policy development, as has the professionalized health-care community, while state legislators have reluctantly followed along. Regardless of which set of actors pulls the strings, however—with the right to die or elsewhere in the policy milieu—it is in this world of mediation that public policy ultimately is shaped.

In the end, none of these policy forces dominate in the policy process. The forces of activism that are responsible for bringing issues to light typically lose some of their momentum once an issue gets before the mediators; just as activism overwhelms restraint to put issues on the agenda, mediation overwhelms activism in formulating policy responses. To complete the circle, the mediators hardly have carte blanche, for the mediation process is held in check by the forces of restraint. Thus, no one should be surprised if very little—if anything at all—gets done in the long run, even when the forces of activism are formidable. For the forces of restraint, the game is not lost when activism overwhelms them, for there is plenty still at stake—indeed, almost everything is still at stake—in the mediation phase of the political power game we know as the policy process.

A Case Study Application

In this book, we present the "right to die" in terms of policy forces in an effort to provide a more realistic and comprehensive analysis of this emerging issue. We do not pretend to offer the definitive and last word on the right to die in specific areas of the policy terrain we cover. In some respects, each of our chapters is worthy of a book-length treatment. Indeed, aspects of some chapters have already been covered in separate volumes elsewhere in the scholarly and popular literature. What we do here is pull together a comprehensive survey of the forces that bear directly on the right-to-die debate. We find that each set of forces we identify— activism, restraint, and mediation—represents an important dimension of the right-to-die landscape as it has existed in the recent past, as it exists today, and as it might possibly exist in the not-too-distant future.

Deathright: Whose Death, Whose Right?

The right to die is all about death but not about all kinds of death. For purposes of our analysis, we conceive of the right to die as an issue that involves primarily those individuals who are seriously ill and have little, if any, hope of recovering to the point where they could enjoy active, meaningful interactions with their surroundings. In effect, we are dealing with individuals for whom medical interventions have reached their limit of efficacy and can only now prolong the dying process. These are the types of cases we will refer to as "right-to-die scenarios" and "right-to-die situations."

Approximately 5,000 people die every day in the United States. For many, death is the result of some catastrophic event. These individuals die quickly: in automobile accidents, on mean streets, while they sleep, on operating tables, and, sometimes, over cornflakes at breakfast. For them, the right to die is hardly an issue: Death just happens. But for an increasing number of Americans, death has become a much slower and more anguishing experience. In such cases, a critical illness or injury has robbed—or is in the process of robbing—an individual of meaningful life. In these cases, the best efforts of health-care providers can only serve to forestall death in the short run and, sometimes, indefinitely. The plight of this group is the subject of our policy analysis.

Simply put, this is a book about an individual's right to choose to die. At present, caregivers often intervene to preserve dying individuals even when there is very little, if any, medically grounded hope for the patient's recovery and return to a productive life (however one measures that). We analyze these kinds of cases, in which individuals at the end of their lives wonder whether they have—or even want—the right to manage their own deaths or have them managed by someone else. Do individuals at the end of meaningful life have a deathright—the right to take the management of death into their own hands? This book is about that question.

Chapter Overview

As the chapters unfold, we attempt to lay on the table the primary forces that mold right-to-die policy across the fifty states. The first and second chapters of the book deal with the forces of restraint in this policy area. Chapter 1 addresses the denial of death that is so central to contemporary American culture. In Chapter 2 we put the American response into a cross-cultural context before trying to explain why Americans are so loath to accept mortality as a natural, expected, and accepted part of life.

Chapters 3, 4, 5, and 6 sketch the forces of activism. In Chapter 3, we discuss the important impact of medical technology in creating right-to-die scenarios. Chapter 4 reviews the erosion of trust that has characterized the doctor-patient relationship in recent decades. Chapter 5 traces the emergence of the rights culture in the United States, a development that has had major implications in many areas of civil rights in the last thirty years. In Chapter 6, we discuss what some have called the "happy-death movement": a loose collection of academic, interest-group, and professional activities designed to advance the concept of a "happy death"—a felicitous end to life for those who find themselves on death's doorstep.

Chapter 7 is the first of two chapters to lay out the forces of policy mediation. We discuss the leading role state-court judges have played in resolving right-to-die questions that have arisen as activism overwhelms restraint. Chapter 8 deals with the response of state legislatures. We find that legislators have been more sensitive than judges to the still formidable forces of restraint: Largely as a result of such restraint, legislators have tended to drag their collective feet on the issue. Chapter 9 then provides a summary analysis of the right to die. We revisit the discussion of the activism-restraint-mediation framework and make some final conclusions.

We have tried to write a book about life and death: policy life and human death. The right to die is currently an issue full of life but far from maturity. It is an issue whose time has come but one for which enduring policy decisions will only evolve with time. We hope our investigation will shed light on the policy process—a process in which policy forces associated with political culture, religious rites, government programs, economic considerations, political will, ethical claims, professionalism, legal analyses, and the legislative process blend together.

The more we understand about the pressures of activism, restraint, and mediation that push, pull, and shape the right-to-die debate, the easier it will be to explain and anticipate the policy process in more general terms. Just as importantly, the more we understand about how policy processes apply to the right to die, the more likely it is that we will be able to affect this and other important policy issues as the years unfold before us.

James M. Hoefler
Carlisle, Penn.

Acknowledgments

This book evolved over the course of several years, and many had a hand in helping in its development. While taking full responsibility for any errors of fact or judgment that remain herein, I would like to take this opportunity to acknowledge those whose advice and support were so helpful in bringing this project to fruition.

First, let me express my special thanks to Brian Kamoie. Brian played an important role as a researcher, critical thinker, and sounding board from the very beginning. He is fully deserving of the mention he receives on the title page of this volume.

I also wish to acknowledge a host of others who played lesser but still important roles in shaping *Deathright*. Pam Byron served as a valuable research assistant throughout the summer of 1992. Harry Pohlman, Gene Hickok, and Arthur Berger read and provided useful comments on early drafts of the work. Susan Feldman, Harry Krebs, Mara Donaldson, Doug Stuart, Steve Fishman, and Mark Ruhl were also among the good colleagues at Dickinson College who helped me think about different parts of the book and the book-writing process. Vickie Kuhn, as always, was a constant source of substantive, administrative, and moral support: Where would any of us in the Political Science Department be without her?

More generally, Dickinson College provided a wonderful venue for reading, writing, and thinking about public policy. The course-release time and research and financial support provided through the college by grants from the Dana and Mellon foundations made the writing of this book much easier than it would have been otherwise. Moreover, the encouragement of seemingly everyone at the college, including President Lee Fritschler, made the writing of this book seem all the more worthwhile.

Greg Lewis and Sandy Schultz and company are also due special thanks. They, together and individually, provided invaluable insights regarding an entire range of right-to-die issues. In addition, I must thank Jennifer Knerr. Not only was she willing to give a fledgling right-to-die manuscript a chance to be something more, she also demonstrated good instincts about the substance of that manuscript and even helped give the work a meaningful title when all was said and done. I am also indebted to Joan Sherman, who combed through the manuscript with great care and sensitivity, skillfully refining and tightening the argument in important and substantive ways at nearly every turn of the page.

On a more personal note, the ongoing support I have received from family and friends has been greatly appreciated. I am especially indebted to Gram, who has been an inspiration to me throughout my life and hers. Last, but not least, I must thank my wife, Susan, for helping to proofread my work, for providing an alternative perspective on various aspects of the book, for scanning the newspapers assiduously for the latest breaking stories, and especially for taking such good care of the girls while I was otherwise occupied at all hours of the day and night. It is so much easier to work with the peace of mind that comes when I think about the loving mother who tends our two beautiful daughters.

J.M.H.

1

Policy Restraint
and the Denial of Death

If you suddenly became unable to make treatment decisions about your health care, would anyone know your choices regarding treatment? Who would you want to make those decisions for you? Would that person or persons know what treatments you would accept or refuse given little or no chance for recovery?

Okay, admit it. It's not something you think about a lot. Heaven knows it isn't pleasant to think about, but the possibility does exist, nonetheless.

—*Health Smart*, 1992

THE RIGHT TO DIE may be among the most legally complex and culturally sensitive areas of civil rights to emerge in our time. The thorny issues associated with a seriously ill individual's right to make a right-to-die decision and the disposition of individuals who are incompetent to make such decisions for themselves promise to keep all parties involved—health-care professionals, medical ethicists, counselors, clerics, families, lawyers, judges, and legislators—busy for some time to come.

As the excerpt from *Health Smart* suggests, Americans do not find these sorts of end-of-life decisions easy to make. Indeed, the sentiments conveyed in this lead article of a hospital newsletter capture quite accurately the profound sense of uneasiness that Americans feel when it comes to the subject of death. Americans find the idea of "managing" death—consciously making decisions that would hasten the moment when one slips over the edge of eternity—hard to cope with. Privately and individually, decisions to end the lives of terminally ill patients have been made for years at hospital bedsides and in doctors' offices. But in public, general questions about when someone should be allowed to die have tended to be swept under the rug. Rather, the question usually is framed: What more can be done to save the life? That, it seems, is the American way.

Evidence of Denial

The shelves of the library are filled with psychology and sociology books that describe how humans, in general, and Americans, in particular, try to cope with the idea of death by denying its reality (Charmaz, 1980, p. 95). *The Denial of Death* by psychologist Ernest Becker (1973) is one of the classic and definitive texts on the subject. In his preface, Becker observes that "the idea of death, the fear of it, haunts the human animal like nothing else ... fear of death is a universal" (p. IX). It is no wonder, he opines, that we hold heroes who defy death in such high esteem. Courageous soldiers on the field of battle, fearless astronauts diving deep into space, survivors of life-threatening ordeals, and daredevils of all descriptions receive our adulation, largely because they have endured in the face of the thing we fear most: death.

Conversely, those who invite death—through suicide—court society's condemnation. Although suicide and attempted suicide are no longer illegal in most states, such acts continue to be considered a sign of weakness or a blight on one's record, something for the family to cover up if circumstances allow. Health-care and social service experts believe that the actual suicide rates for senior citizens may be twice the estimated rate because suicides are so routinely underreported, especially in this age category (Douglas, 1992).

Herman Feifel's (1959) *The Meaning of Death* is another classic work on the subject. Feifel's enduring contribution to the literature is his use of the word *taboo* to describe the status of death in American society. Revealingly, Feifel had to battle against his publisher's "better judgment" to keep that obscene, five-letter word—death—in the title of his treatise (Kastenbaum and Kastenbaum, 1989, p. VIII).

Geoffrey Gorer's classic contribution to the literature, *Death, Grief, and Mourning in Contemporary Britain* (1965), uses the term *pornographic* as a descriptor of the Western response to the subject of human mortality. And of course, there is the best-seller by Elisabeth Kübler-Ross, *On Death and Dying*, that talks about the stages one passes through upon being confronted with the prognosis "terminal." Not surprisingly, given the general tenor of the literature on death, denial is the first stage (the others are, in order, anger, bargaining, depression, and, finally, acceptance). The Kübler-Ross book has been criticized on many grounds since it was first published in 1969, but the notion that denial of death is a widespread phenomenon in contemporary Western civilization has never been seriously challenged. In fact, themes like haunting fear, taboo, pornographic, and widespread denial serve as the foundation for almost everything else that is written on the subject.

Euphemisms

One need not refer to the scholarly literature on death to find out about denial for evidence of our denial is everywhere in our culture, including our language. Proper etiquette requires us to speak in hushed and euphemistic tones when the subject of death comes up. In fact, death has a language all its own: Examples of referring to death without actually saying the word are legion and well known. All we need is a bit of context in order to determine what phraseology is most appropriate.

Cowboys *bite the dust* and after being buried are said to be *pushing up daisies*. Street gang members are *smoked* or *wasted*, although mobsters and gangsters of days gone by were more worried about being *rubbed out, deep-sixed*, or sent to *Davey Jones's locker* with *cement overshoes* on because, for them, *it was curtains*. Today's tough guys *liquidate* or *exterminate* their prey, but farmers simply *kick the bucket*. Aviators do not talk about crashing and burning; for them, *buying the farm* is the accepted expression. Those who have struggled against an illness and lost are said to finally *succumb*, and, if they had found religion by the time of their *passing*, they can be expected to *go on to their final reward* and *meet their maker*. They will find everlasting peace because they have been *called home*.

Professionals who deal with death on a regular basis have their own language, as well. The medical community talks about patients who have *expired*, the clergy speak of *the dearly departed*, and funeral directors refer to *the deceased* in earnest and compassionate tones. And members of the family do not say their loved ones died; rather, they *passed away* or *passed on*. Though some of these expressions are more vivid than others, they all serve to neutralize the event being described, sterilizing it of much of its inherent physiological meaning for the speaker and listener alike. According to Kathy Charmaz (1980, pp. 78–79), such objectifying language builds emotional distance between the speaker and the event in order to reinforce the notion that death is something that happens in the abstract and to others, not to oneself.

The same sort of evasiveness is manifested in other ways, as well. Greeting cards provide one good example. In a study of 200 "sympathy" cards (the term itself is a euphemism), Marsha McGee found that death was mentioned directly less than 3 percent of the time (cited in DeSpelder and Strickland, 1992, p. 22). The words *death* or *died* were absent in another set of 110 sympathy cards studied by McGee. Instead, the verses referred to the dead only indirectly, apparently in order to free the card's sender to choose his or her own favorite euphemism. This is done to avoid violating the cultural taboo against speaking openly and frankly about death.[1]

When one's time finally does come (yet another euphemism), families arrange calling hours in a funeral parlor, a space sometimes referred to as a "slumber room" by those for whom even the word *funeral* is a bit too descriptive and coarse. Beautifully adorned and highly polished caskets (some are sold with innerspring mattresses) are used to frame a body made up to look better than in life. Then, after all is said and done, the deceased will probably be taken to the cemetery—that *final resting place*—where those around the *dearly departed* will pray that he or she *rests in peace*. Clearly, the image being portrayed with all this language and paraphernalia is that death is really just a long nap, rather than the complete and utter end to biological life. The same even applies to family pets: They are not killed; instead, they are *put to sleep.*

Media

The media might seem to present something of a contradiction to our thesis that Americans tend to deny their own mortality. Unlike the greeting cards and personal conversations that skirt the idea of death, television, movies, and newspapers focus on death regularly in all its graphic and violent detail.

News anchors narrate vivid pictures of violent death, then beam their signals into American living rooms, kitchens, and bedrooms on a daily basis. Horrendous crimes, natural disasters, highway and airline accidents, house fires, wars, and calamities of all descriptions are always good material for a lead story; this is the stuff of which the front pages of newspapers are made. News editors serve up mortality plays daily for breakfast, lunch, and dinner. And the more death and violence, the better, especially in competitive markets where the percentage of coverage devoted to gore translates directly into percentage of market share. As the old aphorism in the news business goes, "If it bleeds, it leads."

Brutal death sells just as well in the movie theater as it does in the news. Americans are deluged with tough guys doing jobs—dirty jobs—with death as the common and natural conclusion to much of the action. The Dirty Harrys, the Rambos, the Terminators, and the Elm Street Freddie Krugers of the film world take no prisoners if they can help it. And Americans seem to eat it up. Television's one-hour death vignettes are equally popular. According to one estimate, anyone watching television on a typical weeknight will see a death once every twenty-three minutes on average (Gerbner, 1993). It is no wonder that the children of one family, when informed of their grandfather's death, asked, "Who shot him?" (cited in Humphry and Wickett, 1986, p. 63).

But why, then, given all this exposure, are Americans so afraid of death? Is this not a contradiction? Actually, what we have here is not really a contradiction but a paradox. Print and electronic media commercialize and depersonalize death. Importantly, the players are detached from the viewers: Those who perish are "others," not us or those with whom we have personal contact. Strangers die, not friends or family members. And seeing others die actually reinforces the sense of immortality that is central to the denial reflex. Viewers always emerge whole and healthy—at least physically—after being exposed to violence and death second-hand through news and entertainment outlets. The lesson derived from that kind of exposure is not that death is natural and real but that it is fictional and repressible. Thus, those touched by death in real life feel detached from the process, almost as if they are viewing a movie. They are trained by popular culture to view death as a fiction that they can emerge from unscathed after the credits roll.

There is also a forbidden-fruit attraction to death as portrayed in the media. It is almost as if viewers are driven to peep at the unthinkable, their interest piqued rather than dulled by denial instincts. Indeed, death-related violence is probably second only to sex as a drawing card in terms of the forbidden-fruit premise. As often as not, Americans get some of each in the media: Sex and death are, in this way, a natural pairing. But again, this kind of surreal exposure to death does not help individuals cope with their own mortality anymore than exposure to explicit sexual material helps them to become better lovers. Instead, saturation exposure tends to inoculate Americans against reality, and they become desensitized to the whole idea of death in the process.

In the end, violence-oriented entertainment anesthetizes us to death as a reality in our own lives. As Lynne DeSpelder and Albert Strickland (1992, p. 32) argue, death becomes something that happens to others, not to us or to those we love. Consequently, all this exposure to death fails to prepare us for the real thing. Indeed, we would argue that just the opposite occurs: When death becomes dramatized, fictionalized, and, ultimately, trivialized, we actually become less able to cope with it in real life. And thus we are shocked when death does come.

There is another side to this conundrum about our willingness—even desire—to be exposed to death in the media while denying its reality in our own lives. Deaths in American movies and on American television tend to be "deserved" rather than tragic. Americans long for happy endings where the bad guys die and the good guys—to whom the audience supposedly relates—survive. European filmmakers have noted this predisposition in Americans for years and have felt compelled to alter their products to make them more marketable in the States. In one example, the popular Dutch thriller *The Vanishing* was recut before being released in the United States. In the original version, the boyfriend of a kidnapped woman is buried alive in a grisly and tragic conclusion, but in the remake, it is the kidnapper who is treated to premature burial as part of a "happy" ending.

The Player received a similar treatment. When released in Europe, this movie included a scene involving a mistaken gas-chamber execution. When released in the United States, however, a heroic, last-minute rescue was tacked on. According to the director, "European movie goers accept film as a reflection of life's ups and downs, U.S. audiences want only the ups" ("Film Gets Upbeat Ending," 1992). Romantically optimistic endings, complete with gauzy sentimentalism and "overtly nostalgic tableaux," are actually something of a thematic paradigm in American cinema (Ray, 1985, p. 70). Americans apparently prefer to believe that bad things (e.g., death) do not happen to good people, a premise that was undoubtedly part of Harold Kushner's motivation in writing his best-selling treatise on the subject, *When Bad Things Happen to Good People* (1981). Americans need help in this area, it seems, because the entire premise—that bad things (like death) happen to regular people—is foreign to them.

Pets

Not only are Americans shocked when personally confronted with the death of friends or family, they also find it difficult to deal with the deaths of their pets. This is the whole point of *Pet Loss and Human Bereavement*, (Kay et al., 1984), a book that urges pet-care professionals to become sensitized to the problems that owners have when their pets die. The need for more sensitivity to the bereavement of pet owners evidences the strong bonds that are created between pets and owners in a society that emphasizes individualism and discounts, relative to other Western cultures, the importance of extended family relationships and extra-kinship bonds within the community. In that respect, the United States can be thought of as a lonely society, where pets often fill the emotional void that might otherwise be filled by humans.

That is why we think Americans' response to pet death can be linked to the level of denial they exhibit about human mortality. The existence of pet-loss support groups and pet-grief hotlines, pet funerals, and pet memorial parks all tend to reinforce the notion that, for many, animals have become surrogates for human companionship, thereby making reactions to pet death a corollary for reactions to human death.

Dennis Hoegh knows how seriously owners take the death of their pets; he sells 30,000 caskets and hundreds of cremation urns, plaques, and other memorials each year to bereaved former pet owners. "Pets are a part of the family for many people," he explained, "and when they die, there's a grieving process the owner goes through." Pet turkeys, skunks, snakes, and an ape have been laid to rest in Hoegh caskets, along with Charlie Lindbergh Pheasant, "a competitive fowl who used to run beside taxiing airplanes at the Jacksonville, Florida, Airport as though he were racing them. Charlie became a local celebrity, until he ventured too close to a propeller one day" ("He Fills Need," 1992). Not only was Charlie laid to rest in a donated Hoegh casket, he also had a huge funeral in which the navy marked his loss with the ultimate form of military commemoration: a missing-man formation flyby.

The pet-cemetery business has flourished in postmodern America, with over 400 parks nationwide. Bonheur Memorial Park in Maryland—the final resting place for 28,000 pets, including a goldfish and an elephant—is one of the few facilities in the nation where humans can be buried side by side with their animal friends. As one staff member there suggested, one should "think of [one's] pet as a child with four legs" (Rosenbaum, 1992). For $295, a Bonheur staff member will bathe and embalm the pet, then lay it out in an open casket for private viewing. This charge also includes burial in a deeded lot.

Another such site, the Long Island Pet Cemetery in Wantaugh, Long Island, is the final resting place for thousands of pets, including several horses from New York City's mounted police force. "Here lies Muggsie, 'born a dog, died a gentleman'" is the epitaph on one stone there (Lyall, 1991). One can also find a marker for Worries, a mouse buried in a matchbox. The politically significant dog named Checkers is buried there, as well. According to the *New York Times*, "The grave is covered with flowers, but the Nixons don't visit much" (Lyall, 1991).

Recently, the Long Island Pet Cemetery gained some notoriety when the park's owners were convicted of fraud for mishandling as many as a quarter million pet carcasses since 1984. Some dead pets were burned in mass incinerators, after which portions of the ashes were doled out to unsuspecting owners. Other pet bodies were thrown into a large open pit in the woods. According to news accounts, emotions ran high during the trial: Some pet owners challenged the defendants to fistfights in the parking lot; others scaled the fences of the pet cemetery in a hysterical effort to search for and exhume the remains of their dead pets (Lueck, 1992).

In one lawsuit, plaintiffs who had paid $1,083 in 1989 for the burial of their pet argued that finding out how their ten-year-old sheepdog had been treated had caused them to suffer psychological trauma. In August 1992, a New York State Supreme Court justice appeared to be sympathetic with the nature of the complaint and ordered the pet cemetery's owners to pay the couple $1.2 million for "tossing their dog into a mass grave instead of burying the animal under a headstone with its collar, its toys, and its pink blanket," as arranged for by the owners ("Pair Get $1.2 Million," 1992).

For pet owners hoping to keep their charges alive and out of places like the Long Island Pet Cemetery, there is increasing interest in advanced medical technologies applied for the sake of pets. For example, Buster, a seven-year-old West Highland terrier, racked up $4,000 in medical bills for his owner; Buster's veterinarian used a CAT scan to assay the dog's cancerous throat before ordering a seven-week regimen of chemotherapy and cobalt radiation treatments (Nordheimer, 1990). Americans spend over $6 billion a year on veterinary services, and pets now routinely benefit from some of the most advanced technologies available to humans, including brain and heart surgery, pacemakers, bone-marrow transplants, and nuclear medicine.

"I like to say we work out the bugs on humans and when it's safe enough, we adopt the procedures for animals," quips Dr. Michael Garvey, medical chairman of the Animal Medical Center in New York, where Buster was treated

(Nordheimer, 1990). "If expense is not a consideration, veterinary medicine can do anything on dogs and cats that we can do on human patients." Increasingly, it seems, expense is not a consideration, and pet owners will go to great lengths to prolong the lives of sick pets like Buster, even if only for another year or two. When things look hopeless, many veterinarians now even offer home visits for the purpose of euthanizing beloved pets, in an effort to make death physically and emotionally easier on animals and owners alike.

Cryonics

Less widespread but more dramatic than high-tech pet medicine and the proliferation of pet cemeteries is the growing interest in human immortality. Denial seems to have been taken to its ultimate extreme in cryogenics: Maybe we *never* have to die. Cryonic suspension, touted by some as a shortcut to immortality, involves infusing the body with glycerine, then super-cooling it in a vat of liquid nitrogen, to be maintained at −320°F until medical technology makes thawing a viable option. Glycerine is used as an embalming fluid in order to minimize damage from the crystallizing and clotting of body fluids at very low temperatures. And very low temperatures are used to minimize the deterioration of cell structures within the body's vital organs while the suspended individual waits for medical progress to catch up with his or her hopes.

Cryonicists believe that in the not-too-distant future—optimistically 50 years, more realistically 300 years—the technology required to thaw the body parts, repair any damage that results from the freezing process, and successfully treat the original cause of "death" will have been developed, making death as we understand it essentially obsolete. *The Immortalist,* the appropriately named newsletter of the American Cryonics Society, pulls no punches about the group's mission: The "goal is the preventing and reversing chronic degenerative disease including 'old age' or senile debility leading to indefinitely extended youthful good health" (M. Ettinger, 1992, p. 1).

The Prospect of Immortality, a book by Michigan physics professor Robert Ettinger (1964), is cited by advocates as the founding document of the cryonics movement. The book lays the groundwork for the science and technology used in the 1967 case of Dr. James Bedford, the first human to be cryonically suspended under controlled conditions. Since then, approximately 100 individuals (and several dozen pets) have undergone cryonic suspension.

Today, a half dozen not-for-profit cryonics associations operate in the United States as clearinghouses for information about cryonic suspension; they also provide social support for members and advocate for the cryonic alternative within the public at large. These associations have also begun serving as the legal custodians for suspended bodies in order to prevent the kind of financial foreclosures that have caused the premature thawing of nearly half of all those who have been suspended.[2] These associations typically charge about $135,000 for a full-body suspension. Part of that assessment defrays the costs of the initial infusion and suspension procedure; the remainder is placed in a trust fund. The association then uses the interest to pay the annual cooling and storage charges, leaving the principal intact.

If $135,000 is too steep a price, there is also the head-only option, available for about $40,000, though prices vary depending on the location and the state of health of the head in question. In this procedure, the head is surgically removed from the body and suspended in a hatbox-sized cylinder, in hopes that it will be thawed and reattached to a healthy body at some future time. Even more economical is the brain-only option, available for some $25,000. Of course, in this case, it would be necessary to expropriate an entire body, including the head in which the suspended brain would be surgically implanted after thawing. Approximately 500 individuals have arranged for one of these three options, including a thirty-five-year-old marine captain who, in 1991, signed up for suspension just prior to leaving for the Persian Gulf as part of the Desert Storm contingent (Cieply, 1991).

Another candidate for suspension is Thomas Donaldson, forty-six, a senior mathematician at MIMD Systems in Belmont, California. Donaldson is noteworthy because he filed a lawsuit—the first of its kind—to block state and local officials from preventing him from cryonically suspending his head before being declared legally dead. Donaldson suffers from an inoperable brain tumor and hoped to proceed with decapitation and suspension before the tumor damaged his brain any further. Unfortunately for Donaldson, he lost his case in Santa Barbara County Superior Court, and his appeal was summarily denied.

We should note that the technological feasibility of freezing and thawing is not particularly advanced at this point, and no humans have yet been the subject of experimentation. But advances are being made in this area. Cryonicists proudly note that two animals have been successfully infused with glycerine, cooled to near freezing, warmed, and reinfused with their own blood. At the lowered temperatures, neither animal showed any traditional signs of life (no heartbeat, no respiration), yet both survived the ordeal. Miles, a beagle, was revived after fifteen minutes of suspension, and Daniel, a baboon, was brought back to life after an hour on ice.

Given these successes, cryonicists assert it is only a matter of time until the same can be done with humans. And if bodies are kept at −320°F, cryonicists claim they will have all the time they will need to learn how to avoid death entirely. Even if they are wrong, however, cryonic suspension illustrates well the general predisposition of Americans to deny, equivocate, and even try to cheat when it comes to death: The United States is the only country in the world where cryonic suspension is offered. This is partly because Americans have the technology and the disposable income to spend on such things. And partly, we would argue, it is because they are more predisposed than members of other cultures to deny their own mortality.

Americans Part Ways with Death

Primitives were not particularly bothered by death. Indeed, death was accompanied by rejoicing and festivities in the early days of civilization—celebrations that survive today in the spirit of the traditional Irish wake. This was true even in the earlier days of the American experience. It has been said that death was, for the most part, a familiar friend in previous generations. What, then, has changed to make modern America so uncomfortable with the prospect?

Part of the answer can be found in reviewing the profound changes that have taken place in American death in the past hundred years, changes that have fundamentally altered the nature of dying. Death used to take place in the home. It no longer does. Death used to be common among the young. It no longer is. When old people died in the past, a significant member of the family and a respected member of the community was considered to be lost. Americans no longer seem to feel this way. Life used to be a tenuous commodity, and death might be expected to strike at any time. Americans no longer believe this to be true. And the deathbed used to be a place where family would come together to make peace with the dying individual. The deathbed is now typically located in a hospital or a long-term health-care facility, where the dying individual is physically and emotionally removed from the family.

Funerals have changed dramatically in the last hundred years or so, as well. Rituals and ceremonies that were conducted on the occasion of death used to bring people into intimate contact with the physical realities of human mortality. But the modern funeral is designed to insulate participants from reality and responsibility. Paying others to run our funerals for us means we never have to really cope with the death event. And thus, we never get a chance to prepare for our own inevitable demise.

Profound Changes:
Who Dies, Where They Die, and Why

Who dies in the United States? Where do they die? What are the typical causes of death? Answers to those questions have changed dramatically since the turn of the century. Overall death rates have dropped precipitously. More people are living longer, and fewer are dying at a young age than ever before. As R. Fulton has observed, "Increasing life expectancy and declining mortality rates have produced in contemporary America a 'death-free' generation. For the first time in history a family may expect statistically to live twenty years without the passing of one of its members" (cited in Jackson, 1980, p. 51).

The nature of death has clearly changed in this century. It has shifted from the young to the old, from the home to the institution, from an event that strikes swiftly and surely to a process that can drag on for months and even years. Not surprisingly, these dramatic changes have had an important impact on the ability of Americans to deal with death.

Death and the Home. The shift from a largely agrarian society to our current postindustrial world has had profound effects on the degree to which Americans are exposed to death. In a farm-based, multigenerational household, death—of family members and farm animals, alike—was a natural and common experience to be taken in stride. Ill members of the family were cared for in their homes, where members of the extended family lived—and died—together. In America before the twentieth century, death was an accepted part of the life cycle that spanned the birth-death continuum.

But the separation of work from residence that came along with the industrial revolution made it more difficult to attend to the sick in the home. With industrialization and geographic mobility, "the conjugal family grew more isolated from the threads of kinship, and so fewer relatives were close by in case of illness" (Starr, 1982, p. 73).

The downsizing of family residences became problematic, as well. As one observer wrote in 1913, "Fewer families occupy a single dwelling, and the tiny flat or contracted apartment no longer is sufficient to accommodate sick members of the family. ... The sick are better cared for [in hospitals] ... their presence in the home does not interrupt the occupations and exhaust the means of the wage earners. ... The day of the general home care of the sick can never return" (cited in Starr, 1982, p. 74). As Americans lost touch with caring for the sick, they also lost touch with the entire process of dying. In that respect, our society has regressed.

Today, death is an exceptional event. The classic deathbed scene, with family gathered around to say good-bye, is now largely an anachronism. Americans just do not witness much in the way of death anymore, and as with any emotionally charged phenomenon of this nature, the less contact, the harder it is to cope (Pine, 1980, p. 91). Ultimately, the technological advances and economic developments that have transformed twentieth-century society in the United States have improved our lives in many ways—but our ability to deal with death does not appear to be one of them.

Death and the Young. The medical revolution had its own important impact on the degree to which Americans were exposed to death, especially with regard to children. At the turn of the century, over half of all deaths occurred in children under fourteen. But thanks to successes in conquering childhood diseases, as well as vast improvements in prenatal, neonatal, and pediatric medicine, only 3 percent of all deaths occur in this age group today (DeSpelder and Strickland, 1992, p. 13).

The fact that half of all deaths occurred in youngsters at the turn of the century meant that many families—and probably most extended families—were touched at least once by the death of a child. Indeed, childhood death was a relatively common occurrence. Today, of course, the death of a child is a relatively rare occurrence, which is one reason why, when it does occur, it can have such a devastating impact on parents and siblings. Childhood death has certainly never been easy to accept, but relatively speaking, it was easier to deal with in the past because it was more common, in the same way that it may be easier for a family to accept the death of a child in a Third World country today. When death is a frequent visitor, it does not have such a lasting impact.

Death and the Aged. Today, it is predominantly the old who die. And in many cases, the elderly have largely been disconnected from family in particular and from mainstream society more generally.

The elderly used to represent a vital, integral part of the multigenerational family, with all members living under one roof. In the multigenerational households of the preindustrial United States, aged relatives had important family roles to play as caretakers, counselors, and sources of knowledge. But the industrial revolution brought important changes. The population began migrating to the cities, where living quarters were more cramped than they had been in an agrarian setting. Family businesses and self-sufficient farms gave way to factory work and specialized professions. The need for—and the desirability of—the multigenerational household melted away in the process.

Most modern households consist of only one or two generations: the nuclear family. As a result, those who are most likely to die are less likely than ever to have close intergenerational relationships, and when aged members of the family die today, their deaths have much less of an impact on the rest of the family. The deaths of society's senior members are not witnessed up close and personally as they were at the turn of the century, and Americans get less exposure to death as a result.

The value attached to knowledge and wisdom accumulated over a lifetime has also changed, making the old even more expendable in the fast pace of mainstream society. In the past, anyone who lived to a "ripe old age" was considered wise by definition and treated with respect (Lerner, 1977, p. 444). Today, advances in technology can be disorienting to old people. And changes in the social mores that accompanied the industrialization, urbanization, and then suburbanization of a geographically hypermobile United States have rendered obsolete much of the knowledge that old people were once thought to possess. Grandmothers now thought of as out of touch and grandfathers who are thought of as stuck in the old ways are commonly believed to have lost much of their relevance and importance to the modern American family. Moreover, there is no pressing social need or identifiable benefit for the whole family to live together anymore; Sunday, monthly, or maybe even annual visits are enough.

In addition, the very social status of the elderly has significantly eroded. Seniors of today may be more independent and active, but their lives are disconnected— physically and emotionally—from a mainstream society that is defined by their progeny. Now they live—and die—out of sight, out of mind, and maybe even out of state so that members of the younger generations are not touched by their passing to the same degree that their predecessors were in years passed. Without exposure to death, Americans have become clumsy and tentative about the whole prospect. As the connection between the aged and society has weakened, so, too, has the link between society and death. And that feeds into the denial that is already there.

Old people also became disconnected from workplace society. One hundred years ago, two-thirds of all men sixty-five and over were still in the labor force. But that picture has changed substantially since then. The surge of returning GIs after World War II helped to hasten the retirement of older workers, as the elderly were "shoehorned" out of the work force ("The Forgotten Talent Pool," 1992). The allure of early retirement in an age where increasing emphasis was placed on leisure and creature comforts added to the exodus, as did Social Security rules that tended to penalize those over sixty-five who kept working. By 1950, only 42 percent of those over the age of sixty-five were still part of the full-time work force; today, less than one American in eight continues to work past sixty-five.

For many younger Americans, being retired means being passive, even irrelevant, an attitude that is partly responsible for the declining visibility and eroding social status of older Americans in recent decades. In the nineteenth-century Calvinist tradition, old age was considered a special favor from God. There was also the notion that age provided older people an opportunity to advance their spiritual development. Thus, old people were considered worthy of veneration. But today, the "aged are both avoided and excluded from the subjectively defined worlds of many Americans" (DeSpelder and Strickland, 1992, p. 325). In the end, many of our parents and grandparents die outside the home; we hear about the death when the phone rings and an anonymous third party informs us that grandpa has passed on. And as those most likely to die in America today—the elderly—move out of the workaday limelight, so, too, does the consideration of death.

Increases in Life Expectancy and Decreases in Death Expectancy. As if the impact of changes in the social, economic, and demographic order were not effective enough in distancing Americans from death, a revolution in medicine has had profound effects on the degree to which we are exposed to people who are dying. Life expectancy in ancient Greece was a mere twenty years. Centuries later,

Christ could have been considered a relatively old man, having reached his early thirties in an era when the life expectancy was, on average, only twenty-two. By the Middle Ages, an average Englishman might live to be thirty-one or so, and a resident of the Massachusetts Bay Colony could expect to live to a ripe old age of thirty-five. By the nineteenth century, Englishmen were living, on average, into their early forties. And by 1900, the average American lived to forty-eight. Then the explosion came. In the ninety years since the turn of the century, life expectancy has increased some thirty years in the United States—a sustained increase of about four months in life expectancy for every passing year. Life expectancy had not increased that much in the previous three millennia!

Only part of this dramatic increase can be attributed to increased longevity per se, for, as we have noted, the decrease in childhood mortality has played an important part in the life-expectancy picture. Still, a number of advances in adult medicine in the last few generations have dramatically altered the nature of what kills us, with important implications for the degree to which Americans are exposed to death.

For example, at the turn of the century, illness had a relatively sudden onset, and the sick tended to die quickly. Communicable diseases were the most common cause of death then and for all of recorded history up to that time. In 1900, influenza and pneumonia were the leading causes of death in America, accounting for 12 percent of all fatalities. Tuberculosis followed close behind at 11 percent, and stomach-related disorders ranked third, at 8 percent. These kinds of afflictions, which today are easily treated with modern antibiotics, have now dropped almost completely off the chart as significant causes of death. Chronic, degenerative diseases—age-related afflictions that take a slower and more progressive pace toward death—have taken their place.

As in most other economically developed countries in the world, only about one in twelve people in the United States dies from some form of communicable disease today. Heart disease and cancer now head the list of leading causes of death: Together, these two maladies account for well over half of all U.S. fatalities. Largely as a result of this shift in causes of fatality and thanks to the many advances in medical technology that have redefined the nature of health care in this century, the deathrate in America now stands at a low tidemark of 8.6 deaths per 1,000 individuals per year—only about half of the annual deathrate that existed at the turn of the century (17 deaths per 1,000 per annum). Simply put, there is less death around and, consequently, fewer opportunities to become accustomed to it.

The Deathbed Scene. Just as the prospect of death has become more remote, the location of the deathbed scene has become more distant, as well. Before the turn of the century, a deadly illness ran its course relatively quickly, and there was usually no time and little reason to move the sick to a medical institution, assuming one were even available. Death was a frequent visitor in the home, where 80 percent of all deaths still occurred in 1900. Consequently, it was the rare child who did not come into close personal contact with death, at least once during his or her youth. And, of course, most adults had plenty of experience with it.

Today, the tables are very much reversed. Now, 80 percent of all deaths occur in a medical institution (DeSpelder and Strickland, 1992, p. 19). Death has also been transformed from an *event* into a *process* that takes place over the course of an extended period of time during which the dying individual—usually an old person—is disconnected physically and emotionally from the workaday world in which healthy Americans operate. Death is now very much an extraordinary and disconcerting experience, and, understandably, Americans find themselves struggling to adjust.

Thus, the overwhelming majority of those who die today are institutionalized, chronically ill, and elderly. They are institutionalized because they are chronically ill, they are chronically ill because they are elderly, and they are elderly because they are lucky enough to live in a time when medical advances have eliminated the causes of death that may well have struck them down much earlier in life a hundred years ago. As a result, the traditional deathbed scene of the nineteenth century has largely been replaced with scenes like the one related by Pat Conroy (1987, pp. 146–147) in his best-selling novel, *The Prince of Tides:*

> My grandmother, Tolitha Wingo, is now dying in a Charleston nursing home. ... There are times she does recognize me, when her mind is sharp and frisky and we spend the day laughing and reminiscing. But when I rise to leave, her eyes register both fear and betrayal. She clutches my hand in a hard, blue-veined grip and pleads, "Take me with you, Tom. I refuse to die among strangers. Please, Tom. I know you understand that, at least." My departures kill her a little bit more each time. She breaks my heart. I love her as much as I love anyone in the world, yet I do not allow her to live with me. I lack the courage to feed her, to clean up her shit, to ease her pain, to assuage the abysmal depths of her loneliness and exile. Because I am an American, I let her die by degrees, isolated and abandoned by her family. She often asks me to murder her as an act of kindness and charity. I barely have the courage to visit her.
>
> At the front desk of the nursing home, I spend a great deal of my time arguing with the doctors and nurses. I scream at them and tell them what an extraordinary woman is living among them, a woman worthy of their consideration and tenderness. I complain about their coldness and unprofessionalism. I claim that they treat old people like meat carcasses hanging on steel hooks in freezers. There is one nurse who ... told me, "If she's such an extraordinary woman, Mr. Wingo, why did her family put her in this hellhole to rot away? Tolitha ain't meat and we don't treat her as such. The poor chile just got old and she didn't walk in here by herself. She was dragged in here by you, against her will." ... I am the architect of my grandmother's final days on earth, and because of a singular absence of nerve and grace, I have helped make them

squalid, unbearable, and despairing. Whenever I kiss her, my kisses mask the artifice of a traitor. When I brought her to the nursing home, I told her we were going for a long ride in the country. I did not lie ... the ride has not yet ended.

It is clear that those most likely to die—the elderly—have been segregated from the mainstream to the point where their lives and deaths are not viewed as particularly relevant to the rest of society. Kin, friends, and acquaintances have stepped back from the deathbed, both literally and figuratively, as hospitals and nursing homes now fulfill the role of deathbed host. As a result, the opportunities to be exposed to death are far fewer, less intimate, and more drawn out.

In the end, Americans feel out of place in the foreign, intimidating, antiseptic surroundings of a hospital or nursing home, as they struggle to find the right words during brief and irregular visits. Seeing death in this light, it is no wonder that they have come to fear and deny it. Intimate experiences with death and home-based care for the dying have been traded away for an institutional setting and all the benefits of professional attention and sophisticated technology. But our ability to cope with death has suffered mightily in the process.

Making Arrangements:
The Rise of the Funeral Business

The changes in who dies, where, and why since the turn of the century have put distance between American society and dying. But what happens when we are dead? Answers to that question have changed dramatically in the last century, as well. These changes, too, have built a buffer between Americans and mortality, insulating them from death in ways that makes it harder to accept in the long run.

In nineteenth-century America, family members of the deceased were responsible for washing and dressing the dead body, in preparation for viewing. Public viewing of the body took place in the home, usually in a parlor room that was specifically set aside for just such occasions. Undertakers were available, but often, their role was restricted to renting funeral paraphernalia that could be used to adorn the viewing room. Family members touched and felt the dead body, bringing them into intimate contact with the physiological reality of death. Moreover, a family member, a neighbor, or occasionally a local carpenter was responsible for building a simple coffin. Sometimes, a prefabricated, one-size-fits-all container had to be purchased, and if the body was too big to fit, the legs of the deceased were broken by friends or family members so that the box would, at last, accommodate the corpse. Members of the family would also dig the grave and see to it that it was filled in after its contents were respectfully deposited. Children were present throughout.

During the Civil War, the problems associated with sending dead bodies home—in rotting condition—over long distances helped give rise to the techniques and respectability of embalming. Gradually, from that point on, Americans began ceding responsibility for handling the deceased to members of an increasingly professionalized and commercialized class of entrepreneur: the incorporated funeral director. Today, funeral directors soften the touch of death, making it "friendly," to the degree possible (Aries, cited in Charmaz, 1980, p. 188), by taking full responsibility for everything from the point of death onward.

Funeral directors remove the body from the home or hospital, putting emotional and physical distance between the deceased and his or her family. Then, safely in the basement of the mortuary, funeral directors work their cosmetic miracles to restore the body to a peaceful, almost healthy-looking pose. This, of course, puts even more distance between the survivors of the deceased and the reality of death. Indeed, cosmetic restoration symbolizes our predisposition to waffle about what happens to us at the end of life. Restoring the body—primarily the face—to a vision of an earlier time, before age and disability took their toll, literally masks death, making it easy to set aside the reality of growing old and ill in favor of a more soothing fantasy.

Of course, public viewing has been removed from the home, as well. And as the body is displayed in the commercial parlor, someone else is paid to dig the grave. The excavated dirt is covered up with little green rolls of simulated grass carpeting, lest we dwell during the graveside service on the dirt that will soon cover the deceased. The grave is filled in only after family and friends are safely out of earshot and eyesight, and the body beneath that dirt has been embalmed and sealed in a casket that purportedly prevents decay (as if that should make a difference). This knowledge, too, puts emotional distance between us and the physical realities of death.

Some see the entire American funeral ceremony as having taken on the characteristics of a staged production, with the funeral director (appropriately named) serving as the theatrical choreographer, stage manager, and overall producer of the death-scene vignette (Turner and Edgely, cited in Charmaz, 1980, p. 201). The attentive funeral director ensures that the death scenes are appropriately staged (in the parlor room and at the gravesite) and attends to the props (the casket, candles, flowers, carpet, curtains, and so on) in order to set the appropriate tenor for the occasion. Funeral directors also set the mood by presenting a solemn but supportive demeanor, accompanied by a bit of organ music lilting softly in the background. Casting is something else the funeral director manages, identifying pallbearers and sometimes securing a member of the clergy to conduct the religious portion of the service. And, of course, the funeral director manages the action, positioning the members of the family at the funeral parlor, at the service, and at the gravesite, regulating the flow of visitors, and choreographing the vehicle procession between parlor, church, and cemetery. It is not uncommon for funeral directors to even help visitors with their "lines" when they whisper, "How should I act?" and "What should I say?" before confronting members of the family.

The whole production takes on a fantasylike character. The players are relieved of almost all responsibility in this scenario: They have only to follow directions and to go through the motions without ever really confronting, in a personal and physical way, the body or the event. All this effort is designed to tame death, euphemizing it and sanitizing it of its true meaning in order to make it more palatable, at least in the short run. Of course, in the long run, death becomes more foreign, less natural, and, ultimately, less acceptable to our everyday state of consciousness. Funeral directors make it easy to compartmentalize death by coaching us along and allowing us to turn exposure to death on and off, at will. (A Mississippi mortuary now offers "drive-in" service, in which mourners can pull up to a window—as with a drive-in bank teller—and push a button to select one of two dead people. The selected corpse will be displayed on a color television monitor.) It is no wonder we have become less and less at ease with death over the years.

Summary: Policy Restraint and Death

Changes in funerals, families, and medicine represent a confluence of forces that have dramatically decreased the typical American's exposure to death. This, in turn, has led to a decline in the degree to which Americans seem willing and able to take responsibility for the dying and the dead. Changes in family structures have served to break up the multigenerational household, isolating the old to the point where their families and society have almost no responsibility for their emotional and physical well-being as they approach—and live through—the dying time. And the great advances that have been made in medicine have led to the institutionalization of medical care for those who cannot see to their own health needs, relieving Americans of that heretofore family- and home-based responsibility. Then, when the dying is done, professionally directed funerals relieve us of the responsibility for dealing with dead kin.

All the distance that Americans have put between themselves and death is symptomatic of the denial that is so much a part of modern culture. The euphemisms sugarcoat death, and the overexposure the media provide only serves to objectify death to the point where Americans become numb to their own mortality. Indeed, Americans are so obsessed with and repulsed by death that they cannot even seem to cope with the mortality of their pets. Some have even turned to cryonics—both for themselves and for their pets—in a desperate effort to prevent the inevitable.

In the end, according to David R. Counts (1980, p. 39), "The institutionalization of death and the dehumanization of the dying has become something of a *cause celebre* in North American society." The jobs of caring for the aged and infirm that were traditionally assigned to families have now passed into the hands of strangers employed by bureaucratic institutions. With the transfer of responsibility for caring for the dying goes the ability to prepare for death. "And therein," writes Counts, "lies the problem. It seems not so much that the preparation for death is done badly as that it is hardly done at all."

Part of the willingness of Americans to divorce themselves from death may have to do with its demystification. In cultures where a belief in ghosts and hauntings is prevalent, it is important for friends and family members to make peace with the dying. Attending the deathbed scene and settling old disputes in richly personal encounters is a part of this process. To a degree, this is prompted by a fear that a restless soul, having died without resolving important conflicts with the living, would come back to haunt his or her survivors. The side payments of this belief, of course, are that the dying are not left alone and that the living become accustomed to death. In the less superstitious modern United States, less importance is attached to making peace in any ritualistic way that brings the living and the dying into intimate contact during the dying process. That may help explain why attending to the dying slipped so easily as a priority in American society over the last hundred years.

Whatever the reason, however, it is clear that developments in the twentieth century have fundamentally disconnected life and death in America. This was a radical departure for a society in which care of the dying and disposition of the deceased had traditionally been the responsibility of family and friends. Death was difficult to deny before the modern age since there was simply too much of it around. But geographic mobility increased the emotional and social distance between family members, and industrialization helped put senior citizens—those most likely to die—out to pasture. And urbanization facilitated the scattering of the extended family and precipitated the abdication of responsibility of caring for both the dying (to hospitals) and the dead (to funeral directors).

Charles Jackson (1980, pp. 52–53) sums up developments well when he notes that "in the present century, Americans have been steadily reducing the degree of time and resources they are willing to provide the dead." Largely as a result, he concludes, we end up "treating the dead badly. We avoid them, isolate them, and generally approach them as if their status were an embarrassment ... such treatment is not surprising in a culture which has allowed so much distance to develop between itself and the dead." As a matter of fact, it is to be expected in a culture so obsessed with the denial of death. It is not surprising, then, that public policies having anything to do with death have developed slowly. Indeed, given the tide of denial and the drift of the life-death disconnection in modern American society, it is a wonder that policymaking in the area of death has any vitality at all.

2

Policy Restraint and the Cultural Context of Death

SURELY, THE FEAR OF DEATH is not unique to citizens of the United States. Nor is the avoidance of death a new development. Interest in perpetual life can be traced across cultures and through the ages. The Egyptians, for example, mummified the dead, sometimes alongside their mummified pets. And Ponce de Leon is just one of many who sought a "fountain of youth"—some spa, elixir, life-style, or treatment that would provide a measure of immortality for those who chose to indulge themselves in the hope of everlasting life. So the easy and short answer is no, Americans are not unique either with regard to their fear of death or with regard to their interest in avoiding it.

Americans are unique, however, in the *degree* to which they deny their own mortality. For whatever reason, other societies generally seem to be more at ease with death and dying. A brief survey of other Western and non-Western cultures will put the American treatment of death into context. Then we will turn back to the United States to wrestle with the underlying question of why this is true. The nature of American culture, it turns out, holds some telling clues to the answer.

Other Cultures

Those who study the culture of death note that there seems to be a dividing line between Western and non-Western cultures. Western European civilization as a whole seems more uncomfortable with the idea of death than civilizations that evolved separately from the West. For instance, "the Chinese look upon death not with fear, but with pleasure" (Rzhevsky, cited in Charmaz, 1980, p. 87). Russians likewise seem fatalistic when compared with those living in Western European countries (Charmaz). Indeed, for whatever reason, cultures outside Western Europe seem less troubled by the prospect of death, Becker's claims about the universal nature of death fear notwithstanding. A brief survey of some non-Western cultures will help to illustrate the point.

Non-Western Cultures

Kwasi Wiredu (1990) notes that African societies tend to be deeply communalistic: Africans are defined by their relations to the social order as much as by who and what they are as individuals. According to Wiredu, the Akan society of Ghana is representative of others on the continent in this regard.

The Akan, he states, put great weight on the web of social bonds that link the individual with immediate family members and other kin. Clan members also play a role in looking after the good of the individual. Absent from the Akan culture are the economic and individualistic considerations that make the right to die so problematic in Western societies. The Akan are religious and do believe in a supreme being, but they look to humanistic ethics as guides to behavior when it comes to dealing with death. If questions about a right to die are raised when a seriously ill individual is unable to speak for him- or herself, the Akan defer to the family's judgment.

DeSpelder and Strickland (1992, p. 62) note that the LoDagaa people of Northern Ghana take a similarly communalistic approach to death. They do not fear death but confront it openly in long and elaborate funeral ceremonies. Mass participation by the community is an important feature of mourning rituals, and when young members of the community show signs of fear, they are socialized to accept death by being invited to participate in digging a grave for the deceased.

In the Islamic perspective, as M. Adil Al Aseer (1990) writes, death is viewed as merely a stage in human existence. Though Islamic teachings lay down strict prohibitions against outright suicide, natural death—or death for a good cause—is not to be feared. Indeed, deaths under such circumstances are welcomed. And despite their conservative reputation, Islamic courts have tended to take a progressive "benefits-burdens" approach in considering the preferences of the medical community and family and the good of society in general when weighing end-of-life decisions for terminally ill patients.

The Japanese exhibit what is probably the most interesting approach to death of any of the non-Western cultures typically studied. With its "kingdom of suicide" reputation, Japan tends to go farther along the right-to-die road than any other non-Western society. The Japanese have traditionally been indifferent to death, lacking the tenacity for life that is more common among Western cultures (Kato, 1990, p. 71). Under some conditions, they actually glorify the act of suicide. Examples include hara-kiri, the ultimate act of chivalry, and kamikaze acts, representing the ultimate sacrifice for love of country.

Buddhist traditions help explain the acceptance of death in Japan. A central tenet of Buddhism is captured in the word *mūjo*, meaning impermanence. All things in life, according to mūjo, have a fleeting, almost evanescent, quality to them. A Western phrase that might begin to capture the notion would be "all good things must come to an end"—but mūjo does not have the same grave, foreboding tenor that the Western translation has. According to mūjo, cherry blossoms will fade, pastoral summer days will pass, golden autumn leaves will fall, and blankets of snow will melt with the morning sunlight. So, too, will life fade to death. As such, death is not an extraordinary event but one of many endings in the cosmic scheme of things. In this sense, Buddhism is a very progressive religion, looking forward and accepting change as a natural state of the earthly world (LaFleur, 1974, pp. 229–232), where the fine line between life and death is not particularly distinct or significant. This, of course, contrasts substantially with the more conservative Judeo-Christian tradition in which change and death are both things to resist.

These Buddhist influences have been largely responsible for the Japanese attitude that elevates *sonshi*, or beautiful death with dignity (Kato, 1990, p. 80), to such prominence. In addition, religious influences lead more people in Japan than in any of the leading nineteen industrial nations to believe in reincarnation: 51 percent (cited in Shapiro, 1992, p. 39). The prospect of worldly life after death may very well make it easier for the Japanese to treat death as just another phase of existence. It is only recently—with the Westernization of Japan's culture, where a premium is put on individuality and technology—that euthanasia has become a "problem" for the Japanese.

Western Cultures

Feelings about death in Western cultures seem to be arrayed along a wider continuum than they are outside the West. Attitudes range from the sublime denial of death (as in the United States) to an open acceptance of euthanasia (as in the Netherlands), with attitudes in other cultures falling somewhere between these two extremes.

Europe. No Western culture rivals that of the Netherlands when it comes to acceptance of death for the Dutch tacitly accept euthanasia. Indeed, the Netherlands leads the world in assisted suicides, with an estimated 2,300 cases of mercy killing annually (Katzman, 1992). Although euthanasia had been expressly prohibited by statute until 1993, the law was never enforced by Dutch courts for at least four reasons.

First and maybe most importantly, Dutch physicians have maintained an exalted position in society over the years. Rarely do patients or their families sue physicians for medical malpractice. Second, the Netherlands is a small country with a relatively homogeneous population that has a long tradition of taking liberal positions on issues related to family and morality. The Dutch attitude with regard to the right to die fits nicely into this mold. Third, there is the influence of religion or, rather, the lack thereof. The sway of the relatively conservative Roman Catholic church is not nearly as strong among the Dutch people as it is among other Western Europeans. Indeed, even though 37 percent of the Dutch claim Roman Catholicism as their religion, these Catholics are renowned for their progressive, antiestablishment rejection of dogmatic pronouncements from the religious hierarchy. Add to this progressive Catholic tradition the fact that nearly two-thirds of the rest of the population claim no religious denomination at all and it becomes clear why Dutch soil has been such fertile ground for the euthanasia movement (Humphry and Wickett, 1986, p. 180). Fourth and finally, the judiciary in the Netherlands has a long-standing liberal tradition when it comes to individual rights. Dutch judges (like Dutch physicians) are held in the highest esteem, and when the judiciary speaks, its decisions are rarely rejected by the legislature or by the body politic more generally. So when the Dutch Supreme Court issued its important *Schoonheim* decision on euthanasia in 1976, this tended to carry much more weight than the New Jersey Supreme Court's *Quinlan* decision—a far more modest ruling—rendered the same year (see Chapters 6 and 7 for more on the case of Karen Ann Quinlan). The details of that Dutch case are worth retelling to add some context to the acceptance of mercy killing in the Netherlands.

Dr. Schoonheim was the attending physician for Marie Barendregt, a ninety-three-year-old nursing-home resident who had signed a declaration directing Schoonheim to terminate her life by medical means. Barendregt was bedridden with a fractured hip and could sit up only with help. In addition, she was permanently catheterized and almost totally dependent on the nursing staff for feeding, bathing, and toileting. Through all this, she remained fully conscious, coherent, and adamant about being put out of her misery. After having consulted with his patient, the patient's son, two other independent physicians, and the nursing-home staff, Dr. Schoonheim finally acquiesced. Schoonheim administered a series of three injections, the first of which put her to sleep and the last of which arrested her breathing and caused her death.

Schoonheim was charged and convicted of violating the Dutch Homicide Act. But on appeal to the Dutch Supreme Court, he was acquitted of all wrongdoing. In its decision, the Dutch court laid down several guidelines as operative in this and future cases, making it legal, as a matter of case law, to administer euthanasia as long as (1) there is clear and convincing evidence of a well-considered, voluntary request, (2) the patient is suffering unbearably without reasonable recourse, and (3) the euthanasia is carried out and documented with care by a qualified physician, with the concurrence of a colleague.

This three-part test became codified as a matter of statutory law in the Dutch criminal code in the spring of 1993, decriminalizing an act that had been legal as a matter of case law since 1976 (Simons, 1993). During that time span, prosecutors had occasionally charged doctors with violating the Dutch Homicide Act, and in a very few cases, convictions had been handed down. But in each instance, a higher court overturned the conviction on the ground that the doctor acted out of "higher necessity"—a catchphrase used by the Dutch judges to legitimate what they view to be the inevitably good-faith actions of medical professionals (Fumento, 1991; Newman, 1990).

However, the Dutch position is clearly outside the mainstream of Western political and legal thought. To be sure, Europeans seem more accepting of death than Americans. For example, when William Douglas went to Spain to study the Basques, he found them open, candid, and resigned to the idea of death (Charmaz, 1980, p. 87). And Mary Rose Barrington (1990, p. 85) reports that the public in England is overwhelmingly in favor of euthanizing severely ill patients. Moreover, the fact that doctors occasionally euthanize their patients seems to be widely accepted among the citizens of Great Britain, although the law does not specifically permit this.

Nonetheless, the political order and legal doctrine of most Western countries today also reflect general and enduring cultural predispositions associated with the denial of death and the refusal to even consider managing death by law. Germany, Italy, France, and Spain are more reflective of this conservative mainstream.

Germany must cope with the ghosts of Nazi atrocities whenever the subjects of euthanasia and the right to die are raised, which has a chilling effect on the attitudes of individuals in the German republic. In Italy, France, and Spain, the central role played by the Catholic church has shaded public attitudes in a conservative hue. The Catholic position—that life is God's gift and that humans should not tinker with it—predominates in ways that it does not in the Netherlands. Indeed, although the European denial of death is not as elaborate and manifest as it is in the United States, it is clearly skewed in that direction (with the Dutch position serving as the exception to this general rule).

The Americas. The denial and fear of death are even stronger on the west side of the Atlantic. But one should not think of the North American continent as monolithic in this regard for variations on the denial theme exist both south and north of the U.S. border, as well as within the United States itself.

For example, Mexicans believe there is a deep connection between death and life and are relatively comfortable with the idea of death. Symbols of death are seen everywhere in Mexico, especially in the churches, where bloody representations of Christ and glass-topped coffins of martyrs and saints are commonplace. Mexicans celebrate death and the dead in a national festival known as *Dias de Todos Muertos* ("Days of the Dead"), which provides an occasion for communication with the dead. Some rituals (featuring sugar-candy skulls and tissue-paper skeletons) are geared to appeal to children in order that they might join in the socialization process surrounding death at an early age.[1] The Days of the Dead also present an occasion to picnic on tombstones by day, and gamble and play board games on them by night (Green, 1980), all in a good-hearted attempt to put death in perspective.

Looking to the north, we find that in certain Eskimo cultures, old or sick individuals are allowed to petition for euthanasia by telling their families they are ready to die. Family members then take their dying relative onto "Mother Ice," where the individual is abandoned. Exposed to the elements, death comes in short order. Eskimos believe that anyone dying in this way spends eternity in the highest of heavens (Humphry and Wickett, 1986, p. 2).

Even within the United States, denial is not universal. For example, certain religious and ethnic American subcultures are quite at ease with death. For the Amish, it is simply considered a part of the natural rhythm of life (DeSpelder and Strickland, 1992, p. 46). Putting their own special cast on the whole right-to-die debate, Christian Scientists refuse medical treatments altogether, preferring to let nature—or the will of God—take its course: If death comes, so be it. And some groups of ethnic Catholics (most notably, Irish Catholics) are known for their celebrations after the death of a family member. Even though they may fear and avoid death as much as the next American, many Irish-Americans hold lively wakes, gathering friends and family to share food, drink, and revelry in a sort of death celebration that is very much out of character for mainstream America.

Charmaz (1980, p. 315) also finds that denial of death is less prominent within the African-American and Mexican-American communities. Likewise, Native Americans are relatively accepting of death. They tend to consider it as something neither to be ignored nor feared, and when death comes, Native Americans teach that one should "make room for it" (DeSpelder and Strickland, 1992, p. 58).

Clearly, given all the exceptions to denial (e.g., in non-Western and Dutch cultures) and variations on the denial theme (e.g., in Mexican and Eskimo cultures and in Irish-American, Native American, and African-American subcultures), high levels of denial are not as universal as Becker (1973) suggests. Rather, it is probably safe to say that, as a rule, non-Western cultures are more accepting of death than are Western cultures, and Western cultures are a bit more accepting of death than certain American subcultures. These subcultures are, in turn, more accepting of death than American culture more generally described. Denial exists throughout but at dramatically different levels, with the United States occupying the position at the end of the continuum one might label "greatest sense of denial." A close look at American culture gives us some important clues as to why this is true.

American Culture

There are a number of constants or aspects of culture in America that encourage the denial of death. These constants form a shared consciousness among members of American society, making their culture somewhat unique in this regard. We have sifted the evidence and identified five such constants: individualism, liberty, scientism, the entitlement syndrome, and religious taboo. Each of these cultural thought patterns set Americans up to act the way they do when death is near, making denial easy, natural, and, to a degree, almost inevitable. As a result, what has generally been an accepted phase of life for two millennia in most parts of the world has been transformed in the late-twentieth-century United States into a lonely, disconcerting, and disconnected process to be avoided at all costs.

Individualism: The Lack of Community

Certainly, part of the contrast between the United States and the non-Western world can be attributed to the different roles the individual plays in these cultures. In most Asian and African cultures, the sense of obligation to family and community is a key element of the social order. This contrasts sharply with the American cultural creed, in which individual rights is the concept around which society is organized. The non-Western emphasis on obligation tends to keep the ego in check, and it forces individuals to see their significance as relative to the larger collective. When, on the other hand, societies organize about the principle of individual rights, egos become larger because individuals see themselves by definition as significant in their own right. Thus, the old saw "Western man knows how to live, and Eastern man [and, according to our argument, African man] knows how to die" can be explained, in part, by this difference in the individual's role in the respective cultures.

This also brings up the issue of community. Where community ties are strong, as they often are in non-Western cultures, the reality of death seems relatively manageable. In Japan, for example, the sense of membership in the community runs so strong that traditionally there is very little clear consciousness of personal identity (Kato, 1990, p. 72). The community operates as the body, and as long as the body endures, the death of a single individual is not particularly significant. Moreover, when a community member dies, that death is treated as a community affair, with all the support structures that community involvement suggests.

Sociologists have found that in cultures where the sense of community and interconnectedness is strong, the loss of single individuals touches more people and the loss of single relationships is more easily absorbed. As more people are affected and on more occasions, individuals become accustomed to and thereby desensitized to death. In contrast, in American society, "selves tend to be situated in relatively few, intense, stable relationships" (Charmaz, 1980, p. 281). Death comes less often and impacts more seriously the lives of those who survive. As a result, grief is experienced "less frequently, but more intensely, since ... emotional involvements are not diffused over an entire community, but are usually concentrated on one or a few people" (Blauner, cited in Pine, 1980, p. 91). In support of this hypothesis, Philip Slater found that in cultures where individuality is a high cultural priority, the fear of death logically follows. When the sense of connectedness based on community erodes, as it often does in industrially advanced societies, death fears tend to blossom (Charmaz, 1980, pp. 86–87).

There is another side to individuality in American society that makes death so problematic. The strong sense of individualism that most Americans have may lead them to feel more personally responsible for death, both their own and those of people around them. In societies less driven by individualism, death is commonly seen as the work of God or gods (Kalish, 1980a, p. 1). But in contemporary Western society, where individual autonomy also means that the individual is viewed as being responsible for whatever happens in life, death can produce a profound sense of guilt. Dying is seen as evidence of weakness, and the dying person may feel personally at fault. Family members, friends, and even health-care professionals may also blame themselves for the death.

Ultimately, in a culture that emphasizes the value of power and control of one's own destiny, death, by definition, represents the lack of both power and control, and for that reason it must be avoided at all costs. Moreover, when it is not avoided, Americans tend to see the death as an individual loss that really has very little to do with the community at large. When Americans attend the funerals of others in the community, they do so as individuals out of respect for the dead person, rather than as members of the community out of respect for the whole. It is no wonder that Americans find themselves asking "for whom does the bell toll?" when the church bells chime to mark someone's passing. In societies where community bonds are strong and the nature of the public good is conceived as something more than the simple sum of private passions, the question never comes up because the answer is so obvious: "For whom does the bell toll? Of course, it tolls for thee."

Immortalism: The Endless Pursuit of Happiness

It has been suggested that at least some part of the difference between the way Western (especially American) and non-Western cultures cope with death can be attributed to the manner in which old people are treated in society. In ancient China, the highest achievement in Taoist society was a long life and the wisdom assumed to come with the passing of years. The Aranda people—hunter-gatherers of the Australian forests—accorded supernatural status to those who had achieved extreme old age (Dychtwald, 1989). The Japanese also esteem the elderly, focusing on the value that long life provides for accumulating experience and perfecting spiritual development. By comparison, David Gutman (1991) finds that esteem for elders in America is rare compared with the twenty-six other countries he studied.

The way a culture treats its elderly cannot help but color the way it treats the subject of death. Where the elderly are celebrated, death is confronted head on as an important rite of passage. The culture stays in contact with death in this way, and its members become more comfortable with it as a result. But where the elderly are thought of as irrelevant, death tends to be glossed over as something that happens to others—a deviant behavior that one would do well to avoid, if at all possible. Why do Americans treat their elderly the way they do? We contend that denial of aging—an outgrowth of the liberal "pursuit-of-happiness" axiom that is central to the American political, cultural, and economic creed—is largely to blame.

Americans are proud of their constitutionally grounded rights and have exhibited a general predisposition to celebrate individual liberty, broadly construed, at the expense of almost everything else. The right to free speech (even when libeling public figures in the press), the right to bear arms (without restriction), the right to freely associate, protest, and petition the government (regardless of how unpopular the group or the cause), and the right to privacy (including the exclusion of illegally obtained evidence in criminal proceedings) are just a few manifestations of the rights-oriented culture in which we live. Liberty—the freedom to do what we will in pursuit of our own desires—is an essential element of our political heritage.

Yet, paradoxically, when it comes to death, Americans apparently would rather deny their mortality than champion some abstract right to die. Instead of accepting death, they do everything possible to deny its inevitability. "In this world nothing could be said to be certain, except death and taxes," wrote Ben Franklin in 1789, the year the U.S. Constitution was written. It is interesting to note that two hundred years later, Americans have come to deny the inevitability of both.[2]

It seems that Americans have drawn the line on liberty at death's door. In a culture obsessed with rights and choices, death—the point after which the ideas of rights and choices have no currency—seems pretty much beyond the pale. "In a society that emphasizes the future," notes Feifel, "the prospect of no future at all is an abomination. Hence, death and dying invite our hostility, repudiation and denial, and assume taboo status" (in Weisman, 1972, p. IX).

Attitudes that drive avoidance behavior in America are rooted in the thoughts of John Locke, the British philosopher who is generally considered the primary author of the classical liberal approach to life. Thomas Jefferson gave voice to the American version of liberalism with his Declaration of Independence claims regarding inalienable rights to "life, liberty, and the pursuit of happiness." The logic of liberal ideology, taken to its natural conclusion, argues that death should be avoided at all costs and whenever possible, so that individuals can do with life and liberty what they have the inalienable right to do: seek individual gratification as part of the American dream. Acknowledgment of death implies a sense of limits that flies in the face of American consciousness. Moreover, the contradiction between the life-oriented cultural ethos (activism, hedonism, conquest, liberty) and the death theme (passivity, failure, loss of ability to make choices) intensifies the denial of death (Chang and Chang, 1980, p. 742).

Death is un-American, claims Larry Bugen (1979, p. 257). Basic to our failure to confront death, he argues, is the fact that "American society in its preoccupation with perpetual youth, beauty, and strength, has typically disguised, avoided, denied, and embellished death" (Bugen 1979, p. 252). And there seems to be plenty of evidence to support this claim for our culturally based pursuit of individual gratification is manifest in a variety of curious rituals and behaviors geared toward self-delusion and egoistic aggrandizement.

For instance, Americans treat death as a great surprise when it overcomes a friend or family member, even if the departed was relatively old and ill, as if such a thing were not entirely natural. And, of course, many go to great lengths to camouflage signs of their own aging and infirmity. Widespread use of plastic surgery, wrinkle creams, hair transplants, exercise equipment, and aerobic videos all point toward the seemingly insatiable search for a fountain of youth. Those who design and market equipment, cosmetics, therapies, and procedures that purport to slow (or at least give the illusion of slowing) the aging process have turned the denial of mortality into a multibillion-dollar industry in this country.

Food and Fitness Fads. The proliferation of food fads,[3] diet regimens,[4] weight-loss programs,[5] and eating disorders[6] in the United States also manifests the American pursuit of happiness that leads to the denial of aging and dying. Americans are deluged with advertising that reinforces the desirability of being slim and trim. And if that were not enough to keep the diet business afloat, recent reports speak about doubling the normal life span of laboratory mice with a regimen called "caloric restriction." Some scientists are even wondering if a human life span of 140 years or longer might be achievable through a more controlled dietary regimen (Shurkin, 1992, p. 9). Such talk is music to the ears of many Americans.

More evidence of the American obsession with health can be found in the popularity of various exercise gurus (Jack LaLane, Richard Simmons, Jane Fonda, Cher), exercise programs (aerobics and variations on that theme, including dancercise, jazzercise, low-impact aerobics, and water aerobics), and exercise equipment (thigh and tummy shapers, treadmills, exercycles, step climbers, ski machines, rowing machines). Bodybuilding regimens (weight lifting, power lifting), fad sports (running, power walking, softball, golf, and various racquet sports), and the proliferation of commercial gyms and fitness clubs also provide good indications of American sentiments with regard to health and longevity. Walter Bortz, former president of the American Geriatrics Society, suggests that physical fitness can help stretch an individual's life span to its more natural limit: 120 years (cited in Krucoff, 1992). And once again, it appears that Americans are acting accordingly.

In the end, as J. D. Reed observes, the typical American seems obsessed with the shape of the body: "Paring, preening it, pumping it up and pounding it down, the body national is being rejuvenated with a relentless impatience, slimmed with a fanatic dedication. ... The country runs and runs, from fear of death ... and old age as well" (cited in Stein, 1990, p. 119). And when all else fails, many feel it is necessary to equivocate about their age. They certainly do not broadcast it, and they may even lie about it.

The "Contributions" of Modern Medicine. For those with the money and interest in remaking the body in ways that diet and exercise cannot, modern medicine offers a dizzying variety of procedures and elixirs that can make people appear healthier and younger than they really are. Silicone implants for breasts and hips can add curves to the body where once there were none, and liposuction has become a popular way to do just the opposite. And "face jobs" and "tummy tucks" can surgically nip and gather the skin to create a more youthful appearance.

Interest in synthetic growth hormone therapy is also on the rise. For about $20,000 a year, genetic engineers can produce hormones in the laboratory and inject them into the bodies of aging Americans in hopes of stalling or maybe even reversing the effects of aging. And the compound called Retin-A—the prescription acne medication turned antiwrinkle cream—has kept Americans streaming into dermatologists' offices ever since 1988, when a study in the *Journal of the American Medical Association* reported on the ability of that drug to help restore sun-damaged skin.[7] Shortly thereafter, dermatologists were besieged with prescription requests, and annual sales of Retin-A are now somewhere between $20 million and $60 million.

Minoxidil is another drug with an interesting side effect. Developed initially to control hypertension, Minoxidil was found to stimulate hair growth in some patients and is now sold as a prescription drug to treat hair loss in men. Balding Americans who are considering wigs and weaves and those thinking of surgical hair-plug transplants now have another option.

For older men troubled by failing libido, testosterone-replacement therapy is an increasingly popular antiaging strategy. Injections of testosterone, prescribed by a physician, can help restore the sex drive and treat impotence in men who want to feel, act, and be viewed as "young again" ("Dr. Ponce de Leon," 1990, p. 14).

Those interested in bulking up have sometimes turned to the illegal use of steroids, bought on the black market. According to one report, an estimated 1 million Americans use steroids today (half of them adolescents), accounting for $400 million in annual sales. Although many individuals who take steroids are interested in improving athletic performance, a substantial percentage take them simply to achieve the dramatic enhancements in body shape that steroid use can produce.

In the legal, over-the-counter world, megavitamin therapy has become extremely popular as a strategy for warding off aging. Two books by Durk Pearson and Sandy Shaw (*Life Extension: A Practical Scientific Approach* and the *Life Extension Companion*) spawned a great deal of interest in the ability of vitamins and minerals, taken in large doses, to ameliorate age-related deterioration in physical appearance and abilities. The combined sales of these two books—over 2 million copies, with gross receipts of some $30 million—suggests just how hungry Americans are for information on this subject. Indeed, interest in this and all the other developments in *immortalism* have been sufficient to spawn a loose federation of organizations (such as the Life Extension Foundation of Hollywood, Florida), magazines (like *Longevity Magazine*, with a circulation of a 225,000), mail-order houses, newsletters, and hotlines to keep an eager pool of subscribers abreast of the latest medical developments.

All these figure-altering and age-masking efforts are designed to change or misrepresent the state of one's actual physical condition, and the cost is substantial. It has been estimated that Americans spend approximately $2 billion per year on nostrums to ward off aging, $3 billion per year on food supplements, another $10 billion on efforts to disguise the visible signs of aging (Beck et al., 1990, p. 50), and $33 billion trying to lose weight. To be fair, some of these outlays are spent in an earnest desire to improve health, for the here and now. But at least part of this spending can be attributed to two overlapping motivations: an interest in enhancing longevity and a fear of aging. Both drives, it seems, are typically American, and both forestall private or public discussions about the inevitability of death.

"To be sure," writes Paul Starr (1982, p. 7), "many observers, beginning with de Tocqueville, have remarked that Americans are singularly concerned with their individual well-being. ... Today, were a revived de Tocqueville to observe Americans jogging in parks, shopping in health food stores, talking psychobabble, and reading endless guides to keeping fit, eating right, and staying healthy, he would probably conclude that, if anything, the obsession is now more pronounced." Immortalism is a cultural ethic with Americans, part and parcel of our liberal democratic tradition in which the pursuit of happiness is taken literally by most. It should come as no surprise, then, that Americans as a whole have been slow to consider political issues surrounding death and the right to die as worthy of their interest. The flood of information that they crave—and get—about ways to control the state of their bodies and their lives contributes mightily to death-denying behavior: Why think about death when there is so much one can do to avoid it?

Scientism: An Abiding Faith in Technology

American culture can also be described as *scientistic*. Scientism refers to the predisposition to have an abiding faith in technological advances, almost as a good in and of themselves. Like the sports enthusiast who expresses his or her desire to climb the mountain "because it is there," Americans tend to climb technological mountains, reflexively rather than reflectively, "because they are there," embracing whatever results from the ascent as good by definition. This cultural predisposition to embrace technology, a social by-product of the industrial revolution, is rooted much more deeply in the American experience, tracing back to the frontier days of the eighteenth and nineteenth centuries.

Daniel Elazar, a political scientist who has devoted much of his professional career to writing about America's political culture, sees the idea of "frontier" as central to the American cultural experience. Early pioneers—the first generation of nonnative Americans—opened up what was, for them, an entirely new world by pushing westward across the North American continent. They did this largely out of wanderlust: Travel, adventure, challenge, and the promise of a big payoff were thought of as good things in their own right. For the first several hundred years, the frontier meant the land frontier, and Americans were drawn to it like a magnet. Since the industrial revolution, however, the lust for land development has been slowly transformed into a scientifically based wanderlust. As Elazar (1984, p. 109) puts it, the modern frontier can be thought of as "the constant effort of Americans to extend their control over their environment for [their own] benefit."

That Americans treat technology as a frontier—something both conquerable and worth conquering—is nicely illustrated by U.S. encounters with technology over the years. In 1961, President John Kennedy told Americans that the United States should put a man on the moon by the end of the decade, a goal that was accomplished in dramatic form. And fulfillment of his prophecy only bolstered the already entrenched predisposition to believe in the frontier. Questions about whether going to the moon was really the right thing to do with the billions of dollars spent on that pursuit got very little attention at the time. Instead, it seemed as if the collective American reaction to the idea was "if we *can* (and of course we can), then we should."[8]

There are plenty of other (albeit less spectacular) examples of the frontier phenomenon at work in the American milieu. For example, members of Congress—perennial believers in the technological tooth fairy—passed a number of air- and water-quality laws in the 1970s that presupposed technology developments would make it possible to reach the standards set by federal regulations: If we could go to the moon, surely we could manage the pollution problem. Americans were not quite as lucky with the environment as they were with the space program, however. Instead, science lagged, and air quality, water quality, and fuel efficiency requirements that Congress originally mandated were diluted, delayed, and, in some cases, abandoned altogether over the years. Congress did not get its way for a number of reasons, but for present purposes, it is enough to note the hubris with which that body acted in the first place for it illustrates well the arrogance of the American political culture more generally regarding the faith in technology.

Energy policy—or, better, the lack thereof—represents another good example of the trust that American people and, by extension, the U.S. Congress put in technology. The United States has no real energy policy because Congress is betting that when the fossil fuels really do run out, technology (e.g., cars that run on solar power or hydrogen, or maybe we will jump right to magnetic levitation runabouts a la George Jetson) will step into the breach to save the day. It is no wonder that Americans were so quick to buy into the charade "cold fusion" turned out to be a few years back. They wanted to believe there would be a quick, technological fix, and with cold fusion, they thought they got it.

The same phenomenon is at work in the defense business. Americans celebrated the success of the Patriot missile during the Gulf War, but a General Accounting Office analysis of the missile's performance suggests that it hardly worked at all. Indeed, some evidence suggests that even when Patriots intercepted Scud missiles, the falling debris caused more damage and loss of life than the attacking Scuds would have caused if they had been allowed to fall unintercepted. The public also reveled in the gun camera footage of U.S. aircraft striking Iraqi targets. Played over and over on Cable News Network (CNN), these bomb-damage shots showed direct hits on bridges, vehicles, and factories—never mind the hand-selected, unrepresentative nature of the clips. Also ignored was the fact that some of the footage, described by the top brass as showing "Scud mobile launcher kills," were really just pictures of exploding troop-supply trucks.[9]

The point is that stories that run counter to the American belief system—about space program failures, environmental technology falling short of expectations, ineffective Patriots, and misleading damage-assessment films—get little or no play in the media. This is true partly because they are not as entertaining as the ornamental version of the news. At least part of the explanation for this can be attributed to the fact that accurate stories did not synch out well with American cultural predispositions. Be it a matter of faith, wishful thinking, or scientism, it is clear that Americans would rather believe in technology than face reality.

The same mind-set is at work when it comes to issues of medical technology and, ultimately, the denial of mortality, even in cases where the patient is terminally ill. Why pull the plug or even think about it when procedures that would restore a worthwhile quality of life might be available just around the corner? When one has faith in society's ability to conquer frontiers (in this case, the medical-technology frontier), it makes no sense to even contemplate death: Surely, one of the big university hospitals or one of the well-endowed research clinics will be able to treat the affliction in question. That is the attitude of the cryonicists, and it is shared, to one degree or another, by most Americans in regard to more mainstream medical technologies.

In this vein, Daniel Callahan (1990, p. 50) writes that "a denial of the limits of the possible in effecting cures is thus a central part of the ideology of scientific medicine. It is sustained in part by its actual success in overcoming earlier obstacles and curing illnesses once thought beyond reach, and in part as an act of faith that is at one with the general faith in science." Ultimately, Callahan continues, "there are no fixed limits to the therapeutic possibility of cure ... and thus, no boundaries to the meeting of individual needs." The more we witness in the way of technological progress, the more we expect, to the point where Americans now believe that science will conquer illness, the effects of aging, and even death itself (Charmaz, 1980, p. 90).

The media exacerbate the situation when they magnify and distort the significance of unexpected recoveries and technological advances. Unexpected remissions are attributed to miracle cures instead of random chance, dumb luck, or misdiagnosis of the case in the first place. And that tends to stimulate hopes that doctors can always pull off yet another miracle. By treating spectacular cases as if they have the prospect of becoming the norm, the media create medical mirages that raise the expectations of Americans, fueling their faith and reinforcing existing beliefs about the limitless potential of modern medicine.

We would suggest that, for Americans, belief in technology has become part of a national ideology—a secular religion, even an addiction (Callahan, 1990, p. 92)—in which faith in the goodness and effectiveness of technology operates as the central premise. Ivan Illich notes that Americans have a "deep-seated need for the engineering of miracles" (cited in Humphry and Wickett, 1986, p. 193), and U.S. research institutions and teaching hospitals have engineered one medical miracle after another in response to that need. To speak of managing death in this context would be tantamount to a countercultural surrender, an acceptance of the notion that technology has its reasonable limits. It should come as no surprise, then, that we include scientism as a force of policy restraint in the right-to-die debate.

At the same time, however, Howard Stein (1990, p. 58) believes it is important to realize that "so long as unexamined interests and popular passions govern public policy decisions about the development and use of technology, we will continue to define every problem as a technological one and prescribe solutions in terms of narrow technique devoid and denuded of context. Sometimes a culture's most cherished values are not in its best interest. Sometimes they become a dead end." Scientism is a faith, not a truth, and technology is not always good by definition. Sometimes rockets blow up, and sometimes, perhaps, they should not have been built in the first place. Sometimes the very sick cannot be cured. And it may be that sometimes it does not even make sense to try.

The Entitlement Syndrome. To individualism, immortalism, and scientism, we now add a fourth aspect of the American culture that feeds into the denial of death: the entitlement syndrome. This concept refers to the feeling that Americans have—and deserve—the very best goods and services that the public and private sectors have to offer.

The entitlement syndrome is evident in all aspects of American culture, and medical care is no exception. Not only do Americans have faith in medical technology, they also demand the best treatment that the medical-industrial complex can render—because they feel entitled. Medical ethicist Daniel Callahan is quite clear on this score: "There is, most of all, the power of public demand, which has come to expect medicine to improve not only health, but life more generally, and which has come to see a longer and better life as not simply a benefit but as a deep and basic right" (1990, p. 21). The fact that there is not enough money to pay for all the diagnostic tests, transplants, technologies, and therapies Americans would like to avail themselves of seems irrelevant.

Paul Tsongas, unsuccessful candidate for the 1992 Democratic presidential nomination and benefactor of state-of-the-art treatments for his own rare form of cancer, was often asked what he thought of the Canadian health-care plan as a model for reform. He invariably replied that he was no fan of that system, pointing out that if he were a citizen of Canada when he got sick, he probably would have died. Members of his audience would usually bob their heads in agreement. "Tsongas is entitled to the best, and so are we," those bobs seemed to be signaling, "so don't bother raising questions about limiting access to sophisticated medical treatments." Indeed, one reason why the Canadian model of health care is given so little consideration as a policy alternative in this country is directly tied to the general limits on technology and the waiting lists that are reportedly generated for access to the high-tech medical procedures offered in the provinces to the north. Some say that Americans would not stand for that (Callahan, 1990, pp. 87–88), and they are probably right.

There seems to be a Maslowian aspect to this entitlement phenomenon. According to psychologist Abraham Maslow, we are each driven by a needs hierarchy, and when basic needs are satisfied, the desire for higher-order needs are stimulated to keep us preoccupied. For example, when survival is in question, survival needs predominate. However, once the basics (food, clothing, and shelter) have been secured, worries shift to a second tier of concerns, such as income security and friendship. And once level-two concerns are satisfied, level-three concerns move into the breach. In Maslow's world, individuals are never really satisfied; they just graduate from level to level in an insatiable urge to achieve complete self-actualization.

The same sort of psychology seems to be at work with regard to the right to die. Once one begins advancing up the technological ladder toward ultimate health, concerns about death become displaced to the point where one does not even think about death. It is off the map, and when it tries to pop up on occasion, it is denied. The success of medical progress begets these higher expectations, pushing us up through a hierarchy of desires that are ultimately insatiable (Callahan, 1990, pp. 33, 81).

As A. J. Barsky notes, "There is a progressive decline in our threshold and tolerance for mild disorders and isolated symptoms, along with a greater inclination to view uncomfortable symptoms as pathologic—as signs of disease. ... The standard we use for judging our health appears to have been raised, so that we are more aware of—and more disturbed by—symptoms and impairments that previously we deemed less important" (cited in Callahan, 1990, pp. 54–55). Callahan applies this line of thought to high-tech medicine, as well. A century ago, he argues, before the advent of heart transplants, people never thought that they "needed" a heart transplant; when someone became ill with heart disease, death was simply accepted. But with the development of transplant technology, awe has been converted to need: Now, people "need" transplants, and death is not accepted.

As people get healthier, infirmity becomes that much harder to accept, as well, and death becomes that much more foreign a prospect. In addition, as people get healthier with improving technology, life expectancy goes up. People now live longer, so they desire more technology for a longer time. Callahan calls this the "twice cured, once dead phenomenon" (1990, p. 101). In the past, one got mortally ill and then died; today, according to Callahan, we may be cured of serious illness a number of times before we die. Indeed, when 10 percent of the people account for 75 percent of overall medical costs (Callahan, 1990, p. 101), it is not hard to imagine that some of these people have enjoyed the equivalent of a cat's fabled nine lives.

The nature of the U.S. health-care system also helps to fuel the entitlement fires in other ways. For most Americans, health care is a private-sector commodity. But only a very small percentage of coverage is paid for out of pocket, on a fee-for-service basis. Most Americans are covered by insurance, and the insurers pick up the bulk of the bill for services (after deductibles and copayments). This "third-party" financing arrangement means that care is essentially limitless: an all-you-can-eat health-care buffet, charged on a company credit card. Insurance companies may cap coverage at some point, but for the most part, once the insurance premiums are paid, there is no real incentive for beneficiaries to limit the care they seek. Indeed, there may actually be some incentive to maximize care—to get one's money's worth, as it were. After all, having paid the premiums, one is certainly entitled.

In response to abstract polling questions about end-of-life decisionmaking, Americans overwhelmingly say that they would *not* want to be sustained artificially. But when push comes to shove and death is imminent, Americans tend to shrink from making tough choices about life and death. Instead, they tend to demand that the latest technology be available and employed in every case and to every extent, almost as if access to such advanced medical procedures were a right of citizenship. It is not likely that right-to-die questions will get much of a hearing in an environment like this, where, when it comes to death-defying technology, more is better and—for a number of reasons—we feel entitled to benefit from everything the medical community has to offer. That, it seems, is the American way.

Religious Taboo

The fifth and last dimension of the American cultural psyche that we see as important to the denial-of-death phenomenon is the role that Western religious traditions (primarily Judeo-Christian traditions) have in shaping the response to death. These traditions have generated religious taboos about managing death—playing God, as it were—that undergird the entire culture's predisposition to sidestep public debate about end-of-life decisionmaking. Pressure from religious interest groups plays an important role here, as well. Together, individual religious predispositions and collective interest-group pressures create a formidable force of restraint on the right-to-die policy environment.

Religion is not particularly important in the public life of Americans, generally speaking. Church attendance in the United States has dropped off substantially in recent decades and lags behind attendance rates in other countries. And when it comes to public policy, the United States leads the world in the degree to which matters of church and state are explicitly and constitutionally separated. This does not mean, however, that Americans are irreligious: Survey data actually suggest that religion is very important for Americans in their private lives. According to the *World Values Survey,* "Belief in God is more widespread in America than it is in any of the nineteen major industrial nations" (cited in Shapiro, 1992, pp. 39–40). The overwhelming majority of Americans—98 percent—say they believe there is a god, 70 percent say they believe in the devil, 90 percent say they believe in heaven, and 73 percent say they believe in hell (see Table 2.1).

Importantly, the dominant religious orientations in America—Judaism and Christianity—are in lockstep when it comes to death. Each puts a high premium on the sanctity of life, and each has strong proscriptions against individuals taking death into their own hands. Ancient Greek and Roman cultures tolerated and even embraced euthanasia under honorable conditions (e.g., unremitting pain), but Christianity has traditionally deplored the idea. Christians who attempted euthanasia were excommunicated in earlier days, and those who succeeded were given "an ignominious burial on the highway, impaled by a stake" (Humphry and Wickett, 1986, p. 6). "All things for a reason," argued Christian theologians of the time, believing that the premature taking of a life for any reason would be irreligious.

Early American Protestant beliefs have also helped shape modern American attitudes toward death, according to Charmaz. The Protestant ethos, she writes,

TABLE 2.1   Spiritual Beliefs: Percentage of the Population Saying They Believe in God, the Devil, Heaven, and Hell, 1981–1983

	God	*Devil*	*Heaven*	*Hell*
United States	98	70	90	73
Ireland	97	62	89	59
Canada	93	44	75	42
Spain	92	38	56	38
Italy	88	33	44	33
Belgium	86	24	41	21
Australia	85	42	64	40
United Kingdom	81	34	62	29
Germany	80	18	34	15
Norway	73	30	49	23
Netherlands	71	22	44	16
France	65	18	27	15
Denmark	63	12	17	8
Japan	62	22	37	29
Sweden	60	13	32	11

SOURCE: Shapiro, 1992, p. 40; statistics derived from the *World Values Survey* (1981), Institute for Social Research, University of Michigan. Reprinted by permission.

leads us to treat death as a family secret, almost as if it were something to be ashamed of—something to be "handled" only by relatives and close friends. And if death is to be kept out of public view, surely it is something to be kept outside the reach of public policy.

The influence of the traditionally conservative Roman Catholic church has also had a chilling effect on the right-to-die debate. Some Catholic-based organizations have extended their pro-life position on the abortion question to include a strong pro-life stance on the right to die. Right-to-life organizations have demonstrated both outside and inside hospitals where families have tried to exercise the right to die. On occasion, these prolife groups have gone to court to request that a guardian be appointed to make decisions for seriously ill, incompetent patients, in lieu of family members. Right-to-life organizations have also been active in the halls of state capitols, where the various state chapters of the Catholic Conference have been quite influential. Other Catholics continue to argue that suffering at the end of life may serve a redemptive purpose and that we should not interfere with what they believe is "God's plan."

On top of this, there are general religious taboos in the cultural psyche that argue against dealing forthrightly with the right to die. Americans may not attend church services as often as their counterparts elsewhere in the world, but that does not mean that religious teachings about managing death carry no weight. To the contrary, the religiously legitimated sanctity of life and traditional proscriptions against the management of death are important dimensions of our political culture that should not be overlooked. Even those who do not consider them-

TABLE 2.2   Thinking About Death: Percentage of the Population in Sixteen Western Countries Saying They "Often" or "Sometimes" Think About Death

	Percentage
United States	65.1
Italy	65.1
Australia	61.9
Canada	60.8
Finland	59.7
Spain	59.0
United Kingdom	56.7
France	56.7
Japan	55.2
Ireland	55.2
Netherlands	54.1
Germany	53.0
Norway	52.9
Sweden	51.6
Denmark	51.1
Belgium	46.6

SOURCE: Cited in Shapiro, 1992, p. 42, from Ronald Inglehart: statistics derived from the *World Values Survey* (1981), Institute for Social Research, University of Michigan. Reprinted by permission.

selves religious tend to get weakhearted, on spiritual grounds, when right-to-die scenarios arise.

In sum, the right to die is a sensitive religious issue that causes most to opt for prolonging life, urging that everything possible be done to save the life at stake at the time. The reasons to prolong life would be substantial even if only secular concerns were involved. But when the spiritual life of the decisionmaker is perceived to be at risk, the stakes are raised substantially. In a society that claims to believe so firmly in God and that is so ill at ease with the idea of death to begin with, it is not hard to understand how the religious dimension of American culture operates so effectively in forestalling public debate of right-to-die issues.

Summary: The Forces of Restraint

According to the *World Values Survey,* Americans think about death more than citizens of any other country in the Western world except for Italy (Italy is tied with the United States; see Table 2.2). But our thoughts on death apparently are not constructive. Instead, we euphemize death when it happens to those close to us. And when we watch so many deaths on television and in the movies, death becomes sanitized and objectified: It is something that happens to someone else, not to us. Some even try to avoid it altogether through what advocates purport is something of a frozen fountain of youth—cryonic suspension.

Changes in U.S. society since the turn of the century have put even more distance between Americans and the reality of death. Professionally conducted funerals relieve us of the responsibility for tending to our dead. The breakup of the multigenerational household, together with escalating rates of retirement among the old, means that those most likely to die—the elderly—are increasingly out of sight and out of mind. So, too, are their deaths. And, of course, medical progress has added to the distance between Americans and death. With death rates down and life expectancy up, death is simply not as common an experience today as it was in the past. And when death finally does come, the patient is not at home but off somewhere in an institution of higher medicine. We visit when we can, if we can.

Other cultures do not seem to be in the same situation, and much of the difference can likely be attributed to the importance of the individual in the United States. Where the community is more important than its individual members, death is more likely to be treated openly and supportively as a community phenomenon. And where grieving occurs more regularly and more openly, it is easier to take death in stride with everything else life brings. But in the United States, where individualism is so important, interest in community is traded away for the pursuit of long and healthy (or at least healthy-looking) life. With all the emotional energy Americans spend seeking the twin fountains of youth and youthful looks, it is no small wonder that they have so little time or predisposition to devote to coping with death.

Technology is also important. In countries where technology is not particularly advanced, death is simply a more common experience, witnessed personally on a regular basis. It is considered a frequent visitor and even a friendly visitor at times. But in the United States, technological successes have created an insatiable appetite for curative medicine. In such a nation, where technology is advancing rapidly, it is harder and harder to accept death. The entitlement syndrome and prevailing religious attitudes have also conspired to suppress the right-to-die debate. And thus we argue that American culture itself has been a significant force of restraint in the development of right-to-die policy.

But a survey of these restraint forces tells only half the story. Forty-six states and the District of Columbia have living-will laws on the books today, and the Supreme Court is on record in support of the right to die. Superior courts in several dozen states have come to the same general conclusion. Moreover, the federal government passed a law in 1990—the Patient Self-Determination Act—requiring that hospital personnel inform patients of their rights under state law to refuse medical treatment should they become seriously ill during their hospital stay. And medical ethics committees have been springing up in hospitals across the country. How can all this happen in a land where the people seem so obsessed with the denial of their own mortality?

The answer is tied to the fact that the forces of restraint do not operate in a vacuum. There are also powerful forces of activism at work that have thrust the right to die onto the public-policy agenda, in spite of cultural predispositions to the contrary. The forces of restraint may have delayed these efforts and slowed policy developments that have ensued, but forces of activism have succeeded to the point where the right to die is—or soon will be—a matter of public interest across the country, now and for some years to come.

3

Policy Activism and Medical Technology: Emergence of the Right-to-Die Scenario

In surveying the right-to-die landscape, we see two variations of activism at work, pushing and prodding right-to-die questions onto the public-policy agenda in spite of the forces of restraint. The first sort of activism trickles down from the top, from the medical profession to the patient population. The manner in which hospitals and physicians treat their patients has proved to be an important source of right-to-die activism that we will discuss here and in Chapter 4.

Chapters 5 and 6 present our discussion of the activism that flows in the opposite direction, percolating from the bottom up. We take a grass-roots approach in our search for causes of right-to-die activism that arise almost independently of professional developments in the mainstream medical community. In Chapter 5, we assay the forces of social activism that are closely linked with other social movements, namely, consumerism and the "rights culture" more generally. Chapter 6 wraps up the discussion of activism with a survey of the forces that combine to form what one author has called "the happy-death movement."

Technology plays a Janus-like role in our policy scenario.[1] As discussed in Chapter 2, the increased availability of advanced medical technology feeds into the scientism that is central to American culture. As a result, Americans would rather deny death than contemplate decisions about the right to die. At the same time, however, technology creates scenarios that raise right-to-die questions. Advances in both diagnostic and rescue-medicine technology have helped to create a whole population of individuals who would have died quickly only a few decades ago. Today, the beneficiaries of advanced technology live on—sometimes in seriously degraded states—and that, we contend, tends to force death onto the public-policy agenda.

We also consider the role surging health-care costs play in stimulating interest in the right to die. As technology advances, as the size of the elderly population grows, and as costs skyrocket out of control, policymakers inevitably are increasingly forced to deal with questions of life and death. Whatever the answers, the very fact that questions are being asked suggests that the forces of restraint are being loosened up, making activism not only possible but likely to emerge.

Interventions Create "Would-Have-Dieds"

Interventions of both the diagnostic and rescue-medicine variety have created an entirely new group of individuals: the "would-have-dieds," people who would have died in earlier days. In the past, they would have contracted illnesses without much warning and slipped over the edge of eternity with some dispatch. But today, with the assistance of medical technology, Americans seem able to cheat death, at least in the short term.

Two great revolutions have taken place in American medical technology in the last thirty years (Wildavsky, 1977, pp. 105–124), both of which create their own special population of would-have-dieds. First, there has been a quantum leap in the sophistication and accuracy of diagnostic technology that makes it possible for medical professionals to anticipate, with considerable accuracy, the development of medically threatening conditions. These conditions, if detected early enough, can lead practitioner and patient to remedial strategies well before life is threatened. Beneficiaries of this technology will die another day, and their deaths are more likely to be the result of old age, chronic illness, degenerating health, and, quite possibly, a seriously degraded quality of life in which the lines between life and death are blurred.

The second great revolution has come in rescue medicine. When diagnostic procedures fail, for lack of accuracy or lack of use, to anticipate the onset of a life-threatening medical condition or when serious accidents strike, advances in medical technology make it possible to "rescue" individuals, pulling them back from the brink of death. For example, primary organ failure is no longer the death warrant that it was just a few decades ago. Indeed, many people now rebound from heart, lung, or kidney failure to live on for years and even decades; minutes and hours of life were the most one could hope for when organs failed just a few decades ago. For some of these people, right-to-die questions will be raised only later in life. But other "rescue-medicine would-have-dieds" pose questions involving the right to die immediately. This happens when the biological life has been saved but the resulting quality of life is seriously degraded, that is, when the rescue is incomplete.

Advances in Diagnostics

Tremendous advances in diagnostic testing technologies have been made in this century. The discovery of X rays provided the first real breakthrough over half a century ago. But electronic monitoring of the brain with electroencephalographs (EEGs) and of the heart with electrocardiograms (ECGs), two other diagnostic tools that have proved invaluable to the modern physician, has become commonplace more recently. Indeed, much of the diagnostic technology used today was developed, refined, and marketed publicly only in the last thirty years or so. With the help of these technologies, diagnoses are now made earlier and more accurately, offering a much better chance of successful medical intervention.

Computerized axial tomography (popularly known as a CAT scan or CT scan) is typical of the new wave of computer-assisted imagery that has opened up the inside of the human body for more clinically detailed inspection.[2] Ultrasound, in which high-frequency sound waves are bounced off the body to form echo patterns, is another imaging technology that has been widely used in recent decades.[3] Magnetic resonance imaging (MRI) is among the newest imaging technologies: Although most American hospitals of any size have an MRI machine today, there were only seventy-eight units worldwide as recently as 1984.[4]

Advances in computerization have also led to many advances in scope technology and instrument miniaturization. Today, endoscopies (miniaturized television cameras inserted through the mouth to view the stomach and duodenum area) and colonoscopies (similar equipment inserted through the colon to view the large intestine all the way up to the lower chest area) are done in the doctor's office or on an outpatient basis without much fanfare. And with only a little extra effort, doctors can perform angioplasty, one of the most common heart procedures done in America today.[5] Miniaturization has also brought a whole new classification of operations, known as microsurgery. Athletes with faulty joints were the first beneficiaries, but now such procedures are commonly used in the general population for everything from knee surgery to gall bladder removal.

The diagnostic laboratory is another site where great strides have been made. Advances have been especially pronounced in the areas of hematology (blood studies), general body chemistry, and clinical microbiology. Before the turn of the century, clinical laboratory analysis was unheard of. Today, American physicians order ten billion lab tests annually—about fifty per person per year (Bronzino, Smith, and Wade, 1990, p. 284). Not only do computers make the basic analyses possible, they are now also used to sort, verify, store, and retrieve information. Consequently, more kinds of tests can be run (looking for trace elements, amino acids, cholesterol levels, and the presence of other complex molecules, for example), and the results are more accurate and the analyses more accessible to the clinical diagnostician.

Physicians have the ability to learn more about the individual human condition than ever before, thanks to the diagnostic medicine that has made breast X rays, Pap smears, blood-pressure monitoring, and cholesterol screening an accepted part of everyday life for millions of Americans. Physicians know more about their patient's condition, and they know it earlier. They can also monitor the patient's reaction to different clinical interventions on an almost real-time basis as a result of the strides in monitoring technologies.

Clearly, these advances in medical technology have improved the health of the general population. But at the same time, as formerly fatal diseases are detected and treated early on, medicine will increasingly be faced with an older population whose disabilities are more chronic, more degenerative, and more difficult to defeat. And the would-have-dieds can be expected to take center stage in the right-to-die debate as they age, as their conditions deteriorate, and as hope of a meaningful, productive existence fades in the twilight of their lives. Advanced diagnostics enable individuals to live longer lives, but these same technologies are also responsible for sentencing many to a more lingering death later in life when right-to-die questions are more likely to be raised.

Advances in Rescue Medicine

Perhaps even greater strides have been made in the field of rescue medicine in recent years.

Two hundred years ago, the ministrations of medical professionals were as likely to hasten death as to forestall it. Lewis Thomas (1987, cited in Bronzino, Smith, and Wade, 1990, p. 521) paints this rather gruesome picture:

> By the end of the eighteenth century, getting ill and coming under the care of an energetic physician had become an athletic challenge. The dominant idea then was ... that disease in general was caused by an imbalance in the distribution of fluids within the body. Bleeding, cupping, the application of blistering ointments to the skin over the affected organs, accompanied by violent purging with mercurial or plant cathartics, were the standard features of therapy for any serious illness. The bleeding often involved the removal of a quart or more of blood at one sitting, and the appearance of bluish pallor, a feeble pulse, and profound weakness were taken as signs that the treatment might be having the desired effect.[6]

The account of George Washington's death provides a graphic case in point. Washington, "by all accounts a hale and hearty man in his mid-sixties," developed a sore throat after a tiring horseback ride in the snow on December 12, 1799. A blistering poultice was applied to his neck, and he was repeatedly asked to gargle with a mixture of vinegar, molasses, and butter. Meanwhile, caretakers drew off about five pints of blood, probably half his total blood volume. He died two days later. Among his last words were, "I thank you for your attentions, but I pray you to take no more trouble about me. Let me go off quietly." Indications suggest that what Washington really had was a case of strep throat: It was the shock caused by blood loss that most likely killed him (Bronzino, Smith, and Wade, 1990, p. 521).

The primitive state of premodern medicine precipitated brief encounters with death during which few questions about the appropriate response (save for acceptance) had a chance to germinate. Medical technology based on crude and often misguided principles, the home-based health-care model that emphasized palliation more than cure, and the late detection of fatal conditions (most people with chronic, degenerative conditions were dying quite a while before anyone knew it) all led to a relatively short period of infirmity before death took its toll. The simple understanding of death as the lack of a heartbeat, and the high incidence of acute disease and serious injury are other factors that led to a relatively brief deathbed scene (if one even made it to the bed). This all caused most people to adopt a fatalistic acceptance of death (Lofland, 1978, p. 18). After all, what other options were there?

Today, the progress of intervention technology has fueled a curative, activist orientation among health-care professionals who place a high value on prolonging life. As a result, individuals are rescued from a brief encounter with death only to suffer a lingering exit later in life.

Kidney Technology. Some of the earliest and most dramatic advances in rescue medicine have been made in the area of organ failure. Three decades ago, people died if their major organs failed. But now, with some luck and a third party willing to pay, organ failure can be transformed from a death warrant into an entirely manageable condition.

The first of the modern organ augmentation technologies came with the development of the kidney machine at the end of World War II. The very earliest dialysis machines were cumbersome, experimental contraptions that really did not do much to extend the life of those with end-stage renal disease (ESRD). The real turning point for ESRD came with advances made by a team of Seattle doctors led by Dr. Belding Scribner in the early 1960s. Scribner and his colleagues developed a kidney shunt that could be implanted in the body permanently, making it possible for ESRD patients to literally "plug in" to dialysis machines. Dialysis had been available for short-term kidney failure since the early 1950s, but with improved machinery and implanted shunts, it became a long-term therapy with widespread application.

Then came the development of cyclosporine and other immunosuppressive drugs, also in the 1960s, making kidney transplants a realistic long-term alternative to dialysis. By the end of that decade, kidney transplants had become commonplace, and by 1985, physicians were transplanting upwards of 8,000 kidneys a year.[7] Of course, that means that kidney transplantation is responsible for adding 8,000 names to the would-have-died list annually. And many of these rescue-medicine would-have-dieds—just like diagnostic would-have-dieds—must live through a slower, more degenerating death some years down the road, when ethical questions about the right to die inevitably are raised.

Advances in ESRD treatments raised real-time ethical problems, as well. For example, dialysis was expensive when first developed, and only a few machines were available to serve the many patients who could benefit from treatment. Who would decide who should have access to this lifesaving technology? And what criteria would be used? These were the kinds of questions that physicians and researchers had traditionally decided among themselves, within the professional fraternity. But the Seattle physicians who pioneered dialysis procedures in the early 1960s seemed uniquely aware of the sensitive nature of the resource-allocation decisions that would have to be made. This sensitivity is evidenced by their decision to distribute responsibility beyond the medical profession by empowering a new kind of medical decision-making structure: the ethics committee.

This committee, composed of community members, would be asked to decide what individual characteristics to consider when selecting candidates for treatment. Even after the physicians excluded out-of-state residents (a questionable criterion in itself), children, and patients over the age of forty-five, there were four potential candidates for every dialysis machine available. What should be done? Was it appropriate to screen individuals on the basis of parenthood, profession, or some amorphous "worth to society" classification? Or should medical suitability be the sole criterion for deciding who would get dialysis? Should the ability to pay be a factor?

In effect, by creating an ethics committee to decide such life-and-death questions, the Seattle physicians were throwing up their hands and acknowledging openly (maybe for the first time) that medical professionals no longer had or wanted to have a corner on the decision-making market. Once that gate was opened, however—once doctors forfeited their hegemony over medical decision-making and conceded their fallibility (or at least their insecurity) about making life-and-death decisions—there would be no turning back. Beginning with Scribner's ethics committee, the general public became increasingly comfortable with the notion that people outside the medical fraternity were capable of providing some input regarding life-and-death situations. Medical decisionmaking would never again be quite the same.

Kidney transplantation raised its own set of ethical dilemmas in which not one, but two lives would be seen as hanging in the balance: the life of the donor and the life of the recipient. Interest in dying donors would fuel public-policy concerns in developing brain-death criteria; when is it safe, for example, to harvest the organs from a dying donor if time is of the essence? Interest in healthy donors would raise ethical issues, as well. Would they be coerced by family members to give up one of their kidneys to save the life of another family member? Would some individuals be induced by financial exigency to sell a kidney on the black market in order to raise some quick cash?[8] What about parents who purposely conceive a child in order to harvest organs or other tissue to save the life of another offspring? These kinds of issues simply touched too many raw nerves to be decided within the medical profession. Members of the general public—ethics committee members, the media, judges, legislators, and interest-group activists, to name a few—would find themselves sucked into the vortex of difficult resource-management questions raised by kidney technology.

Hearts and Lungs. Although not as many ethical issues arise when it comes to hearts and lungs, progress in the technology used to augment the functioning of both organs has added considerably to the would-have-died population. As such, we cannot overlook the potential of advances in this area to stimulate right-to-die activism.

Pacemakers, developed in the 1960s, have certainly done their part in this regard. A half million Americans are walking around today with surgically implanted pacemakers, and implantation operations are being done at a rate of 200,000 a year, making this the most common cardiovascular therapy in America. Half of those with implants are living eight years or more, and all who live have been spared a brief encounter with death.

Portable defibrillation equipment has also added substantially to the would-have-died rolls.[9] Also a product of the 1960s, electronic defibrillators are now available in most ambulances and are largely responsible for the dramatic increase in heart attack survival rates in recent years. Only about one in ten individuals rescued with electronic defibrillation ever leave the hospital alive, but all who are rescued in this way are saved for another, later death.

Respiration technology, featuring artificial organs that pull those with lung failure back from the brink of death, has also played a role here. Iron lungs were first developed in the 1950s as an aid to polio victims. These large and cumbersome "tanks" are not nearly as common today as the more practical, positive-pressure ventilators that were developed in that watershed decade for medical advances, the 1960s. With these machines, a flexible plastic hose is "intubated" through the patient's nose or mouth or placed permanently through the trachea to provide the breath of life to those with malfunctioning lungs.

All these advanced medical procedures and technologies—dialysis, organ transplants, defibrillation, and artificial respiration, to name just a few—have two things in common. First, they were all developed in the last thirty years, and second, they all create a population of would-have-died individuals and ultimately prompt consideration of right-to-die issues.

Interventions Create "May-Have-Dieds"

Sometimes, rescue medicine falls short of its goal: to return the patient to a reasonable quality of life. Sometimes, all it does is preserve life in a technical, biological sense, with both the current quality of life and the chances for an improve-ment in quality of life diminished to the vanishing point. Sometimes, all the res-cue medicine in the world can only maintain an individual in what is clinically referred to as a "persistent vegetative state" (PVS). The PVS condition has been a factor in fully 40 percent of all right-to-die cases aired in state and federal courts to date (see Chapter 7), providing empirical evidence that right-to-die activism has been precipitated by recent advances in medical technology. Progress in neonatology that helps severely ill children survive, at least in the short run, has also been the subject of widespread ethical and legal debate.

The Persistent Vegetative State

The persistent vegetative state is characterized by massive and irreversible brain damage that leaves the individual unable to sense or respond to his or her sur-roundings. The cerebral cortex, sometimes referred to as the "gray matter" and considered the seat of all emotions, sensations, and understanding that distin-guish human from subhuman life, no longer functions in patients diagnosed as being in a PVS. Such individuals may experience sleep cycles, and while "awake," they may blink their eyes and contort different parts of their bodies, but they are unable to sense joy or pain. Indeed, PVS patients cannot process or respond to any of the stimuli the surrounding world provides. Unable to swallow, such indi-viduals are usually fed and hydrated through a tube surgically implanted in the stomach wall. This sort of artificial nutrition and hydration (ANH) has itself be-come commonly available only in the last twenty years or so.

It has been estimated that approximately 14,000 individuals are maintained in a PVS in the United States at present, and most could be maintained in that condi-tion indefinitely.[10] Most typically, PVS results from either head injury or hypoxia (a condition caused by a prolonged lack of oxygen to the brain), although some instances of PVS also have been induced by hypoglycemia (insulin overdose). Cli-nicians contend that patients who exhibit no response to their environment for a month or more are extremely unlikely to ever regain consciousness.[11]

Certainly, opinions will vary, but many argue that the slim hope of returning to a severely degraded existence, when combined with the acute financial and emo-tional burdens imposed on the patient's family (individuals whose well-being was presumably important to the now-unconscious patient), makes PVS one of the most disturbing and compelling right-to-die scenarios created by advanced med-ical technology.

Right-to-die questions are even raised when the patient is not technically in a PVS. In particular, we are thinking of those who, near the end of life, lie tubed and restrained in a strange place, surrounded by foreign equipment and unfamiliar faces. According to Henry Glick (1992, p. 209), as many as a million Americans are now being artificially sustained by medical machinery in various states of unconsciousness. Bronzino, Smith, and Wade (1990, p. 544) bring the issue into focus when they point out that:

> Clearly there are circumstances where this kind of vigorous struggle is appropriate and in keeping with medicine's longstanding humanitarian commitments. But when it becomes the predominant response to death, as many believe it has, genuine problems are posed. The most worrisome is the danger—which already may be a reality—that a whole class of patients, particularly elderly patients whose lives are at a natural and inescapable end, will be kept alive by mechanical means long beyond what can be of any benefit to them. ... Technology is particularly well suited to keeping the body going when life is threatened. But it is not particularly well suited to the needs of persons who are not benefitted by having their bodies kept alive.

In times of illness, when one is likely to be insecure and vulnerable, the patient may end up feeling assaulted by the same technology that, in health, had been revered. Conscious patients may complain about the humiliation associated with being treated as inanimate objects that are poked, prodded, stuck, eviscerated, implanted, and evacuated according to schedules set by someone else. Unconscious patients simply stare while members of the family feel the humiliation. As medical ethicist Joseph Fletcher puts it, "The classical deathbed scene, with its loving partings and solemn words, is practically a thing of the past. In its stead is a sedated, comatose, betubed object, manipulated and subconscious, if not subhuman" (cited in Cohn, 1989). And as medical technology creates a natural constituency of may-have-dieds and their families, the right to die is added to the public agenda.

Neonates

Rescue medicine also has made great progress in the world of neonatal health care. Indeed, caring for premature, low-birth-weight babies is one area in which some of the greatest strides have been made. In 1961, newborns in the two- to three-pound range had only a 50 percent survival rate. Today, 80 percent survive, and those who do have fewer medical complications. The very low-weight babies—those under two pounds—had only a 10 percent chance of survival thirty years ago; today, half of them live.

When to Continue Treatment, When to Withdraw? Neonatalogists may have been less interested than those in the organ transplant world in having their own resource-management decisions opened up to public scrutiny, at least at first. As David Rothman (1991, p. 160) notes,

> Issues of life and death remained relatively obscure in the 1960s, largely because doctors, inside the closed world of the intensive care units, turned off the machines when they believed the patient's death was imminent and irreversible. "Very few hospitals," reported a committee of neurologists in 1969, "had any regulations on the matter of

discontinuing the medical aids to respiration and circulation. No one has encountered any medicolegal difficulties. Very few have sought legal opinions." The intensive care units were a private domain, whatever the formal definition of death, and doctors exercised their discretion.

All this changed in 1969, however, with the exposure of the Johns Hopkins University Hospital case in which a baby was allowed to starve to death. The case involved a newborn infant who was transferred to Johns Hopkins for surgery to correct an intestinal blockage. The parents, upon being informed that their child suffered from mental retardation, refused to give permission for the surgery. Consequently, "the infant was moved to a corner of the nursery, and over a period of fifteen days, starved to death" (Rothman, 1991, p. 191). According to Johns Hopkins physicians, this was common practice for children with spina bifida, a congenital condition in which a gap in the spinal column causes paralysis, incontinence, and, frequently, mental retardation. Babies with this condition simply were not treated aggressively. Often, they never even left the delivery room; their charts would read "stillbirth."[12]

A few physicians were deeply troubled by the Hopkins incident, however, and re-created the scenario in a film that was ultimately shown on national television, accompanied by inflammatory newspaper headlines like "Drs Watch as Sick Baby Starves." The story (as retold by the media) laid bare the inner sanctum of physician decisionmaking for all to see and judge, and many Americans did both. As a result of the widespread publicity, symposia and conferences were held all over the country to debate the issues surrounding the case. Significantly, these conferences were not dominated by physicians as they might have been ten years before. Instead, philosophers and ethicists, theologians, lawyers, patient advocates, public-policy analysts, and private individuals could all be found elbowing their way to the table.

A few years later, a situation that was the flip side of the Hopkins case was brought to the public's attention by the parents of a one-pound, twelve-ounce infant boy, delivered after only twenty-four and a half weeks of gestation. Robert and Peggy Stinson coauthored *The Long Dying of Baby Andrew* in 1976 to express their outrage at having no control over the fate of their severely ill offspring after he was admitted to the neonatal intensive care unit (ICU) at a teaching hospital in Philadelphia. They requested that heroics be stopped but were tagged as uncooperative parents by the teams of interns who rotated through the ICU every month or so. And so it went: Baby Andrew lived, with the help of the best technology, for six months, but his story, as told by his parents and reported in the media, had a much longer life and a much more telling impact.

Not all agreed with the Stinsons' decision or even with their account of what took place. But few could argue with one conclusion drawn from their story: "It's not the technology per se that inspires fear—it's the mentality of the people employing it. Fallible people lose sight of their fallibility in the scramble to push back the frontiers of knowledge, to redesign nature and to outwit death" (cited in Rothman, 1991, p. 215). The blurb on the jacket of the Stinsons' book, by Hastings Center cofounder and director Daniel Callahan, described the incident more succinctly as "technological enthusiasm" prevailing over "human care." Agree or not, it was clear that such cases would continue to be aired in public and that the right to die would slowly come to the forefront as a result.

A Special Case: Anencephaly. Some children born with organs that are malformed, partially formed, or, in some cases, entirely missing can still have a fighting chance for life, thanks to the transplant and life-support technology available in modern neonatal intensive care units in the United States. But not much can be done for anencephalic children—those born with underdeveloped brains. There are about 4,000 such births a year, about 1 for every 850 healthy births. For infants born with anencephaly, some portion of the brain stem may exist, but the largest part of the brain, the cortex, is either severely underdeveloped or absent altogether. The expected life span of anencephalic children is extremely short: The vast majority are stillborn, and of those who are born alive, fully 95 percent die within a week (Krauthammer, 1992). Only a very few of these babies survive for more than a few months.

Nearly all severely anencephalic babies are maintained in something akin to a persistent vegetative state. Like their adult counterparts, these infants have no ability to sense their environment. The maintenance technology is well developed, and that allows anencephalic children to live on even when a caring family is not sure that the life being maintained is worth living. And so, the right-to-die question pops up once again.

Another right-to-die issue mixes the rights of anencephalic children with the needs of potential organ recipients, both situations produced by modern medical miracles. The case of Theresa Ann Campo Pearson is illustrative.

A month before the Campo baby was due to be born, routine prenatal tests revealed that she suffered from anencephaly. With this knowledge, the parents, Laura Campo and Justin Pearson of Ft. Lauderdale, Florida, decided to proceed with the pregnancy, already in its eighth month. Knowing their baby had no chance to live, they had decided to attempt to donate their baby's organs to those needing transplants. On March 21, 1992, at the Broward General Medical Center, Theresa Ann was born. As expected, her brain was severely underdeveloped; it included a partially formed stem, which controlled her breathing and her heartbeat, but nothing else. There was no cortex, and an incomplete skull left a gap where several bones should have been. Although her body and organs were fully formed and healthy, Theresa Ann was incapable of experiencing consciousness, pain, emotion, or thought without the cortex of her brain. In effect, her condition was the congenital counterpart of a persistent vegetative state. Also, like any other anencephalic infant, Theresa Ann's life span was expected to be only several weeks at the most.

The baby's parents were confident in their decision to donate her organs to others in need of pediatric transplants, but legal restrictions challenged their ability to carry out that decision. Before Theresa Ann could be considered eligible to donate her organs in her home state of Florida, she first needed to be declared legally brain dead. As in most states, the legal definition of death in Florida requires the "irreversible cessation of all functions of the entire brain, including the brain stem" ("Baby Born Without Brain Dies," 1992). Because Theresa Ann technically did have some brain activity in her partially formed brain stem (controlling reflexive movements), she was considered ineligible as a donor. The parents knew Theresa Ann was terminally ill with no chance for a meaningful life and were hoping that their child could leave her "mark on society in this world and hopefully allow another child to live" ("Organ Donations Barred by Judge," 1992). To keep that hope alive, they decided to take their case to court.

Theresa Ann's parents went to court alone, however. Fearing potential ethical and moral controversy, medical and legal professionals involved in organ-donor and transplant organizations declined to join the family's legal effort. Although commending the parents' intent, doctors were afraid they might be accused of being too quick with the knife, an accusation that would only reinforce the already widespread misperception that the procurement of organs was sometimes performed before a person was really dead. Joining Campo and Pearson in an effort to change brain-death policy would only serve to further undermine the public's trust in the nation's organ-donor program, they thought, and that program was already facing difficulties in securing donations (Chartrand, 1992).

Meanwhile, as the Campo-Pearson legal challenge involving Theresa Ann played out in the Florida courts, Theresa Ann's condition was allowed to decline, along with the viability of her organs from a transplant standpoint. Finally, a circuit court judge decided to refuse to waive the brain-death definition. A few days later, the Florida State Supreme Court rejected the family's appeal for an emergency hearing, claiming it did not have the constitutional authority to hear the case. Theresa Ann was subsequently removed from a ventilator, which she had been placed on to sustain her when her vital organs began to fail. Later that afternoon, at 3:45 P.M. on March 31, 1992, Theresa Ann Campo Pearson died of respiratory failure. She was nine days old. As feared, her organs had deteriorated beyond the point of usefulness: In spite of all of her parents' efforts, not one organ could be donated to any of the more than 30,000 patients on the national organ donation list (Kolata, 1992a; "Waiting List Soars," 1993).[13]

Settling the May-Have-Died Question

The Campo case and the situation of the 14,000 PVS patients in the United States raise an important question: What does it mean to be "alive" when medical technology can take the place of vital organs despite an irreversibly nonfunctioning brain? Those in a PVS and severely brain-impaired neonates do not live life as we know it. Instead, they exist in only the most marginal of human conditions, unable to sense the world around them and without realistic hope for improvement. But can they be considered dead from a medical, legal, or ethical perspective? The ethicists are still debating the issue, and, for the most part, the answer from legal and medical circles is a conservative one: They are alive as long as any brain activity exists at any level.

It was long believed that the heart was both the seat of the soul and the key to life (Kastenbaum and Kastenbaum, 1989, pp. 32–36). This is clearly reflected in the fact that the heart is the human organ most written and sung about as the source of our humanity. Conversational language and popular sayings also reflect this long-standing conception ("she has a heart of gold," "his heart is in the right place"). But this did not resolve the issue of when death occurred for premoderns for the prospect of burying the dead alive, even though the heart has stopped beating, has haunted humans for centuries. Indeed, the traditional deathwatch, where friends and family watch over the apparently dead body for some extended period of time, has its genesis in this fear.

As mentioned in Chapter 2, the predeath watch was designed to comfort the dying patient, while at the same time giving family and friends an opportunity to make peace with the soon-to-be-deceased person (lest a restless ghost come back to haunt them). But the postmortem watch was intended to give the apparently dead individual one last chance to show some sign of revival. As if this were not security enough, it was not uncommon for nineteenth-century coffins to be equipped with elaborate rope-and-bell mechanisms, contraptions that would allow a seemingly dead individual to signal those above ground that he or she had been prematurely interred. Lack of heartbeat and breath were taken as the obvious signs of death then, just as they are today, but enough cases of spontaneous resuscitation had been rumored and recorded to give premoderns some pause.

Still, it was only recently that attention officially shifted to the brain as the organ that could ultimately signal death. This shift took place for at least two reasons: the advent of the EEG, which made monitoring of the brain's functioning possible, and the advent of organ transplants, which made monitoring of brain activity necessary.[14] Thus, brain death was something that could be and needed to be established. To be sure, the vast majority of deaths are still certified by checking for pulse and respiration. But in the case of may-have-dieds, especially if the individual is slated to donate organs, cessation of brain activity has become the more widely accepted standard.

The concept of brain death stems from a 1959 article by two French neurophysiologists, Mallaret and Goulon. These physicians studied patients on artificial life supports who showed no electrical brain activity and were therefore considered to be "beyond coma" (Kastenbaum and Kastenbaum, 1989, p. 34). Studies involving the brain-death concept continued throughout the 1960s, but no definitive standards emerged until a committee of Harvard Medical School faculty members convened in 1968—nine years after the French published their study—to codify clear, brain-oriented criteria of death.

The Harvard criteria included a four-part test for clinical death. The first three parts had to do with the more standard definitions of death (i.e., the individual should be unresponsive to stimuli, unable to move or breathe independently, and lack observable reflexes), and the last criterion dealt with the new brain-death concept itself. According to the Harvard criteria, to be declared dead an individual should display an absence of brain activity, signified by two flat EEGs (showing an absence of "peaks and valleys" that indicate electrophysiological activity) taken twenty-four hours apart.

This four-part test was slowly absorbed as a standard protocol of medical practice during the 1970s. And in 1981, a slightly modified variation of Harvard's test was adopted as the Uniform Determination of Death Act (UDDA) by the President's Commission for the Study of Ethical Problems in Medicine and Biomedical and Behavioral Research (1981). In its report, the commission recommended adoption of the UDDA as a public-policy standard of practice for the United States. Subsequently, the National Conference of Commissioners on Uniform State Laws, working in collaboration with the American Bar Association (ABA) and the American Medical Association (AMA), passed a very similar code. Most states took this policy lead and adopted some form of the uniform code as the legal standard for their own laws.

This did not settle the matter, however, for a good deal of controversy remains with regard to what specific brain area should be monitored for electrical activity. Like premoderns who held deathwatches and built coffins rigged with alarm bells, many postmoderns—the Harvard group, the uniform commissioners, the AMA, and the ABA—continue to advance a conservative, "comprehensive brain-death" criterion, just to be sure. This standard requires that electrical activity be absent from *each* region of the brain, including the cerebral cortex (the thinking center), the cerebellum (a small lobe at the base of the brain that controls balance and the coordination of voluntary movement), and the brain stem (which connects the base of the brain to the spinal cord and is responsible for regulating respiration, heart action, swallowing, and other such reflex functions). Activity in any one of these areas would be evidence of life, according to the comprehensive brain-death standard.

Others argue, however, that individuals with an inoperative cortex are unable to think or sense their surroundings as part of a conscious experience and have therefore lost their characteristic humanity. According to this more liberal interpretation, an individual with a dead cortex can be considered physiologically dead even though some reflex activity remains. The conservatives have prevailed to this point almost without exception, and the comprehensive brain-death approach informs the legal codes of most states. It was the standard applied in the case of baby Campo, and it is the interpretation most commonly accepted in hospitals across the country, as well. In the larger scheme of things, however, the very fact that the issue is debated at all is important evidence that right-to-die activism is afoot, despite all the cultural forces of restraint that operate in American society today. Advances in medical technology have created a population of may-have-dieds, and that has made death an important subject of public-policy concern.

Who Will Pay?

With who-gets-what-treatment questions flying in every direction by the 1970s, it was only natural that the question of who would pay should emerge. End-stage renal disease provided the first large-scale opportunity to ask that question. The perfecting of permanently implanted shunts early in the 1960s made dialysis practical as a long-term way of life for thousands. Later in the decade, the development of immunosuppressant drugs made transplants a viable option, as well. But dialysis and transplant technology were (and still are) extraordinarily expensive. And that led to a further question: Would Americans stand idly by while thousands died from a treatable condition for lack of money?

The Case of ESRD

Not surprisingly, given their characteristically weak-kneed reaction to dilemmas that deal with death at any level, Americans, speaking through the policy process, answered this question in the negative. Rather than decide which individuals to subsidize and which to let go, Americans tried to sidestep this discussion entirely by making ESRD technology universally available. And so, both dialysis and transplantation became the first "extreme" medical technologies that government subsidized as an entitlement.

Approximately 70,000 Americans receive either kidney dialysis or kidney transplants in any given year, and much of this care is funded by Medicare (the tab runs about $2 billion per year). Although Medicare is designed primarily as a public health-care plan for the elderly, the age rules were suspended for those with kidney disease: Anyone with ESRD potentially qualifies for coverage. Although kidney patients constitute only about one-quarter of 1 percent of all Medicare beneficiaries, they consume 10 percent of inpatient expenditures and 13 percent of outpatient expenditures annually (Evans, cited in Blank, 1988, p. 6).

From the very start, Congress seemed bent on avoiding life-and-death questions altogether by spending whatever was necessary to cover everyone—death denial and policy restraint at its finest. It is more important for our present purposes, however, to note that questions about the medical management of death have at least been raised and discussed at the federal level of government. This suggests that a new threshold has been crossed: Medical management of life and death is an item falling squarely on the public-policy agenda.

The ESRD experience also set the stage for government to start asking tough questions about the distribution of its health-care resources. Few could argue the absolute benefits of providing dialysis and transplants to those who would otherwise die. But in a world of increasingly scarce resources, the ESRD experience made it clear that the federal government could not provide everything that was technologically feasible to everyone who could potentially benefit. Life-and-death decisions would have to be made consciously at some point, and death would have to be managed, like it or not, because the Medicare budget simply would not accommodate many more stretches like the one it made in covering ESRD.

The Elderly

Like ESRD patients, the elderly also consume a disproportionate amount of public health-care resources. On average, public-sector spending on health care for those in the twilight of life far outstrips public-sector support for those below the age of sixty-five.[15] On the one hand, increased levels of spending on the elderly are to be expected because older people have a higher morbidity rate. On the other hand, however, the government underwrites only 27 percent of health-care costs for those under sixty-five but covers fully 64 percent of costs for those over sixty-five (Hahn and Lefkowitz, 1992, p. 13). It is this differential in percentages of support—not necessarily the differential in absolute spending—that has led some to take a closer look at the kinds of services all these outlays are buying.

High-tech Care. Much of the spending for elderly health care is devoted to routine procedures under Medicare and reimbursement for long-term care under Medicaid. But a significant percentage of this spending goes for procedures that do little more than forestall an inevitable death. According to the Health Care Financing Administration (HCFA), 28 percent of the Medicare budget (about $30 billion annually) is spent on individuals in their last year of life, primarily in the final thirty days (N. Clark, 1992). Admittedly, even from a probability standpoint, it is not easy to determine who is in the last thirty days of life. And certainly, a share of the outlays in the last thirty days are devoted to providing comfort care. Still, a significant portion of that spending (conservative estimates put the number at around $5 billion) is devoted to providing those at the end of life with the latest in state-of-the-art medical care.[16]

Other studies conducted by HCFA reveal that Medicare reimbursements are consistently six times higher for those who die in a hospital than for those who survive hospitalization, a fact attributed by some to the high-tech services provided dying patients in their last weeks and days of life. Ultimately, it seems that health-care spending in the United States is skewed to a degree toward the seriously ill elderly—individuals who will die regardless of interventions. In the eyes of some, this is a luxury that the health-care finance system is less and less able to afford. As a result, fairly or not, life-and-death issues are being raised in the context of debates about how much health care the elderly are entitled to receive.[17]

One critic of the status quo, Richard D. Lamm (a former governor of Colorado), put the point sharply in 1984 when he stated in a public address that elderly, terminally ill persons have a "duty to die and get out of the way. Let the other society, our kids, build a reasonable life" (Worsnop, 1992, p. 149). Others have been more cautious in advancing the same conclusion. In 1977, a year after California took the plunge as the first state to pass a living-will law, Robert A. Derzon, chief administrator of HCFA at the time, opined that "cost-savings from a nationwide push toward living wills is likely to be enormous" (Worsnop, 1992, p. 148).

Thomas H. Murray, director of the Center for Biomedical Ethics at Case Western Reserve University in Cleveland, agrees that right-to-die developments could potentially help control health-care spending, although he also worries about the abuses that such developments could invite (Worsnop, 1992, p. 150). The bottom line, regardless of which direction the debate goes from here, is that the United States spends enormous amounts on those at the end of life, while other health-care needs go begging. That has led some to explore the right-to-die argument for relief, thereby creating a measure of right-to-die activism within some circles.

Nursing-Home Care. Clearly, whether one agrees with Lamm's hard-line, "duty to die" assessment or not, the elderly are putting a strain on the health-care system today. Only about 5 percent of the nation's 28 million elderly are in nursing homes at any one time (Eckholm, 1990), but total public outlays for nursing-home care have more than doubled from $11 billion in 1980 to $25 billion in 1990. These outlays are projected to double again in the 1990s, reaching $53 billion ($193 per capita annually) by the year 2000 (Callahan, 1990, p. 273). This is a strain that, rightly or wrongly, will inevitably prompt questions about the right to die among nursing-home residents, members of their families, and the tax-paying public more generally.

Projected demographic shifts and health-care trends only promise to magnify the strain on the health-care system in the years to come. In 1970, 10 percent of Americans were over sixty-five; now that number is up to 12.5 percent and climbing steadily. By 2010, the percentage of Americans over the age of sixty-five could reach 20 percent as baby boomers swell the ranks of the nation's elderly population. A small minority of this entire age group will require nursing-home care, but 23 percent of those over the age of eighty-five—the fastest-growing of all age groups in the United States today[18]—will find themselves residing in such institutions.

Dementia. More important than the raw increase in numbers, however, may be the degree of infirmity experienced by this elderly population. Not only are the superannuated more likely to require nursing-home care, they are also much more likely to suffer from advanced stages of dementia. Only about 10 percent of elderly Americans suffer some form of mental disability, but Peter J. Cross and Barry J. Gurland (cited in Blank, 1988, p. 127) estimate that between 20 percent and 30 percent of those eighty-five and older will suffer some form of such afflictions (the National Institute on Aging and the Alzheimer's Association peg the level at 50 percent). If current trends hold true, another half million individuals with terminal dementia will be added to the list of 1.5 million patients in that condition already in the United States (Blank, 1988, pp. 125–126).

Dementia (a chronic illness category in which Alzheimer's disease is the most common variety) is a serious disease that now ranks as the fourth leading killer of adults, with a tally of 100,000 deaths annually. To be sure, the cost of caring for individual patients in this condition is not particularly high when compared with the kinds of high-tech treatments now employed as a matter of course in many American hospitals. Nonetheless, the combined costs of caring for those suffering from such afflictions is considerable, varying from an estimated low of $24 billion (Office of Technology Assessment, cited in Blank, 1988, p. 126) to a high of $88 billion (Gelman and Hager, 1989, p. 45).

Dementia is an irreversible process that becomes increasingly expensive to treat as the quality of the patient's life erodes. It is a debilitating, often dehumanizing condition for which there is no known cure. It slowly robs the individual of memory and the capacity to function, making him or her increasingly dependent on others for the daily necessities of life, including feeding and toileting, in what some have described as an "endless funeral." Ultimately, the overall costs of caring for growing numbers of patients suffering from dementia, combined with the mentally and physically dehumanizing and irreversible nature of the condition, are leading some to ask if incurring greater expenses to maintain an irreversibly degrading and dehumanizing quality of life makes sense anymore. Many are beginning to wonder, as America ages and the ranks of the infirm elderly swell, if this situation does not invite—and even demand—a serious public-policy discussion about life and death, including the right to die.

Costing Out the PVS Problem

Certainly, health-care spending that raises right-to-die questions is not limited to geriatric care. It seems that seriously ill Americans in general receive more than what is considered a fair share of health-care resources in other countries. According to 1982 figures, the United States devoted 15 percent of expenditures to support care rendered in the ICUs of American hospitals, where 5 percent of the 1.4 million hospital beds are located. That contrasts sharply with Great Britain, where only 3 percent to 4 percent of outlays are expended for intensive-care procedures and only 1 percent of beds are devoted to the ICU.[19]

There is, in addition, a small but growing population of individuals mired in the limbo referred to as a persistent vegetative state. Generally, estimates of the current PVS population in the United States hover around the 14,000 mark. Whatever the exact figure, however, it is clear that this group of individuals—for whom care can be very expensive, with little if any chance that medical interventions will have any positive effect—is growing in number.

Estimating the cost of care per PVS patient at $50,000 per year (a conservative guess if much advanced technology is required), this group consumes about $7 billion in resources annually. As already noted, those in a PVS do not meet the standard brain-death criteria now in use, so they are kept alive by artificial means indefinitely, usually at the request and sometimes the demand of the family (Blank, 1988, p. 131). Historically, physicians have chosen to treat these patients aggressively, and insurers have simply paid the bills without question, disbursing the costs among policyholders in the form of higher premiums and higher deductibles. Some patients in a PVS with ESRD are even transported three times a week from a long-term care facility to a medical center to be dialyzed, even though they have no sense of what is going on around them and no hope of recovery. More and more, however, physicians are taking a more critical look at the care they provide. The case of Helga Wanglie is illustrative.

Helga Wanglie was eighty-six when she slipped on a rug in her Minneapolis home, falling and breaking her hip in December 1989. After being successfully treated, she was discharged from Hennepin County Medical Center and moved to a nursing home. However, in January 1990, she developed respiratory complications and was readmitted to the hospital so that she could be placed on a respirator. In this condition, she was still aware of her surroundings, able to acknowledge pain and suffering, and able to recognize her family. In early May, after five months of unsuccessful attempts to wean her from the respirator, she was transferred to a long-term care facility that specialized in treating respirator-dependent patients. She subsequently suffered a heart attack there.

Though resuscitated, Wanglie had been deprived of oxygen for several minutes during the attack, leaving her with severe and irreversible brain damage. On May 31, 1990, she was readmitted to the hospital, where she continued to use a respirator. She also received antibiotics for recurrent pneumonia, along with artificially provided food and fluids through a tube implanted into her stomach. After repeated evaluations, her condition was diagnosed as PVS with the complication of permanent respirator dependency (Cranford, 1991, p. 23). In this condition, Wanglie was totally unaware of her surroundings and unable to recognize her loved ones, including her eighty-seven-year-old husband of fifty-three years, Oliver. Doctors who examined her said there was no hope that she would ever regain consciousness (Walsh, 1991).

Like most Americans, Wanglie had left no previous written record of what kind of care she wanted, and due to her unresponsive condition, she was no longer in a position to indicate her preferences. Because of her dismal prognosis, the medical staff suggested that the family reevaluate continuing the extensive care required to prolong her existence. Relatives claimed to understand Wanglie's virtually nonexistent chances for recovery, but nevertheless, they opposed termination of treatment, "hoping for a miracle" (Walsh, 1991). Angered by the medical staff and others who saw her continued treatment as futile, her husband stated, "She told me many times that if anything happened to her, she didn't want anybody or anything to shorten her life. I intend to keep that promise" ("Doctors Want to Pull Plug," 1990).

Doctors responded to the Wanglie family's intransigence by affirming their commitment to saving and preserving life when possible, while countering that, in Helga Wanglie's case, they would have to go beyond the limit of "reasonable care" to maintain her existence. In short, medical staff members and hospital administrators agreed that continued treatment would not be "in the patient's personal or medical interest" (Walsh, 1991). Since the family remained unconvinced, hospital administrators and the medical staff, in an unprecedented move, took the case to court, where they requested the appointment of an independent guardian. An editorial in the *New England Journal of Medicine,* which supported the institution's position, opined that "the hospital's plea [was] born of realism, not hubris. ... It advances the claim that physicians should not be slaves to technology, any more than patients should be its prisoners. They should be free to deliver, and act on, an honest and time-honored message: 'Sorry, there's nothing more we can do'" (Miles, 1991, p. 514). Oliver Wanglie, a retired lawyer, filed a countersuit against the hospital with the support of his family, requesting that *he* be named guardian.

In a May 1991 hearing before Probate Judge Patricia L. Belois, Steven H. Miles provided testimony for the parties bringing suit against Oliver Wanglie. According to Miles, the physician who served as ethical consultant to the hospital in the case, family members are the "preferred surrogates" for comatose patients. At the same time, he noted, "physicians have a duty to overrule families in certain circumstances. I believe a doctor cannot be obligated and should not be obligated to provide medical care which cannot serve a patient's personal, medical interest" (Walsh, 1991).

The Wanglies persisted, however, in demanding that all medical treatment to keep Helga alive be continued. Describing her as a devout Lutheran who reportedly told relatives that she favored every effort to maintain life, her family claimed to be certain that, by insisting that life-support measures be continued, they were fulfilling her wishes. Oliver Wanglie argued that no one was better suited than he to decide his wife's fate and that the belief in sustaining life at all costs was something they had discussed and shared ("Judge Rejects Request," 1991). William Lubov, the court-appointed attorney for Helga Wanglie contended, in classic, individualistic form, "I couldn't disagree with the opinion of the family more, but I feel even more strongly that the right of the individual to choose is paramount" (Walsh, 1991).

In a ruling issued July 1, 1991, Judge Belois of the Hennepin County Court rejected the hospital's position and gave Oliver Wanglie guardianship over his wife, who was then eighty-seven. Helga Wanglie and her family won the legal battle, but shortly thereafter, she lost her battle for life: She died of multisystem organ failure on Independence Day, 1991. Her medical bill was approximately $750,000.

The insurance company in the Wanglie case, fearing negative publicity, decided to assume responsibility for these costs without a fight. But more and more health insurers are beginning to take a critical look at the kinds of care they are willing to underwrite. There has been a surge of interest in managed care and coverage cutbacks in recent years that may ultimately nudge the PVS population out of line for coverage, leaving Medicaid (after the family spends down their assets to the poverty level) as the sole source of continued support. Again, with pressures on public health-care budgets already strong, right-to-die questions—and maybe even Lamm's more radical "obligation-to-die" questions—cannot help but arise.

Malpractice

Malpractice is another element of the cost containment crisis in U.S. health care that might eventually lead individuals and policymakers to consider right-to-die alternatives. According to the AMA, only a little over three malpractice actions were filed per year for every 100 physicians in 1982. But by 1989, that number had more than doubled, jumping to 7.4 claims per year for every 100 physicians. Jury awards have skyrocketed, as well: The average jury award to plaintiffs for malpractice actions is now $300,000. To compensate for this, insurance companies boosted malpractice premiums in that same time period by 167 percent (Olen, 1991). Today, physicians collectively pay about $4 billion a year for medical malpractice coverage, and hospitals pay another $2 billion for the same purpose.

The average fee paid by individual American physicians for liability insurance in today's market tops the $15,000 mark, with specialists paying much higher rates. For example, Chicago obstetricians and neurosurgeons pay upwards of $150,000 per year (Domenici and Koop, 1991). Eleven cents of every dollar paid to a doctor goes for such insurance, and the AMA estimates that another $15.1 billion (about 2.5 percent of all medical spending) is spent every year on "defensive medicine"—therapies and tests that are ordered more out of concern about a potential malpractice suit than out medical necessity.

This has all led some in the medical community to start sharing treatment plan decisionmaking with their patients. Putting patients more directly in control of treatment decisions may take some of the burden off the physicians, and presumably this would reduce some of the doctors' liability in the process. When the medical decision-making structure is opened up, the family and the patient become coauthors of the treatment plans that are chosen. As such, family members may be less likely to cry foul when things do not turn out as planned. And even if they do cry foul, they may be less likely to win their cases in court if judges and juries find the plaintiffs' fingerprints are all over the medical record.

Ultimately, shared decisionmaking may cause malpractice premiums to stabilize. It may even lead to an attenuation of defensive medical practices. Both are potential benefits that will be difficult to resist in the years to come. But however that plays out, we should note, for present purposes, that inviting patients into the medical decision-making matrix on a regular basis cannot help but fuel a measure of right-to-die activism. If patients get used to being asked if they want to go ahead with procedure A or surgery B, they cannot help but become more interested in making choices at the very end of life, when they must decide whether they will continue to live or not.

Summary: Medical Technology and the Emergence of the Right-to-Die Scenario

The emergence of kidney dialysis and organ donation dilemmas, together with the definition of death and neonatal-care conundrums, forces discussion of death as a matter of public policy. Academics, the press, state legislators, and the American people have come to expect that these sorts of situations will be fair game as a matter of public discourse. Add into the mix the raft of new ethical dilemmas (surrogate motherhood, the disposition of frozen embryos when parents die or divorce, "morning after" birth control pills, and so on), and we end up with a society just ripe for public policymaking in the medical ethics arena.

Indeed, the whole business of ethics in medicine has become so volatile and the interest is so intense that a whole new academic animal—the bioethicist—emerged to deal with the conundrums that seem to pop up almost daily, beginning in the 1960s. Bioethicists would demand seats at the decision-making tables around the country as policies were formed to address medical-ethical dilemmas, and they would create their own decision forums by founding centers and schools of public-policy study and analysis. Ultimately, these academics would begin to set the ethics agenda for the nation at large as the years progressed.

Certainly, much of the foment regarding ethical questions about life and death can be traced to the fantastic advances in medical technology that have taken place in the last thirty years. But costs are also cropping up, promoting activism, as well. In fact, more money is spent on health care in the United States than anywhere else in the world. Fourteen percent of America's mammoth gross national product (GNP)—about one dollar out of every seven—is spent on health care.[20]

Our nearest spending competitor is Canada, where only about 9 percent of the gross domestic product (GDP) is devoted to health care. To some, the U.S. rate of increase in spending is even more frightening: Health-care spending has grown half again as fast as the rate of inflation in most years since the 1970s, and there seems to be no end in sight to that phenomenon (Melville, 1992, p. 14).

Especially troubling to some is the fact that a disproportionate amount of that spending goes toward maintaining and occasionally trying to rescue those at the very end of life. This is not particularly surprising, considering how much Americans seem obsessed with the denial of death. Ironically, however, health-care dollars spent during the last days and weeks of life are partly responsible for the increasing interest we have witnessed in right-to-die issues in recent years. Some have begun to question the amount of money spent on rescue medicine for the dying when health-care costs are spiraling out of control and when other medical needs (e.g., prenatal care and preventive medicine) are so apt to go unaddressed. A look into the future suggests that, unless spending priorities are changed, the situation will deteriorate even further as the baby-boom generation passes from middle age into the more medically dependent years of retirement. There should be no doubt that baby boomers will increase the drain on the health-care budget when they retire, just as they increased the drain on the education budgets when they went to school in the 1960s and 1970s.

In the end, whether explicitly acknowledged or not, the underlying pressures of cost containment will provide a good deal of impetus for raising right-to-die questions in the coming years. As George Lundberg notes, "There will never be sufficient money or services to provide everyone with the care they may want" (cited in Rothman, 1992, p. 32). Likewise, John Kilner discounts the popular American myth that there are enough resources to underwrite the cost of treating every terminal disease. Choices must be made, he argues, and better sooner than later. Following up, Callahan (1990, p. 21) notes that "the very nature of medical progress is to pull to itself many more resources than should rationally be spent on it." Rationing is inevitable, these authors contend, and those who are already on death's doorstep for one reason or another are the logical source for potential savings because expenditures here are (arguably) not nearly as important in the big picture as expenditures on those who potentially have many productive years of life ahead of them.

Underlying all this is a debate between individual rights and entitlements versus the collective good. It should be no surprise that the right-to-die debate is so problematic in the United States, where public policy and tradition usually favor individual liberty and downplay social goods. When it comes to death, the expectation that individuals have everything coming to them is the prevailing ethos, all in accordance with individualism and the entitlement syndrome (e.g., as with

Medicare covering dialysis and transplants). Meanwhile, the collective well-being associated with the judicious discussion of death-related issues tends to take a back seat. A number of authors are now sensing a sea change in attitudes, though, with more and more people finding aggressive medical interventions less acceptable than a quiet and humane death (Rothman, 1992, p. 37). As society learns to accept and live within limits, it seems only logical to assume that the right to die will likely come into much clearer focus as a viable alternative for both individuals and policymakers alike.

4

Policy Activism and Medical Professionalism: The Doctor-Patient Disconnection

WE HAVE DISCUSSED the ways in which substantial advances in medical technology over the last few decades have created right-to-die scenarios. As Lyn Lofland (1978, p. 74) notes, "Dying now, as it never has been historically, is something one can 'be' long enough for that period of 'being' to be viewed as problematic." But there is more to right-to-die activism from a medical perspective than technological progress and the issues of scarce resources. There has also been a "revolution in attitudes toward medical practitioners and medical institutions, a revolution marked by a decline in trust in the doctor" (Lofland, 1978, p. 107). This decline in trust is the underlying force of activism surveyed in this chapter.

When trust declines, patients become more willing to question their doctors as sources of authority, and questioning leads to demands from patients and their families that they be included as partners when it comes to making health-care treatment decisions, even when—or especially when—death is a real possibility. We do not mean to suggest that activism is in full swing, with patients and their families leading an insurrection against physicians and hospitals. We do argue, however, that trust has eroded and that this erosion in confidence is beginning to manifest itself as right-to-die activism.

Hospitals Come of Age

Dramatic changes in American institutions of higher medicine—the hospitals—have increased the quality and sophistication of health care substantially since the turn of the twentieth century. At the same time, these advances also have added substantially to the social distance between caretakers and patients. And as patients have become increasingly estranged from their institutions of higher medicine, they have become increasingly suspicious of what goes on there.

Hospitals in Historical Context

The modern hospital, as we know it today, has only existed for a few score years. Through the 1800s, hospitals typically provided only food, shelter, and nursing care to dislocated indigents. Very little in the way of clinically sound treatments were available there (Bronzino, Smith, and Wade, 1990, p. 5), and rarely would a member of the middle or upper classes be found among the patients of one of these institutions.

Throughout the period, hospitals were primarily religious and charitable places for tending the sick and the poor on a long-term basis. Patients had the status of children, and caretakers played the role of parents who, as often as not, lived on the premises. Those who were cared for in these hospitals had to help with the nursing, washing, ironing, and cleaning, all of which were considered part of their "family" chores.

Hospitals were dangerous places before the turn of the twentieth century. Even though individuals with infectious diseases were not accepted by these institutions, contagions contracted within hospitals spread easily among patients and staff in less-than-sanitary settings. Mortality rates of 25 percent among the patient population were not uncommon, nor was it extraordinary to find mortality rates of 10 percent per year among the medical staff (Bronzino, Smith, and Wade, 1990, p. 8). Not until Florence Nightingale's crusade against unsanitary conditions in the hospital in the late 1880s was it acknowledged that "deaths were caused more frequently by hospital conditions than by disease" (cited in Bronzino, Smith, and Wade, 1990, p. 9). Even then, hospital conditions only improved slowly, when they improved at all.

As a result, most health care was delivered in the home, where family and friends acted as the nursing staff, and "illnesses not cured by home remedies were left to run their frequently fatal course" (Bronzino, Smith, and Wade, 1990, p. 10). Such was the state of American health care prior to the turn of the century.

Hospitals in Transformation

The beginning decades of the twentieth century were boom times for hospitals. The number of institutions grew dramatically at that time. In 1872, there were only 178 hospitals in the United States. But by 1910, that number had grown to 4,000. The number swelled another 50 percent to 6,000 in the following decade (Starr, 1982, pp. 73, 178). Much of this explosion in the number of hospitals was fueled by an ever-expanding client base of middle- and upper-income individuals.

Pain control was one reason for this growth. Before the turn of the century, the only drugs available to manage pain—alcohol and opiates—were available at home, without prescription (President's Commission, 1983, p. 17). Thereafter, thanks to the great advances in organic chemistry in the early years of the twentieth century, it became possible to isolate and in some cases synthesize the active ingredients of drugs that, until that time, were available only in their natural herbal or vegetable form. Organic chemistry also made it possible to control and monitor drug use to optimize desired effects and minimize perverse side effects, and the hospital was the easiest and most logical place to do that.

Surgery was another reason for the increase in hospital clientele. Before the 1900s, most operations took place at home or in the doctor's office. But surgery began coming into the hospital around the turn of the century, when—with appreciation for antiseptic conditions and the monitored, controlled use of ether—it became a practical, viable option.

X-ray technology was yet another important aspect of the hospital metamorphosis.[1] Early X-ray machines were available only in hospitals; because they were bulky and expensive, they usually had to be collectively purchased and centrally located. The availability of X-ray machines—these windows on the body—drew many middle-class and upper-class families out of their domiciles and into the hospital for the first time.

This new technology also required more education on the part of the professional staff, and it was probably more responsible than any other technological development for prompting physicians to become more specialized in their training. Development of the X ray also led to a whole new classification of health-care workers: medical technicians. Not surprisingly, radiology was among the first specialized departments to emerge in the modern American hospital, the new nerve center of medical activity where "family" could no longer be used as a metaphor for describing caretaker-patient relationships. Instead, with the beginnings of specialization of tasks, the increasing acceptance of the dispassionate scientific method as a model for care, and the proliferation of regulations regarding sanitation, the hospital began to mimic the bureaucratically organized factory that was emerging at about the same time.

Slowly but surely, as the industrial revolution progressed, the hospital began to lose its character as a family-oriented, long-term almshouse for the indigent. The modern institution took on the characteristics (and, inevitably, some of the impersonality) of the factory assembly line, with its system of raw material inputs (admissions), production (medical interventions), and product outputs (discharged patients). Ultimately, these reformed institutions of higher medicine began to operate on Weberian principles of organization, including clear divisions of labor, chains of command, specialization, marketing, and concern with the bottom line (Starr, 1982, pp. 145–148).

Religiously oriented patrons of the poor yielded to "professional healers," and indigent inmates were joined by middle- and upper-class patients as impersonal provider-client relationships emerged where once there was only paternalism and charity. Spirituality and philanthropy yielded to medical science and the market-place. The communal character of the hospital was stripped away in the process and replaced by the less personal structure of a business organization.

Modern Developments

The 1930s and 1940s brought more important changes to the hospital. The advent of sulfanilamide in the mid-1930s and penicillin in the early 1940s made it possi-ble to manage bodily infections for the first time. And in the 1930s, another tech-nological advance—refrigeration—enabled hospitals to store large quantities of blood. The combination of blood reserves and infection control proved a boon for surgeons and patients alike, and operations went from harrowing, death defy-ing experiences to regularly successful, mainstream aspects of hospital service.

At about the same time, however, as ethnic and religious hospitals began to lose their distinctive character, they also began losing touch with their community roots. As Rothman (1991, p. 130) writes, "The ethnic hospital survives in name only. It is now in all senses a public space, with the same personal ties to its pa-tients that a busy midtown hotel has to its guests." In the past, hospital staff in many big and even small city institutions were chosen largely on the basis of eth-nic or religious qualities: Catholics staffed and ran Catholic hospitals that primar-ily served the ethnic Catholic community, and Jewish hospitals were staffed, oper-ated, and populated primarily by ethnic Jews.[2] Today, technical merit is the primary criterion for selection and advancement within hospital hierarchies, both secular and religious, so that the staff in either kind of institution is likely to be as diverse as the larger community it serves.

The good news is that hospitals now strive to hire and promote the very best clinicians available, personal characteristics aside. The bad news is that those looking for an institution that will attend to their special ethnic or religious pre-dispositions will be disappointed. Jewish hospitals may still offer kosher food, and Catholic hospitals may still schedule daily services in the hospital chapel, but both the staff and clientele of the modern medical institution tend to be heterogeneous groups. Importantly, when a hospital loses its ethnic or religious cast, it also loses its ability to bridge the social distance between itself and its natural pool of cli-ents, becoming a more sterile and foreboding institution in the process.

Those who wish to be treated in the community or neighborhood hospital are apt to have their share of disappointments, as well. Many rural, small-town, and neighborhood hospitals have closed their doors in the last few decades because the cash flow in these smaller institutions was too low to allow for the purchase of sophisticated equipment.[3] And even if they can buy this kind of equipment, smaller institutions that have managed to stay open may not be able to compete with big-city medical centers in the range, number, and pedigrees of specialists. This has forced those in the community to travel farther to regional medical centers for their hospital care, and the distance traveled is both geographic and social now that hospitals have changed from safe havens to strange places.

To exacerbate the situation, hospital stays have become shorter in recent years. In the 1920s, the average stay in general hospitals was just a little over eleven days (Rothman, 1991, p. 126). Today, inpatient stays average less than a week, and many interactions that had previously required hospital admittance are done on an outpatient basis. There is good reason to celebrate this development (e.g., lowered costs and increased productivity), but an unintended side effect is that patients have less time to become familiar with hospital surroundings and personnel. As a result, hospitals have begun to hire patient representatives and social workers in the last few decades. Patient advocacy has become an entirely new career track for employees of an institution whose clients need someone to help them navigate the increasingly turbid bureaucratic whirlpool that the modern American hospital has become.

Max Weber has described how bureaucratization in the West is largely responsible for "removing social functions from the family and household and implanting them in specialized institutions autonomous of kinship considerations" (Blauner, 1966, p. 384). Clearly, this has been the case with hospitals. As they transformed themselves from palliative almshouses for the poor to bureaucratically organized institutions of higher medicine, hospitals also began assuming responsibility for those who die. Whereas only the indigent died in an institutional setting in the early 1900s, fully 80 percent of all Americans die in health-care institutions today—65 percent in hospitals, 15 percent in nursing homes (President's Commission, 1983, p. 17). Thus, hospitals have become increasingly strange and foreboding places at the same time as they have become the primary site of American death. That, we argue, is one reason why patients are more and more likely to challenge their hospitals on a raft of issues, including those that bear directly on their right to make end-of-life treatment decisions.

Physician-Patient Relations

Although important, the transformation of the American hospital is only one factor in the activism associated with provider-patient relationships. There have also been dramatic changes in the way physicians relate to their patients. In the past, doctors were typically friends of the family, but medical care today is more accurately characterized by impersonal relationships, in which physicians tend to be strangers whom we are suspicious of rather than friends we can trust.

The Golden Days
of Physician-Patient Friendship

"We spent the rest of the afternoon climbing up and down stairs and in and out of his patients' houses. I can remember being offered tea, cakes, or cookies by people anxious to hear what he had to say and grateful for his presence. And my father—he seemed to know everyone's friends and relatives. He was full of reminiscences which he and his patients shared. Each visit was an occasion for warm conversation in addition to the medical treatments" (recollections of a physician's son, cited in Rothman, 1991, pp. 112–113).

As this premodern account of the relationship between a physician and his patients suggests, there was a time in the not-so-distant past when doctors and patients were much more intimately involved in each other's lives than they are today. These social relationships between patient and practitioner grew out of both commercial and professional expediency.

The case for commercial expediency is clear. There were no credentialing agencies for physicians in the premodern United States, and physicians did not have much in the way of specialized knowledge to peddle. Medical practice at the time consisted largely of a commonsense application of homespun nostrums, and much of the potentially lucrative work was parceled out to other members of the community: Barbers let the blood, midwives delivered the babies, and those who developed reputations as bonesetters attended to the fractures.

As with a carpenter or a plumber, the ability of a physician to attract business was largely a matter of goodwill in those times. Indeed, it is no overstatement to suggest that community ties of friendship and acquaintance were, for the nineteenth-century physician, a matter of professional survival (Rothman, 1991, p. 110). The renowned physician Oliver Wendell Holmes, Sr., laid out the situation bluntly in his 1871 address to the graduating class of Bellevue Medical School. He spent most of his time instructing the class of fledgling practitioners on the art of patient relations, imploring them never to forget the "physician in our city whose smile was commonly reckoned on being worth $5,000 a year to him [quite a sum in 1871]" (cited in Rothman, 1991, p. 111).

To build and maintain a practice, physicians had to be responsive, caring, and trustworthy. Professionalism required intimacy, as well, for knowledge of a family's medical and personal history was an important tool—maybe the most important tool—in the doctor's proverbial black bag. Prior to the advent of X rays, advanced medical imaging, and computer-assisted lab testing, personal contact with the patient was often the doctor's most useful diagnostic aid.

Knowing this, patients also sought to reinforce family ties with physicians, against the time when a member of the family would fall ill. It was a two-way street: Physicians were intimate with families because intimacy provided a commercial and clinical basis for the practice, and families courted physicians, sharing their medical histories and family secrets along the way, so that the doctors could be more effective when illness struck. This shared knowledge was usually so detailed and complete that office records "were rarely kept, being considered unnecessary by the solo practitioner who knew, and had no trouble remembering the patient, family, and their illnesses without taking notes" (Stoeckle and Billings, cited in Rothman, 1991, p. 118).

These sorts of personal relationships continued even with the industrialization and urbanization that were moving into full swing around the turn of the twentieth century. This was a period in which doctors, like hospitals, were chosen for their religious or ethnic characteristics. Physicians had either demographic qualities or interpersonal skills (preferably both) to bank on, both of which engendered trust in patients. And home visits continued to be the norm, right through World War II.[4]

Passing of the Golden Years

Of course, all that has changed. Physicians no longer visit homes, and patients rarely consider their medical caretakers to be friends of the family. Encounters with health care are now routinized and bureaucratized. Technologically sophisticated instrumentation has taken the place of the personal conversation and the laying on of hands as the primary diagnostic aid. In the process, health care has been transformed from a domestic, almost spiritual concern into an impersonal, secular undertaking, and the erosion of trust in our health-care providers has been an inevitable result.

The Doctor Is In. In the 1930s and 1940s, dramatic advances in communications technology began to change the nature of physician-patient relationships in a tangible way. The telephone was a boon for physicians hoping to build a steady practice. Telephones made it possible for patients to see the doctor at the office at a prearranged time. The patient, knowing the doctor would not be out on some other call, was willing to make an office visit. At the same time, the telephone made the office practice more profitable for the doctor, who could arrange a steady stream of appointments rather than relying on an uneven trickle of home-visit requests.[5]

Telephones eliminated much of the uncertainty for both doctor and patient, thereby making office visits much more attractive, if less personal, than home visits for both parties involved. As people seeking care came to physicians, rather than the other way around, doctors could see more patients. But seeing more patients and seeing them in the office rather than in the home taxed the emotional capacity of the physician to the point where personal friendships could no longer be maintained with the entire clientele. Social distance increased, and as a result, the trust patients had in their physicians began to erode.

The Birth of Specialization. Certainly, changing the site of health-care services from the home to the office revolutionized the physician-patient relationship. But other, more subtle revolutions in the profession, begun much earlier, also blossomed and had an even more profound effect on that relationship.

The seeds of this transformation date back as far as the Renaissance. Until that time, the Hippocratic school dominated the practice of medicine. Practicing and training others on the Greek island of Cos around 400 B.C., Hippocrates, the founding father of modern medicine, taught his students that disease was not the hand of evil gods at work but a natural and rationally comprehensible phenomenon. The Hippocratic approach was holistic in nature and viewed the whole body as a dynamic organism whose state was directly affected and, to a degree, controllable by the environment in which it operated. That all began changing with the coming of the Renaissance, however, as anatomists began to deconstruct this holistic Hippocratic paradigm.

Dissection of human cadavers came into vogue during the fifteenth and sixteenth centuries as a way of understanding disease. (Leonardo da Vinci began depicting the human body in anatomically graphic detail about the same time.) This shift from Hippocratic holism to Renaissance specificity led physicians to stop asking, "How do you feel?" and begin asking, "Where does it hurt?" Anatomists of this period began to perceive disease as a malfunction of the body at a localized site, and they tried to understand in detail the operation and malfunction of various sites within the whole.

The mechanistic conception of the body advanced by the seventeenth-century French philosopher René Descartes was very much in harmony with the small but growing trend toward the specialization paradigm. Descartes argued that the human body was a physical entity subject to the mechanical laws of nature. As such, it could be viewed as nothing but a complex "earthly machine" in which inputs must equal outputs and where effects had discoverable causes which could be remedied with "the same precision and certainty as the disorders of a clock"; this view, according to J. M. Boyle and J. E. Morriss, "was destined to become a fundamental root metaphor for medical science [so that] today, the image of the person as a machine is retained" (cited in Bronzino, Smith, and Wade, 1990, pp. 542–543).

The seeds of specialization, planted in the fifteenth and sixteenth centuries and nurtured along by Descartes in the seventeenth century, were slow to germinate. But by the mid-nineteenth century, they had begun to take root, and they were ready to blossom as a new kind of anti-Hippocratic orthodoxy in professional medical circles in the 1900s (Bronzino, Smith, and Wade, 1990, pp. 537–539). No longer would the body be viewed in holistic terms; instead, it would be seen in mechanistic terms, as a collection of separable, identifiable, and dissectable parts. Little by little, as the new orthodoxy took hold, physicians would stop looking at patients as people to be cared for and start conceiving of them as a collection of parts, some of which needed to be fixed. This orthodoxy of specialization and compartmentalization may have been good for modern medicine,[6] but it also increased the social distance between patient and doctor.

Embracing Tools. Another important professional transformation began during the Renaissance: a shift in the medical profession's view with regard to "tools." An antitechnological bias in medicine can be traced to the medieval universities of the thirteenth century, where formal medical training took place in an environment in which theologians eschewed the use of medical instruments as degrading. Scholars of all types learned to operate with their heads, not their hands, lest they lower themselves to the level of tradesmen, with whom the use of tools was associated (Reiser, 1984, cited in Bronzino, Smith, and Wade, 1990, p. 540).

But Renaissance anatomists who dissected cadavers required tools to accomplish the task and analyze what was found, and with the acceptance of these instruments, the antitechnological bias began to dissipate. It was no coincidence that the first great "modern," university-based medical schools emerged in Europe during the Enlightenment. These institutions began to push an appreciation of empirical data (pulse rate, temperature, and so forth), collected using the hands and other tools, as important indicators of disease.

By the nineteenth century, when the drive to improve diagnostic techniques had become fairly well established, members of the medical community had set aside most of their apprehension about working with their hands, and they began to embrace technology wholeheartedly. The stethoscope, ophthalmoscope, and laryngoscope, all developed in the mid-1800s, made embracing technology both easier and more necessary. At the same time, however, these new diagnostic tools made it possible, preferable, and maybe even inevitable that the practitioner and patient would become more distant from each other.

As Stanley Reiser has observed (cited in Starr, 1982, p. 136), this new diagnostic equipment encouraged the physician to "move away from involvement with the patient's experiences and sensations, to a more detached relation, less with the patient but more with the sounds of the body"—sounds the patient could neither hear nor interpret. This reduced the dependence of the physician on the patient's statements and increased the asymmetry of information (and power) between the two individuals. The nature of private medical practice—and the nature of the doctor-patient relationship—would be forever changed as a result.

Modern Developments. The ongoing shift from home-based to office-based medical practice, together with the application of increasingly specialized knowledge and the use of increasingly sophisticated tools, continued to have an important effect on the doctor-patient relationship as the twentieth century progressed. As the physician's practice grew in efficiency and numbers, his or her economic reliance on any one patient or family diminished. The physician no longer needed that "$5,000 smile" that Holmes had talked about, nor was there a need to be so friendly, and the social gulf between patient and practitioner began to widen further.

By the 1960s, house calls represented less than 1 percent of patient-doctor contacts. Office visits made it possible for physicians to maximize their incomes by seeing more patients in less time, and it also enabled patients to avail themselves of the increasingly sophisticated equipment that began to adorn the physician's office (Rothman, 1991, p. 128). For physicians, pausing by a patient's sickbed to ask a question or give reassurance changed from standard practice to an indulgence to an anachronism: Why speak to the patient when so much more can be learned through diagnostic equipment? Such conversations had become add-ons, something physicians ought to do as a moral, not medical, obligation (Rothman, 1991, p. 132). No longer would doctors "see" a patient. Now, with the acceptance of the scientific method and the accompanying array of diagnostic equipment, the physician had only to "examine" the patient (Starr, 1982).

Trust in medical professionals eroded even further with the advent of Medicare and Medicaid in the 1960s. These two public programs gave an impetus for government to conduct large-scale assessments of the quality of health care being provided. When substantial variation in therapies and outcomes were reported (such as variations in the frequency and success rates of surgeries for different physicians and hospitals across the country), doubts about doctors and doctoring were inevitably raised. The fact that different doctors came to different conclusions, with widely varying outcomes, flies in the face of the notion of physician omniscience, and that only accelerated the erosion of confidence already in progress.

Several other factors came into play about this time, as well. Physician income exploded in the decades following World War II. Doctors had always been respected members of the community, but the quantum jump in salary added a socioeconomic distance between patient and provider that had not existed before. Solo practice began to decline in these middle years of the twentieth century, as well. Group practice, a veritable oddity in 1940 (involving only 1 percent of all physicians), had become a popular option by the 1980s, when fully one-quarter of all practicing physicians were members of a medical group. Administrative staffs also increased dramatically, as physicians sought to optimize their clinical contact time while they struggled to manage the crush of insurance and government paperwork. Instead of the quaint Rockwellian image of the country doctor going door to door, the modern physician is more likely viewed as a well-to-do baron, lording over a large staff of paraprofessionals and secretaries in well-equipped, imposing office spaces.

A substantial amount of the work doctors do has moved out of the office altogether and into the hospital. In the 1930s, only one doctor in sixteen worked full-time in a hospital, and 40 percent of the patient-doctor encounters still took place in the home, including half of all births attended by a physician. Doctors typically saw fifty patients a week in those years. But by the 1950s, one out of every six doctors worked full-time in a hospital, and only one in ten visits took place in the home. By then, 96 percent of all babies were being delivered in the hospital, and doctors were seeing twice as many patients a week (Starr, 1982, p. 359). As these trends in venue and volume continue, it becomes increasingly clear why doctors are viewed as having changed from family friends into medical strangers.

The continuing rise of specialization and commensurate decline of general practice also has exacerbated the situation. No longer is a patient treated by one general practitioner (GP); instead, a series of specialists now enter the picture, making it difficult for patients to feel at home with any of them. In one study, conducted between 1928 and 1931, 81 percent of patient visits were made to general practitioners (Rothman, 1991, p. 114). Even as late as 1940, 70 percent of all patient encounters were logged with GPs. But by the 1960s, less than a third of all physicians identified themselves as general practitioners (Rothman, 1991, p. 129), and that percentage has now dropped below the 25 percent mark.[7]

Patients and specialists tend to be strangers almost by definition since patients only go to a specialist when first encountering a particular sort of disorder and stop going when the problem has been addressed.[8] As a result, specialization cannot help but diminish and discount the interpersonal involvement between patient and physician.[9]

Avoiding Death Widens the Gulf

Many factors in the historical development of the doctor-patient relationship over the years help explain the disconnection that seems to characterize that relationship today. In addition, a number of current issues revolving around specific physician predispositions to avoid the issue of death bear directly on that disconnection, making the division between patient and caretaker even more profound. Medical training (which tends to discourage compassion and encourage autonomy), the ethos of not telling the truth about death ("surely, the patient can't take it"), and adherence to the technological imperative ("do everything possible for the patient") all are responsible, to one degree or another, for driving the wedge between physicians and their patients even deeper. When doctors act autonomously, denying death and applying technology at every turn, they breed distrust and contempt in their patients. Doctors are challenged at the bedside and with increasing frequency in the courtroom as a result, as right-to-die activism boils up and over.

Physician Training and the Denial of Death

Physicians generally do not deal well with the subject of death, and that behavior, we contend, has enhanced the disconnection between physicians and their patients. The wider the gulf becomes, the more likely it is that right-to-die questions will spill out of the hospital room and onto the floors of the legislatures and courts. A number of explanations for this have already been offered. We now add to that list by suggesting that modern medical training is at least partly to blame.

Prospective physicians enter medical school already socialized in the ways of denial shared by the culture at large, and there is little done to break down that denial in medical school.[10] In fact, just the opposite seems to occur. Original tendencies toward denial are reinforced during training and enhanced into a more sophisticated and deep-seated predisposition to shunt considerations of death aside once doctors are out of school and engaged in active practice.

Few medical schools in the United States have made courses in death and dying an integral part of their curricula, leading some to argue that physician training is inadequate (Carse and Dallery, 1977, p. 329). The majority of medical school students get only brief discussions of dying in clinical courses that primarily deal with biophysical considerations, leaving aside entirely the psychosocial dimensions of death.[11] Even when courses on death are offered, they are often underenrolled electives that end up canceled for lack of interest, in an overall training regimen where "death is scientifically attacked and humanly denied" (W. Smith, 1985, p. 285).[12]

As if the lack of coursework on the sensitive treatment of death and dying were not enough, the medical training itself tends to drive out whatever compassion student physicians bring to their chosen career (The Boston Women's Health Book Collective, 1984, p. 567). The process really begins in undergraduate education, during which premed students are saddled with one of the most rigorous academic programs on campus. Studies suggest that, as a result, such students tend to socialize less than their peers.

Opportunities for social life are even fewer in medical school, which places enormous pressures on students to absorb a great deal of technical material. The coursework is covered in a compressed amount of time, largely through one-way lectures that reinforce absolutism and discourage critical thinking. Study demands force students to lead insular lives, and characteristics that might help physicians relate to their patients—empathy and compassion, for example—are conspicuously absent, if not consciously discouraged. Adversarial relationships rather than collaborative ones are emphasized with peers as well as patients when the time comes to move out of the lecture hall and into the clinical ward during residency.

Stein (1990, p. 182) describes the life of a resident in harsh detail:

One is exposed to the constant prospect of public humiliation through the press of sleeplessness, long periods of little or no food, long hours of work, harsh training rituals, and the urgency to perform impeccably and come up with the right answers in the eyes of numerous superiors. In this environment the individualist physician identity is forged, and the drive for self-reliance, the need for absolutes, the renunciation of uncertainty, the fear of failure, and the need to be decisive and virtually self-sufficient are established.

Others describe resident programs as "grueling ... often demanding as much as thirty-six hours at a stretch and hundreds of hours per week in constantly under-staffed conditions. Sleep deprivation leads to testiness that becomes second nature for many even after residency is over and normal sleep patterns return" (The Boston Women's Health Book Collective, 1984, p. 568). Work loads demand that fast judgments be made again and again, and over time, making snap judgments becomes second nature, a habit that may endure even after residency, when time to think and consult is not in such short supply. In the end, despite the idealism that most medical students bring to their training, the physical and mental stress of the training regimen produces fully certified physicians who are "more cynical, detached, and mechanistic than at entry" (The Boston Women's Health Book Collective, 1984, p. 570). As Derek Bok, former president of Harvard University, has commented, the physician's ability to communicate actually deteriorates as a result of the process.

It seems as if modern American medical training breeds an ethic of "detached concern" (Lief and Fox, cited in Bugen, 1979, p. 179) that emphasizes saving lives rather than focusing on the care for and disposition of dying patients. Physicians are trained to treat patients as objects to be fixed, in accordance with the classical Cartesian mentality. Thus, these professionals become skilled at applying technology and dealing with body physiology, but as a group, they are not especially skilled in or comfortable with attending to the emotional needs of their patients. The treatment of body physiology is certainly superior today, but emotionally, individuals may feel they are not getting everything they want from the medical care they receive. In short, medical training may produce, from the patient's perspective, a collection of caretakers that are best described as strangers and mechanics, rather than friends and humanists.

Truth Telling

The avoidance of death is manifest everywhere in the behavior of health-care professionals. Studies reveal that nurses take longer to answer bedside calls of terminally ill patients (DeSpelder and Strickland, 1992, p. 132). Other studies show that physicians avoid patients altogether once they begin to die (Bugen, 1979, p. 179;

also see Schulz and Aderman, 1980, p. 134). When death does finally come, some hospitals use "false-bottom gurneys, which transport the corpse to a nondescript exit, camouflaging its odious human cargo. Death is compartmentalized, shut away from public view" (DeSpelder and Strickland, 1992, p. 130).

This behavior has perhaps been explained in repeated studies that suggest that medical professionals tend to define the dying as deviant and avoid them as a result (Wheeler, 1972, Feifel, 1959, and LeShan, 1972, cited in Chang and Chang, 1980, p. 744).[13] But from the practitioner's perspective, it may be hard to find the time and emotional reserves necessary to provide a more realistic and humanistic treatment of death.[14] Others explain the physicians' lack of sensitivity and their predisposition to set discussions of death aside to "conventional wisdom." Indeed, the ethic of medicine, from Hippocrates onward, was that physicians should "keep bad news to themselves—to be purveyors of hope, not doom" (Rothman, 1991, p. 122). As Hippocrates himself put it, the doctor should go about his or her duties "calmly and adroitly, concealing most things from the patient while … attending to him. … Reveal nothing of the patient's future or present condition" (cited in DeSpelder and Strickland, 1992, p. 352).

Speaking on this subject before a group of young physicians, Oliver Wendell Holmes, Sr., echoed this traditional wisdom by counseling that "your patient has no more right to all the truth you know than he has to all the medicine in your saddlebags. … He should get only just so much as is good for him. … It is a terrible thing to take away hope, every earthly hope, from a fellow creature" (cited in Rothman, 1991, p. 122).

We can see the manifestations of that tradition today, even though most studies on the subject tend to suggest that the conventional wisdom is flawed. The literature on death and dying is rife with research and clinical reports about the beneficence and propriety of revealing information about the patient's condition to the patient and his or her family. Indeed, most researchers suggest that detachment and denial are exactly the wrong approaches to take. Instead, the overwhelming consensus suggests that informing severely ill patients—truthfully but gently—about the gravity of their condition is the best course of action (Schulz and Anderman, 1980, p. 136). Yet the tradition of equivocation and even prevarication continues.

Some physicians, no doubt, worry that patients will be unable to cope with bad news (Glaser and Straus, cited in Schulz and Anderman, 1980, p. 139).[15] Others defer to family members who may want to bolster the patient's hopes by shunting discussions of death aside. Understandably, many may not want to deal with what is painful and discomforting information to relay—"you are going to die." Whatever the reason, however, studies beginning in the 1950s show that physicians did not talk about death with their patients.[16] The situation had changed relatively little by the mid-1970s. According to John Hinton (1976, p. 129), relatively few doctors were telling their patients that there was virtually no hope for recovery. And

G. J. Annas (1975, pp. 9–10) notes that surveys consistently revealed that over 80 percent of physicians routinely failed to inform patients that they were terminally ill.

Some suggest that such attitudes are beginning to change.[17] In reality, however, even if they are, behavior is lagging behind for the lack of direct acknowledgment of the impending death continues to be a prominent characteristic of interaction between staff and dying patients (Charmaz, 1980, p. 134). And that seems to be at the root of some of the mistrust that has evolved between caregivers and their charges. If physicians had been honest about the subject of death all along, their patients may have given them the benefit of the doubt. In a way, by ducking the tough questions and answers, physicians have effectively encouraged right-to-die activism.

The Technological Imperative

Scientism, the belief in the beneficence and efficacy of technology, is alive and well in the medical community (just as it is in the general population), to the point where death has become a completely unacceptable alternative in the eyes of some (maybe most) physicians. As Bronzino, Smith, and Wade (1990, p. 544) note, "Modern medicine [has an] apparent obsession with death prevention. For many in the modern health care system, every death, even when it is by no means premature, represents a failure. The understandable desire to avoid this failure motivates physicians to act aggressively to keep their patients alive." In a similar vein, Bugen (1979, p. 253) suggests that "every death corresponds to a failure, either of the individual physician, or more commonly of medicine as a whole. ... In his dedication to the ideals of the scientific community, the physician responds with vigorous application of diagnostic tests, technological gadgetry, and heroic therapy in order to prolong life."

This general need of physicians to treat every affliction with an aggressive use of sophisticated procedures—however small the potential benefit, however high the real emotional and financial costs—is so endemic to the profession that Robert Blank (1988, p. 13) finds the predisposition is worthy of a label: "the technological imperative."

Dr. Steven Schroder, an internist and head of the Robert Wood Johnson Foundation, toured teaching hospitals in Europe, and his reactions to the differences in treatment on either side of the Atlantic sum up the technological imperative quite succinctly. In Europe, "the patients were different," he noted. "They were healthier and they were younger. The common patient in an ICU in a major U.S. hospital is an eighty-five-year-old whose heart is failing, whose lungs are failing, who is in need of artificial respiration." Schroder asked European doctors about the difference, and he reported that many gave the same reply: "'I trained in the U.S.

Your teaching hospitals are excellent, your technology is superb, but you don't know when to stop'" (cited in Stout, 1993).

According to Alonzo Plough (1986, p. 7), there are at least two reasons—both related to the technological imperative—why doctors tend to overuse technology. First, there is a professionally inspired and reinforced sense of perfectionism that is drilled into medical students almost from the first day they attend classes. Doctors are trained to heal, cure, and use all the resources at their disposal to forestall death. Indeed, as Karen Michaelson (1988, p. 13) states, "Some physicians may feel it is malpractice not to use available technology." Moreover, when a doctor contemplates providing anything short of an aggressive, comprehensive response to a medical condition, fears of tort liability inevitably surface.[18] It is a no-win situation for the physician, however, for aggressive treatment may just fuel a family's hopes when no hope is warranted: Bringing vast arrays of medical technology to bear on the patient creates expectations. In such an environment, death is thought of not so much as a natural event but as a medical failure, prompting those outside the hospital to sue for malpractice when death finally does come.[19]

Second, there may be defense mechanisms at work within the physician's psyche. As Stein (1990, p. 46) says, "Patients often do not respond according to practitioners' timetables or recover to the degree clinicians hope and expect. Failure to achieve a 'cure' or a 'fix' often precipitates an attempt by the clinician to restore his or her sense of self-esteem. ... The flight from despair can lead to relentless activism, ostensibly on behalf of the patient, to protect the physician from depression." Ultimately, the "refusal to accept therapeutic defeat can ... lead to therapeutic mania, to subjecting the patient to what is significantly called heroic surgical attack" (Main, cited in Stein, 1990, p. 46). In the end, a physician is likely to use a variety of techniques to avoid dealing with a patient's death, including "prescribing life-sustaining techniques he knows will not provide a cure" (Schoenfeld, 1978, p. 53).

Regardless of the explanation or mix of explanations for this behavior,[20] the medical community has come to a point where it operates on the basis of what Paul Starr (1982, p. 390) calls "therapeutic relentlessness." He goes on to note that "in its commitment to the preservation of life, medical care ironically has come to symbolize a prototypically modern form of torture, combining benevolence, indifference, and technical wizardry. Rather than engendering trust, technological medicine often raises anxieties about the ability of individuals to make choices for themselves" (Starr, 1982, p. 390). Increasingly, these elevated levels of anxiety have fueled significant "counter-technological" efforts to "demedicalize" the two most profound life events any of us will ever face: childbirth[21] and death[22] (Starr, 1982, p. 391).

In sum, American physicians are trained to regard state-of-the-art medicine as the only acceptable form of patient care (Bronzino, Smith, and Wade, 1990, p. 253). But the technological imperative is nothing more than evidence of scientism in the medical community. The behavior of medical practitioners and the professors who train them simply reflect our culture, including "its values, beliefs, rites, and symbols. Central to the culture is faith in progress through science [and] technology" (Knowles, 1977b, p. 58).

But where scientism in the general population acts as a force of restraint, in the medical community it acts as a force of activism because the indiscriminate use of technology creates right-to-die scenarios that widen the social gulf between patients and caretakers. American physicians do a great deal of good; nothing said here is meant to obscure that reality. But sometimes, the technological imperative encourages physicians to overtreat patients who are already at the end of meaningful life. Consequently, unless doctors change their ways, patients and their families will find themselves even further at odds with the medical community, raising right-to-die questions when in the past—in the days when trust and friendship prevailed—they simply accepted whatever treatments were offered, under the "doctor-knows-best" principle.

Doctors and Death in Retrospect

Benevolent abdication on the part of patients was once the rule, and medical paternalism was embraced by both parties of the doctor-patient relationship. But little by little, the close bonds that had existed between patient and physician have broken down, and not much of the 1800s-style affinity exists anymore. Given this, it should surprise no one that many Americans living near the Mexican border now routinely cross over into Mexico for medical care. Most cite the high cost of care in the United States as the primary reason for defecting to the south, but a substantial 20 percent of them also mention the personal attention they receive from Mexican doctors and clinics (Hilts, 1992). No one wants to trade away modern technology for the 1800s' version of medical care. But at least some, it appears, would like to again have a taste of the friendly, personal relationship that existed between doctor and patient 100 years ago.

Few would disagree that modern medicine has accomplished a great deal as a result of the shift from holism, homespun nostrums, and charity care to specialization, professionalization, and technological sophistication. At the same time, however, there have been significant and unanticipated side effects. Most importantly, clinical humanism has been largely traded in for a more dispassionate approach, in which the body is viewed as a mechanistic system. It is all part and parcel of the scientific revolution, with emphasis on quantifiable data, objective analysis, and specialized knowledge about things empirical. In adopting this new orthodoxy, however, physicians have become more detached from their patients, and patients have become more leery, in turn. This environment, in which many patients are ready to call physicians' directives into question, is ripe with possibilities for right-to-die activism.

The Future of Medical Decisionmaking

Looking ahead, one sees change in the offing. Many physicians are still holding firm to the old ways, prevaricating about the terminal conditions of their patients and making unilateral decisions to proceed with aggressive treatment, even if there is little hope for recovery. Yet, the physician's grip on the old ways seems to be slipping. Increased attention to informed consent, do-not-resuscitate (DNR) orders, and the emergence of ethics committees are testament to that. Given physician recalcitrance, however, it will be a while before new decision-making structures that empower patients and their families are fully and effectively in play.

Physician Autonomy: Holding Firm

According to the second report of the Kennedy Commission on biomedical ethics, convened by the federal government in 1978 to study medical decisionmaking, the relationship between physicians and patients should be marked by mutual respect and shared decisionmaking. In such relationships, it is incumbent upon medical professionals to convey all relevant information to the patient, then proceed no further until consent has been given. Unpleasant information should never be withheld, and the final decision regarding medical treatment—including the right to decide the course of treatment in cases in which life itself is at stake—should ultimately rest with the competent individual. In cases where the patient is not competent to decide, decisionmaking should be dispersed among interested second parties (e.g., physicians, family, and maybe friends of the individual) and disinterested third parties (e.g., members of a hospital ethics committee).

The report's rhetoric was quite explicit, but it did not have the full, intended effect on members of the medical community. Although courts, legislators, and some members of the medical community regularly cited principles laid out in the Kennedy Commission report, commission pronouncements got very little attention in the mainstream medical journals. According to Jay Katz, "the old attitudes and practices persist, for medicine lacks a tradition of communicating uncertainties to patients and sharing decision making" (cited in Rothman, 1991, p. 250).

To be sure, doctors today are more likely than ever to discuss the big-ticket items (such as decisions regarding respiration and DNR orders) with patients and their families. But medical professionals continue to "reserve for themselves more technical (and covert) decisions [regarding treatment]" (Rothman, 1991, p. 254). Diana Crane (cited in Blank, 1988, p. 88) stated, "Consultation with the family is used in part as a method of ensuring that [family members] will accept the decision and not take legal action against the physician later." In short, most observers conclude that physicians today have not really accepted the ethic of shared decisionmaking prescribed by the Kennedy Commission.

In fact, according to one study, 60 to 90 percent of physicians would still rather withhold information about the condition of a terminally ill patient (Humphry and Wickett, 1986, p. 64). Another study, conducted in the early 1980s and reported in the *New England Journal of Medicine,* found that only one in five physicians consulted the family of elderly and ailing patients about end-of-life decisionmaking, and only one in ten physicians discussed resuscitation with the patient, even when the patient was fully competent (cited in Humphry and Wickett, 1986, p. 119). As we have noted previously, today's physicians are much more willing to discuss treatment decisions with their patients, but this new attitude has been slow to come, when it has come at all, and changes in behavior have sometimes lagged far behind changes in attitude.

The Absence of First Principles. Part of the resistance to change may come from the typical physician's predisposition, inculcated during medical training, to rely on the inductive, case-based approach to treatment decisions, in which clinical anecdotes rather than any enduring, first principles or ethical rules guide decisionmaking.

Physicians decide which anecdotes to apply and how, rejecting general rules and principles in the process. It is a mode of thinking that empowers physicians, who are, they would argue, the only ones with enough personal knowledge and technical expertise to draw appropriate conclusions regarding diagnosis and treatment. As Rothman (1991, pp. 1–2) notes, physicians have always "made their decisions on a case-by-case basis, responding to the particular circumstances as they saw fit, reluctant by both training and practice to formulate or adhere to guidelines or rules."

Ethics was traditionally thought to mean a doctor operating in good faith for the benefit of the patient as best as he or she saw fit. And the idea of anyone, including ethicists or authors of presidential commission reports, making guidelines for medical treatment decisions that diminished the power of the physician was always considered anathema. "In fact," according to Rothman (1991, p. 9), "many medical schools long resisted the formal teaching of ethics, not because they believed that ethics could not be taught, but because it had to be taught at the bedside, by starting with the individual case ... by role modeling, by students taking cues from individual physicians."

Studying general principles was no way to understand medical ethics. Rather, one learned what to do by watching other physicians deal with real-life situations; it was implicitly understood that the physicians being observed were right by definition. The only first principle here was that there are no first principles, save for the trust patients should have in the good intentions of physicians to exercise their autonomy judiciously. As British psychologist John Hinton (1976, p. 140) puts it, "The doctor must, himself, assume final responsibility in some very hard decisions when the end of a patient's chronic, incurable illness is nearing." The Kennedy Commission may have viewed patient autonomy and informed consent as the cornerstones of the ethical practice in medicine, but physicians have tended to see things differently.

Patient Abdication. Some have suggested that patients do not want decision-making authority, forcing doctors to fill the decision-making vacuum. Crane reports that one of the research physicians she interviewed made the following remarks: "You can't let the family influence you. But it is necessary to handle them with diplomacy, so they will go along with your decisions. I steer them to my way of thinking. They don't want to make the decisions themselves" (1975, p. 193). If this respondent is correct, then maybe some of the fault does lie with patients and their families—individuals too squeamish to get involved beyond signing consent forms. There are many who support this line of argument.

According to C. G. Schoenfeld (1978, p. 53), "Patients tend to regard their physicians as parent substitutes." Or, as Anna Freud (1976, p. 200) states, "The patient ... will do his best to push [his doctor] into the place of parental authority, and will make use of [his doctor] as parental authority to the utmost." Doctors represent, for most people, "some combination of man-of-science, father-confessor, advisor, and even a bit of magician. Just as a sick child looks to his parents, so a sick adult looks to his doctor to make him *all better*" (Strauss, 1977, p. 2). Consequently, "patients and family members tend to be persuaded by the mode of treatment or plans that the physician proposes" (Charmaz, 1980, p. 119).

Another piece of the puzzle of patient abdication must involve patient denial. In a 1984 study, R. N. Eidinger and David Schapira found that only half of the 315 cancer patients interviewed could accurately report the severity of their medical condition, despite clearly being told about it (Schapira, 1990, p. 4). Yet, over 90 percent of the patients in the study expressed a desire to know everything possible about their condition. These patients apparently denied the information they received, making it necessary for the physician to step into the breach.[23]

But dependency is not the only explanation for patient acquiescence. Another factor probably has something to do with the great power that devolves to physicians by virtue of the tremendous asymmetry in information that they enjoy vis-à-vis the patient. As the President's Commission (1983, pp. 44–45) notes, "How information is communicated and continuing care is provided can forcefully induce a patient to make certain choices. In many medical care situations, patients are dependent and professionals are relatively powerful."

The precept is understated for it would be hard to overestimate the real power physicians possess when they sit down to describe for the patient the diagnosis, the prognosis, the levels of pain and discomfort involved in prospective courses of treatment, and the degree of medical certainty about chances for a successful return to a reasonable quality of life. There may also be a tacit communication that the patient has no (or little) choice: "Though coercive treatment is rare, care givers can—unwittingly or not—exert undue influence on patients by means of subtle or overt manipulation" (DeSpelder and Strickland, 1992, p. 352).

Physicians Loosen Their Grip

Obviously, physicians retain a great deal of power in their relationships with patients. But the seeds of a physician-patient disconnection have been sown. In years past, doctors were shielded by the privacy afforded by the patient's own bedroom. As Rothman (1991, pp. 1-2) states,

> Well into the post-World War II period, decisions at the bedside were the almost exclusive concern of the individual physician, even when they raised fundamental ethical and social issues. It was mainly doctors who wrote and read about the morality of withholding a course of antibiotics and letting pneumonia serve as the old man's friend, of considering a newborn with grave birth defects a "stillbirth" and sparing the parents the agony of choice and the burden of care, of experimenting on the institutionalized retarded to learn more about hepatitis, or of giving one patient and not another access to the iron lung when the machine was in short supply. Moreover, it was usually the individual physician who decided these matters at the bedside or in the privacy of the hospital room, without formal discussions with patients, their families, or even with colleagues, and certainly without drawing the attention of journalists, judges, or professional philosophers.

As Rothman goes on to note, however, "By the mid-1970s, both the style and the substance of medical decision making had changed. The authority that an individual physician had once exercised covertly was now subject to debate and review by colleagues and lay people." In fact, the practice of medicine has changed so substantially in the last few decades that physicians today might be excused for thinking that they now operate in glass houses. Performing as if under a microscope, they are second-guessed at every turn. Perhaps this is, in part, why there is such strong dissatisfaction among members of the profession. In the mid-1980s, one survey revealed that 40 percent of all physicians would choose not to go to medical school if they had known beforehand what they learned about their profession after graduating.

Chief among the physicians' complaints is the erosion of physician autonomy that Rothman speaks about. Even simple admissions often must be preapproved by a third-party payer as a part of a "managed-care" process in which all major medical expenses are screened to reduce excessive or unnecessary use of the health-care system. Managed care is a large ($13 billion in 1991, see Freudenheim, 1992a) and growing segment of the health-care industry in the United States today, and as more third-party payers resort to this concept in an effort to control costs, the second-guessing of physicians will only escalate.

In addition, most hospitals have been forced by concerns over rising costs to form their own utilization review (UR) committees, which study treatment records on a daily basis. Patient stays that are longer than expected and diagnostic tests that seem excessive or out of the ordinary raise warning flags that lead administrators to ask physicians to defend their "nonstandard" treatment plans. Patient-abuse hotlines, bioethics committee consults, malpractice suits, internal chart reviews by the quality assurance staff, and external reviews by peer review organizations (PROs) combine to give physicians less and less room to operate as the semiautonomous centers of power that they were just a few years ago.

Federal directives attempt to limit physician autonomy, as well. A good deal of publicity swirled around the case of a child with Down's Syndrome who died in 1982 after relatively routine surgery had been withheld—a case reminiscent of the 1969 Johns Hopkins case in which withholding treatment from a severely disabled newborn was at issue (see Chapter 3). In response to the 1982 case, the Reagan administration issued what became known as the "Baby Doe directive," forbidding the "discriminatory failure to feed and care for handicapped infants." This regulation and subsequent revisions were contested in a series of court cases before the issue finally culminated, in a legal sense, with the Supreme Court case of *Bowen* v. *American Hospital Association et al.* (1986). This ruling, in a significant manifestation of right-to-die activism, affirmed parents' rights to make treatment decisions for their children in such cases (Levin, 1988, p. 191). The physicians first were told by the executive branch that they must provide care, then were told by the judiciary that the parents had the power to decide. No one even considered leaving the decision in the hands of the physician.

Populist predispositions fueled by consumerism and the role of rights in the American political culture (the subject of the next two chapters) have also played a part in eroding physician autonomy. In the end, it may be that patients are slowly assuming control as physicians, begrudgingly, let go of the technological imperative. Evidence of this progress in the devolution of decision-making authority can be seen in at least two areas. First, the do-not-resuscitate order has become a common, patient-directed "treatment plan" in hospitals today. Second, ethics committees have been formed in hospitals all across the country: groups of medical professionals and lay people from the community who come together regularly to discuss and set policy on questions of an ethically sensitive nature.

DNR Orders. The resuscitation of individuals whose hearts have stopped has been attempted for centuries. But only in the last twenty-five years have procedures been codified and refined to the point where resuscitation is a commonplace occurrence. Standard resuscitation protocol now may involve cardiac resuscitation, including chest compressions (cardiopulmonary resuscitation, or CPR), electrical shocks (electrical defibrillation), and intravenous medications designed to stimulate a heartbeat or regulate heart rhythm. Resuscitation may also include artificial ventilation, either mouth-to-mouth or by means of a mechanical respirator that forces oxygen into the lungs via a tube inserted through the nose or mouth.

Cardiac arrest occurs at some point in every dying process, whatever the underlying cause of death. This makes almost everyone a potential candidate for artificial resuscitation. But as resuscitation procedures were perfected, it became clear that it did not necessarily make sense to initiate resuscitation efforts in every instance. As early as 1974, the American Heart Association and the National Academy of Sciences issued policy statements to that effect, arguing, for example, that resuscitation was not indicated in cases where the patient was terminally and irreversibly ill.

In recognition of that philosophy, hospitals had, through the late 1960s and early 1970s, operated under their own, usually informal DNR policies, in which the patient had little if any input (Rothman, 1991; see also Quill, 1993, p. 29). A grand jury investigation of La Guardia Hospital in that time frame revealed the existence of a card-and-dot system: Each patient had his or her own index card, and those whose cards had a purple dot were not to be resuscitated. The cards were kept by nurses and disposed of after the patient either was discharged or died. La Guardia had no policy to obtain consent or even inform DNR-coded patients or their families; decisionmaking was unilateral, haphazard, and secret. Shortly thereafter, New York Hospital was sued for refusing to resuscitate a female patient who had been "purple dotted." Not only had New York Hospital refused to initiate resuscitation, personnel also prevented the patient's nephew—by coincidence, a doctor himself who was at the bedside during his aunt's cardiac arrest—from coming to her aid.

Stories like these caused sufficient activism in the medical and legal communities to initiate a dialogue on formalizing DNR policies, with patient consent as an operating first principle. Such policies began appearing in 1976, as the concept of "informed consent" began to carry more weight in both medical and legal circles. Slowly, purple dots on index cards, word-of-mouth orders, and pencil notations that could be erased later were replaced with public documents that spelled out in some detail what the doctor had told and heard from the patient. With advice from their physicians, patients could begin thinking about negotiating their own deaths, a concept quite foreign at the time.

At first, the legal status of the formal DNR order was somewhat dubious, and DNR policies were being written in individual hospitals across the country with little guidance. Gradually, however, standards began to emerge, and the Joint Commission on Accreditation for Hospital Organizations (JCAHO, or "Joint Commission") set some guidelines for hospitals to follow.[24] Today, approximately 6,000 hospitals across the United States are required by the Joint Commission to have DNR policies on the books that comply with both JCAHO guidelines and any more restrictive state laws that exist.[25] As a result, the right to be allowed to die (i.e., not to be resuscitated) is out of the closet and part of the formal operating procedures of every JCAHO-accredited hospital in the nation today.[26]

But when it comes to CPR, the technological imperative apparently continues to hold sway for all indications are that this procedure is substantially overused. About one-third of all patients who die in the hospital—many of whom are elderly and in the final stages of terminal conditions—receive CPR at some point in their dying.[27] If successfully revived, these patients are typically transferred to expensive intensive care wards where dying is forestalled temporarily, at great emotional cost to the family and great financial cost to society ("Cost of Heart Revival," 1993). At the same time, greater concern with cost containment and the impetus to advance patient discretion inherent in JCAHO directives, federal reports, court decisions, state laws, and elsewhere promise to keep the right to die moving forward, via increased attention to DNR orders.

Ethics Committees. As we have noted, ethics—the deductive study of first principles—was once thought not to exist in medical circles. But today, ethics committees have been formed in most hospitals across the country, another new fixture in the medical profession that reveals the shift away from physician hegemony in decisionmaking.

The concept of ethics committees, first popularized by Dr. Scribner's dialysis team in Seattle in the early 1960s, really did not gain widespread acceptance until after the *Quinlan* decision, delivered by the New Jersey Supreme Court in 1976 (President's Commission, 1983, pp. 443–444). In the text of that decision, the court envisioned that ethics committees, composed of both professional and community representatives, would primarily be consultation devices, used to flesh out issues and suggest appropriate courses of action by building consensus rather than mandating binding decisions along majority-rules lines.

Interest in the idea of ethics committees built slowly, and the early committees that did form were not exactly what the New Jersey justices had in mind. According to one survey, less than 5 percent of U.S. hospitals had ethics committees in place by 1983 (seven years after *Quinlan*).[28] Moreover, these early committees were dominated by health-care professionals, particularly physicians, and tended to shut out patients and their families. Early ethics committees were not particularly busy, either: Most reported considering only one ethics case a year, and some reviewed no cases at all.

The ethics committee idea was encouraged when the President's Commission for the Study of Ethical Problems in Medicine and Biomedical and Behavioral Research came out with its report in 1983, imploring physicians to take up the cause in greater numbers and with more energy (President's Commission, 1983). The rash of infant-care cases that were reported by the media during the early years of the 1980s—including the one leading to the Reagan administration's "Baby Doe directive"—added even more urgency to the need for such committees. President

Ronald Reagan's secretary of health and human services also pushed the idea until the professional medical organizations—most importantly, the American Medical Association and the American Hospital Association—finally acceded to the idea and endorsed the ethics committee recommendation.

By 1985, the percentage of hospitals reporting the existence of ethics committees had jumped to 30 percent, up from 5 percent just two years prior (Humphry and Wickett, 1986, p. 201). Today, the Joint Commission expects *all* hospitals to have some sort of deliberative and representative ethics body in place. It is difficult to tell how much of an impact these bodies have had to date, but their very existence signals that changes are in the wind.

Establishing New Directions

Only thirty years ago, it was thought that a physician must do everything possible to save a patient, in accordance with the Western ethical system of individualism that placed infinite worth on human life. The goal of medicine, in light of the technological imperative, was to prevent death at all costs (Sprung, 1990). As recently as seven years ago, the withdrawal of artificially provided nutrition and hydration was viewed as "a gross deviation from legal and medical standards" (Sprung, 1990, pp. 2212–2213). Today, however, both premises have fallen, and a new medical and legal consensus has emerged.

Much of the foundation for the medical consensus that is emerging can be traced to the work of the President's Commission and its influential report, *Deciding to Forego Life-Sustaining Treatment,* issued in 1983. This report advocated a number of reforms in the delivery of health care, including codification of DNR procedures, constitution of ethics committees, and creation of advanced directive laws.[29] The President's Commission also advocated hospital "right-to-know policies" (presaging passage of the federal Patient Self-Determination Act, discussed in Chapter 6) that spell out a patient's rights under state law and hospital policy.[30]

In the same vein, Dr. Michael H. Myerson is one among many in the medical community who have begun giving voice to a whole new way of thinking about doctor-patient relationships. Myerson argues that doctors need to improve their understanding of the interplay between health and human rights. As a first step toward that end, doctors must begin considering "their patients as knowledgeable allies, not as passive recipients of care, and involve them fully in the entire care process, including decision-making about treatment" (cited in Altman, 1993b).

In addition, there are indications that important changes are afoot in medical education, as well. The first development of significance is the increase in the number of females entering medical school. Empirical evidence suggests that women enter the profession with different assumptions and expectations than their male counterparts. And some research studies indicate that females ultimately behave more sensitively and compassionately than males as physicians.[31]

Thus, "female physicians may be more adept than men at cooperating with newly inquisitive patients and less willing to play the omniscient lord of the body" (Angier, 1992). If this is true, the growing presence of women in the medical profession will have a salutary effect on the degree to which physicians share decision-making responsibilities with patients and acquiesce to patient wishes in the end.

We can also point to the radical reforms now taking place in American medical school curricula. At Dartmouth, medical students spend less time in lectures and labs and more time dealing with real-life medical problems in the community. Furthermore, they are now required, with the help of faculty mentors, to teach preventative medicine and advise distressed families on their health-care problems. Also, to add a measure of sensitivity to the traditionally dispassionate approach to physician training, Dartmouth medical students are allowed and even encouraged to express their emotions during anatomy classes where cadavers are dissected.

Much of the impetus for these changes stems from the activities of former Surgeon General Dr. C. Everett Koop, who returned to his alma mater on a self-described mission to bring humanism back into medical training. Central to his thrust is the notion that students should get involved with patients early, before they begin to see them as abstractions and cases ("Dartmouth Redesigns Medical Training," 1992). Indeed, Martha Weinman Lear (1993) reports that 117 of the 126 accredited medical schools in the United States now require some study of physician-patient relationships.

At Emory University and elsewhere, medical schools are moving away from the passive model of learning that tends to be sterilized of human content. In this curricular reform, group thinking and problemsolving are emphasized over the staid and traditional one-way lecture that reinforces hierarchical tendencies to believe only medical professionals can find the right approach in individual cases. Harvard has been experimenting with this same reform since 1985. As at Emory, Harvard has been placing students in small groups rather than large lecture halls, encouraging them to develop problem-solving skills by studying hypothetical cases in an environment that stresses consensus-building instead of clearly delineated, right and wrong answers ("Dartmouth Redesigns Medical Training," 1992).

Remaining Ambivalence and Ambiguity

Cultures of any kind change slowly and incrementally, so we should not expect the traditions of physician autonomy, built up and reinforced over centuries, to crumble overnight. The dichotomy between physician beliefs and physician behavior is symptomatic of both a changing ethos (the attitudes, at least, are changing) and an entrenched tradition (which, in large part, still drives behavior).

Generally speaking, physician attitudes seem to echo the professional wisdom espoused by the President's Commission report, the AMA's Council on Ethical and Judicial Affairs (American Medical Association, 1989), and a slew of state-court decisions in the last fifteen years. These sources of guidance, together with Joint Commission directives (Joint Commission, 1992), the Patient Self-Determination Act, and a host of liberal state laws, have led M. Z. Solomon et al. (1993, pp. 14–15) to suggest that "there is now a body of literature, policy, law, and regulation that presents a generally agreed upon set of basic principles, as well as procedural recommendations for incorporating those principles into clinical practice."

For example, the overwhelming majority (87 percent) of health-care providers in a recent study by Solomon et al. (1993), including 687 physicians and 759 nurses, agreed that "all competent patients, even if they are to be considered terminally ill, have the right to refuse life support, even if that refusal may lead to death." At the same time, however, only 36 percent of the same group were satisfied that patients were informed of their alternatives, and less than a third thought that patients got the help they needed to make decisions about care alternatives. It should come as no surprise, given these numbers, that fully 55 percent of the health-care providers polled believed that, at least sometimes, patients were overtreated with burdensome procedures. (Only 12 percent thought that health-care providers occasionally gave up too quickly.)

The Solomon study involved some in-depth, follow-up interviews to detect the real motivations behind this apparent paradox, and it found a number of explanations. Some doctors expressed a fear of tort liability.[32] Others worried about the "public nature" of patient autonomy: It opens up physician behavior to public scrutiny in ways unheard of just a decade ago. Nancy Dubler (1993, p. 24), in a commentary on the Solomon study, points out that a lack of education is a primary cause for the disjunction between attitudes and behavior: "How can we expect staff to be comfortable with a process for which they have little or no training and which seems fraught with moral, legal, and regulatory dangers?"

Solomon argues that ignorance lies at the root of the disjunction between physician attitudes and behaviors, as well. It seems that many physicians are either unaware or ill informed about current professional and legal thinking on end-of-life decisionmaking: Physicians' attitudes mesh quite well with the professional and legal consensus, but the doctors do not know it. Consequently, they wrongly fear that acting on conviction will lead them into uncharted territory.

Even when DNR orders and living wills that would seem to protect the physician are executed, relieving him or her of some liability, physicians may not comply with patient wishes (Danis et al., 1991). Sometimes, when families contradict the patient's wishes, physicians take their views under consideration, giving them great weight. At other times, the physicians may give their own ethical principles priority when they conflict with patient wishes. This was often the case, according to the Danis study, when a patient's advanced directive was too restrictive to allow a simple or basic procedure that would yield the patient substantial benefits from the physician's perspective. The reverse may also be true: Despite an advance directive requesting that treatment be provided, physicians may judge that treatment would be of little benefit to the patient in the given circumstances and unilaterally decide to withhold or withdraw treatment.[33]

Summary: Change Is in the Offing

Clearly, the medical decision-making landscape looks substantially different today than it did just a few years ago. Before the 1960s, physicians enjoyed a substantial degree of autonomy in making treatment decisions for, rather than in conjunction with, their patients. In the 1960s and 1970s, however, that centuries-old tradition of sub-rosa discretion began to erode as changes, both in the medical profession and in society more generally (see Chapters 5 and 6), conspired to "make the invisible visible" (Rothman, 1991, p. 3). Ultimately, as the social and medical ferment continued into the 1980s and early 1990s, medical decisionmaking has become radically transformed from what once was wholly a matter of professional concern into what has increasingly become a matter of individual choice. This leads us to believe that the forces of right-to-die restraint are slowly being overwhelmed as public-policy activism takes control.

The bottom line is that change is in the air, brought on by forces that have put pressure on members of the medical profession to ease their stranglehold on patient care and treatment decisionmaking. The days of the autonomous physician, ruling by fiat without much consideration of the patient's wishes, are slowly drawing to a close. These days are numbered for two kinds of reasons. First, the dramatic changes in the medical profession itself have led to a breakdown in patient trust and an increased expectation that patients will be involved in formulating treatment plans. Second, there have been changes in society. Expectations about what is appropriate and acceptable in medical-care decisionmaking have undergone a fundamental transformation at the grass-roots level, and it is these developments to which we turn in Chapters 5 and 6.

As these strains of activism converge, the time may soon come when even the most autocratic physicians find themselves mimicking the Wizard of Oz, who, at the end of the story, begs Dorothy and her friends to "pay no attention to the man behind the curtain." Of course, despite his entreaties, the wizard's days of autonomy were over when the curtain was pulled back for all to see. For physicians, like Lyman Frank Baum's wizard, there can be no turning back.

5

Social Activism and Health-Care Consumerism

IF THE MEDICAL ACTIVISM discussed in Chapters 3 and 4 can be thought of as policy-making agitation of a trickle-down sort, then the grass-roots forces discussed here and in Chapter 6 might be thought of as activism of the percolator variety, bubbling forth from the mass of nonprofessionals upward. This chapter is about activism that flows from the general predisposition Americans have to embrace individual rights. In this context, the right to die can be understood not as some ghoulish aberration but as a natural extension of rights Americans already expect to enjoy. Chapter 6 will deal with the agitation for rights as they apply to the business of dying specifically.

Emergence of a Rights Culture

Americans have always cherished their civil rights, especially those protected by the first amendments to the U.S. Constitution—the revered Bill of Rights. But sensitivity about this subject increased substantially within the body politic during the 1960s when interest in an entirely new layer of individual rights sprang forth. This new genre of civil rights was not explicitly expressed anywhere in the Constitution's words per se. Instead, they became part of the legal and cultural fabric of American society as "penumbral rights," an amorphous set of guarantees that many came to think of as existing in the shadow of the Constitution. These guarantees took shape largely as promises that individuals would be treated fairly in their interactions with "the establishment," if establishment is broadly defined to include all sorts of authority figures and power brokers in both the public and private sectors. The increasing predisposition of individuals to claim these rights is a phenomenon we refer to as the emergence of a rights culture.

The 1960s was a decade in which the establishment (i.e., middle- and upper-class Anglo-Saxon males who tended to hold the reins of political and economic power) was perceived as evil, almost by definition, by many who were not a part of that establishment. Many lost faith in government because of the Vietnam War, which seemed to spin out of control with no end in sight. Activism in the area of race was another manifestation of an emergent rights culture, and Americans, primarily those of African-American descent, began questioning and often rejecting the status quo. The women's movement got an enormous boost in this decade, as well, as Americans—especially female Americans—began rejecting sexual mores and gender stereotypes that tended to relegate women in the United States to a second-class status.

These were the years when a number of other groups within American society also began to assert their claims to rights, including those who advocated the causes of farm workers, blue-collar laborers, prisoners, homosexuals, tenants, children, the poor, and disabled persons. Not surprisingly and certainly not coincidentally, these were also the fledgling years of the consumerism movement. This basic rights crusade, grounded in the complementary demands associated with product safety for consumers and product liability for corporations, cut across racial, gender, and age boundaries to radically alter the nature of the U.S. marketplace.

Producers were put on notice in the 1960s when President John Kennedy announced his "consumer bill of rights," a document that codified for the consumer the right to have safe products and product choice and the right to petition for the redress of consumer-oriented grievances. The document was an official reflection of the times, though, more than a bold new assertion for consumerist sentiments were already gelling in the country at the time. No longer would American consumers be satisfied with what laissez-faire capitalism was dishing out. Instead, they would demand greater levels of corporate responsibility in such areas as environmental protection, product safety, product labeling, and honesty in advertising. Health care was just one more area of consumer interest in which expectations were raised.

To ensure that the corporations would do their part, Americans began to demand more government oversight. As a result, the Food and Drug Administration (FDA) started playing a more activist role with regard to drug trials and product labeling. Ralph Nader's stinging indictment of the Chevrolet Corvair and the subsequent formation of consumer-rights advocacy organizations (groups that became known as "Nader's Raiders") were important policy forces, as well. Nader and his followers were skillful at manipulating the levers of power in Washington to ensure that government bureaucrats and federal legislators toed the line on product safety in ways unheard of just a decade before.

Then, in 1972, the consumer movement got another boost when the Consumer Product Safety Commission (CPSC) was created as an independent regulatory agency. The CPSC was charged with the responsibility of reducing the risk of injury to consumers from products sold to them. In addition, the commission was empowered to conduct product-safety research and set safety standards in such areas as flammable fabrics and poison-protective packaging. Its other responsibilities included conducting consumer-education programs and establishing a clearinghouse for injury information. Today, it would be difficult to imagine a world in which the federal government did not engage in such activities. But at the time, all these activities—risk management, consumer education, and safety research— were revolutionary roles for the government to play.

A host of federal "truth in" regulations were also passed in these years: truth in advertising, truth in lending, truth in labeling, and truth in packaging were among them. Empowered with these new rules, consumers launched an onslaught of tort litigation that has carried through to the 1990s unabated. There was significant activity at the state level, as well, as state offices of the attorney general were transformed from entities almost entirely concerned with violent and organized crime into hotbeds of activity on the consumer-rights front. The change had more than a little to do with the realization that consumer expectations were running high and that there was a good deal of political hay to be made by bringing corporate scoundrels to justice.

In the end, the collective activity of fifty state offices of the attorney general, other state agencies involved with consumer interests, and the federal CPSC and other like-minded agencies created a whole new market environment for American producers and consumers. Slowly but surely, the old adage so appropriate in the freewheeling laissez-faire days of the earlier twentieth century—caveat emptor, let the buyer beware—began giving way as a descriptor of consumer-producer relations. Today, the aphorism caveat venditor—let the seller beware—reflects more accurately the character of the modern marketplace.

In retrospect, it is fair to say that by the 1970s, some of the more radical sentiments of the stormy 1960s had been mollified. Still, the smoldering embers of that turbulent decade remained: Even if the establishment was no longer thought of as necessarily evil by definition, neither was it deemed right by definition. Instead, the actions of members of the establishment would be judged on a case-by-case basis, receiving neither the immediate rejection of the 1960s nor the benefit of the doubt that was so freely accorded it in prior decades. Consumers, including consumers of health care, would no longer stand idly by, accepting without question whatever goods and services were being offered. They would demand that the government protect them, and they would insist on being able to protect themselves. Producers of all kinds of goods and services, including physicians and hospitals in the case of health care, would lose power in the process. Ultimately, this redistribution of power in the medical marketplace led Americans to start demanding more control over the way the health-care system treated them, both in life and in death.

Health-Care Consumerism

The emergence of a rights culture that fueled the consumerism movement in the 1960s quite naturally spread to the health-care arena. Consumerism called into question the traditional relationship between physician (seller) and patient (buyer). In the late 1960s and early 1970s, activists in the health-care rights movement were demanding that more attention be paid to informed consent, the right to view medical records, and the extension of due process protections when individuals were involuntarily committed to institutions. Each claim robbed from physicians some of the authority that they had exercised exclusively in days past.

The Physician-Patient Relationship

The relationship between Americans and their physicians is somewhat unique, according to Paul Starr (1982), because physicians have traditionally been held in high esteem. This is not always true in other cultures. In the former Soviet Union, for example, the fact that 70 percent of physicians were women did not reflect the advances that women had made in that society so much as it reflected the relatively low esteem in which doctors were held in that country. In contrast, American physicians have been the most respected of all professionals in the United States, at least since the turn of the century.

Doctors have mastered knowledge in an area of great importance to Americans—the preservation of life—and this expertise gives them a great power advantage from the start. As Marie Haug and Bebe Levin (1983, p. 11) note: "In a society where vigorous health is a central value, and where death is to be forestalled at all costs, power will accrue to persons whose skills are believed to conquer disease and prevent premature demise." Command of an esoteric language has only added to the physician's mystique.

The traditional imbalance in power between physician and patient is compounded by the fact that most individuals who come in contact with doctors are in a relatively weakened state to begin with, making them more vulnerable than they might otherwise be to the exercise of power and authority. They may be in great pain or in shock. Or they may be at their wits' end, desperate for a medical fix. As such, patients are put into a subordinate role vis-à-vis their doctors.

This is true even during regular medical checkups. Due to advances in diagnostic technology, physicians can find all kinds of terrible things wrong even with seemingly healthy individuals, and that, too, puts the patient at a distinct power disadvantage. Clearly, the advent of high-technology medical equipment—both of the diagnostic and the rescue-medicine variety—has widened what Talcott Parsons has called the "competence gap," from which physicians draw considerable authority and power.

At the same time, physician hegemony is on the wane. In the previous chapter, we charted the changes in physician behavior that led to an erosion of the trust that had characterized the doctor-patient relationship before the turn of the century. Here, we note how patients themselves have chipped away at physician autonomy through the medical consumerism movement. This new philosophy of patient empowerment challenged the doctor's right to make unilateral decisions and demanded that power be shared in a relationship that shifts the focus from physician autonomy to physician obligation and from patient compliance to patient rights. It is a new kind of bond in which faith and trust have been replaced by caution and doubt (Haug and Levin, 1983, p. 10). As a result of this shift in philosophy, recipients of health care today are more likely to be "wary consumers" rather than "grateful supplicants" (Rothman, 1991, p. 128).

Part of this radical transformation in physician-patient relations can be attributed to improved education nationwide, as measured, in part, by the number of years of formal education completed. In addition, there is another, more informal dimension to education—education that is facilitated by the stream of popular literature on health that has emerged in the last few decades. Health and fitness magazines, consumer reports, books on every popular health subject imaginable, and medical columns in newspapers have advised increasingly health-conscious consumers about new treatment options and their side effects, old treatment protocols found to be ineffective or even dangerous, and new ailments that were formerly misdiagnosed as something else. These publications have also encouraged readers to press physicians for candid answers and to shop around for a second (or third or fourth) opinion if they are unsatisfied. All this information and encouragement has empowered patients by bringing the authority of the physician into question, putting doctors on the defensive for the first time since being challenged by their medical school supervisors.

The advances of medical technology and proliferation of treatment options have also cut into physician credibility. Many patients today have some form of chronic or degenerative illness, such as cancer, heart disease, diabetes, or kidney disease. Although much progress has been made in treating these ailments, there is still a measure of disagreement in the medical community with regard to the standards of care that should be rendered in specific cases. The proliferation of specialists only exacerbates the problem for each different specialist seems to put a different spin on diagnosis and treatment. Such disagreements lead to a further breakdown in the faith the patient has in any particular physician (Haug and Levin, 1983, p. 33). Long, drawn-out illnesses also give patients more time to think about and question their treatments. As noted in Chapter 3, George Washington had only a few days to disagree with his caretakers before death arrived, but most of us will have months or even years to think about the care received while dying.

Then there are the medical ethicists who chime in with policy pronouncements about the importance of patient autonomy in editorials and news articles, during policy symposia that they arrange, and before congressional committees. One such opinionmaker is Willard Gaylin, president of the Hastings Institute, a center devoted to the study of medical-ethical issues. Gaylin testified that "patient-consumers must no longer trust exclusively the benevolence of the professional. ... Basic decisions must be returned to the hands of the patient population whose health care future will be affected. ... We should all share in the decision making" (cited in Rothman, 1991, p. 188).

The electronic media have played an important role, as well. Gone are the candycoated images of trustworthy doctors as packaged in the character of Dr. Welby. (Could there be a better, more seductive name for the doctor portrayed in this stereotype?) In the place of these fictional dramas about good doctors practicing good medicine, we now find real-life exposés about bad medicine, served up almost nightly on the news and covered more extensively on "60 Minutes," "20/20," "Frontline," "48 Hours," and the like. The daytime talk shows—hosted by Phil Donahue, Oprah Winfrey, Sally Jesse Raphael, and Geraldo Rivera—then add their explosive spin to the health-care issues currently in vogue. These television programs broadcast stories about physicians having sex with patients, overcharging, prescribing drugs with tragic side effects, conducting experiments on humans without fully informed consent, performing unnecessary surgeries, as well as absentee doctors (who are out on the golf course while residents perform their operations). Some programs narrow in on specific physicians who have committed other ethical transgressions, like the fertility specialist who, in 1991, confessed to using his own sperm to artificially inseminate over seventy patients without their knowledge.

Even though the overwhelming percentage of physicians may be selfless, ethical, upstanding practitioners, these stories of deviance cut deep into the faith Americans put in the medical profession, and that initiates a cycle of skepticism-based activity as these reports of abuse feed into themselves. Exposés increase doubts in the patient population, which, in turn, increase awareness and encourage individuals to raise issues of safety and trust. This then causes more complaints and revelations of more problems and ultimately produces even more exposés. And the cycle starts again. Once begun, this engine of policy activism is difficult to stop as long as there is fuel, and, apparently, there is fuel aplenty.

As a result, "doctor's orders," a command that had previously carried great weight in American society, is beginning to lose its power. Today, the compliant "you're the doctor" acknowledgment of authority is being replaced by the more challenging notion (sometimes expressed but usually only thought) that "maybe I should get a second opinion." In searching out these second opinions, some patients turn to paraprofessional and nontraditional health-care providers for assistance. This, too, cuts into traditional physician credibility and manifests its decline.

Alternative Approaches to Health Care

Haug and Levin (1983, p. 21) note how the growth of paraprofessional fields has been an important factor in the demystification of medicine. Tasks once done solely by physicians are now delegated to nurse practitioners, midwives, and physicians' assistants, especially in health maintenance organizations (HMOs), where cost control is a primary concern. The operating philosophy of the HMO requires providers to husband resources and deliver services at the lowest possible level of technical sophistication. That means greater use of paraprofessionals to perform the less technical procedures and tasks related to diagnosis and treatment. The HMO philosophy of capitated coverage—annual flat-fee coverage, as opposed to bills paid on a rolling, "fee-for-service" basis—may also mean increased patient self-care, with a special emphasis on disease prevention.

In both paraprofessional care and self-care, individuals become aware that someone other than a full-fledged physician can provide quality care, adding to the notion that maybe the legendary stature traditionally accorded the physician is not particularly well deserved, after all. In addition, it may be easier for patients to question a paraprofessional rather than a physician about their medical care. HMOs, nonexistent twenty years ago, cover nearly 20 percent of the population today. It would be surprising—indeed, incredible—if this exposure did not undermine faith in physicians to some degree.

There is also a surge of interest in caring for oneself that arises independently of the HMO philosophy. Part of this development can be traced to the 1974 bestseller *The Type A Behavior and Your Heart,* written by cardiologists Meyer Friedman and Ray Rosenman. These doctors argued that personality traits such as impatience and irritability increase a person's risk of heart disease, which led them and their readers to believe that the health of the heart could be changed by personality-altering behaviors. *The Relaxation Response,* a 1975 best-seller by Herbert Benson (another cardiologist) and Miriam Klipper, arrived just in time to follow up on Friedman and Rosenman's work. The first book described why some people are at risk for heart disease. The second, a behavioral guide to heart disease risk reduction, capitalized on the interest in transcendental meditation (TM) that had become something of a cultural fad in the 1970s.

In 1979, Norman Cousins, longtime editor of the *Saturday Review,* made a significant contribution to the self-care movement when he told of how taking vitamin C and watching comedies on television led to his seemingly miraculous recovery from what was thought to be an incurable disease. That same year, Jon Kabat-Zinn, a professor of medicine, established a stress-reduction clinic at the

University of Massachusetts Medical Center—the first hospital-based program to use a combination of medication and yoga to reduce stress. The use of prescription drugs at the clinic was a traditional approach that kept physicians firmly in control, but the yoga was something patients could do at home, without any prescription. This helped to bring yoga—like TM—into the mainstream of American life as a preventive, self-directed approach to health. Biofeedback, in which individuals are trained to become aware of their heart rate and blood pressure in order to control them through conscious mental effort, was another self-care alternative that became popular during these years.

More advances were made along these lines in the 1980s. Stores started putting blood pressure and pulse-monitoring machines in their lobbies, and bars started installing Breathalyzer machines. Also in this decade, the *Physician's Desk Reference* (*PDR*) became available for purchase by the public (see, e.g., *Physician's Desk Reference*, 1992). In years past, the *PDR*, a compendium of legal drugs available in the United States (including recommended doses, generic information, and potential side effects), was a carefully guarded trade secret of physicians. Now, patients armed with their own copies of the *PDR* are able to second-guess the physician, about both the dosage and the choice of drugs. The *PDR* also made it possible for patients to become more aware of potential side effects—yet another potential ground on which to call doctors into question.

The rise of the home-health-care business, an industry response to the escalating costs of institutional care, has also been a significant development in the popularization of medicine. Home health care, in which treatments and therapies are provided in the home (with the assistance of visiting paraprofessionals as needed), shifts the locus of control and responsibility from bureaucratic institutions to the domestic scene. More importantly, it shifts the locus of authority away from professional physicians and toward paraprofessionals and individuals—the patients and their relatives. Home health care has gone from an anomaly to a $3.2-billion industry in the last decade or so, and forecasters are calling for steady growth in the future (Freudenheim, 1992a). By providing health-monitoring equipment, intravenous nutrition and drugs, and other sorts of portable technology to individuals in their homes, these companies are helping to sever the already frayed tether of dependency between patient and doctor. Home health care takes the mystery out of treatment and puts control in the hands of the lay public, whose toleration for autocratic physicians cannot help but begin to ebb in the process.

Self-care resource groups have also proliferated in the last two decades. Networks, coalitions, advocacy groups, alliances, and associations of every size, shape, and persuasion have grown up around every health-care cause imaginable. Some of these groups provide educational materials and hold information sessions. Other groups focus on coping skills for patients and families. Some provide a forum for sharing the trials and tribulations of a particular affliction. And others do a little bit of all these things.

Occasionally, groups will espouse a very broad mandate, such as those organizations that focus on women's health-care issues in general. Other groups concentrate their attention on specific afflictions—the Malignant Hyperthermia Association of America, for example, which educates and provides support specifically to those who suffer from malignant hyperthermia (MH), a potentially life-threatening sensitivity to anesthesia. Whatever the goal, however, and whatever the health issue, self-care resource groups empower individuals in battles with both their afflictions and their physicians.

In addition to self-care and paraprofessional care, there is also a surge of interest in "alternative medicine"—medical philosophies that fall outside the mainstream established by the American Medical Association. One development worth noting is the renewed interest in homeopathic medicine (Gorman, 1992).

Homeopathy, an approach to health care that originated with German physician Samuel Hahnemann (1755–1843), operates on what its practitioners call the "law of similars." The principle holds that a substance that causes the symptoms that the patient suffers from will cure the patient if given in extremely diluted solutions. Interestingly, although nobody knows how homeopathy works, practitioners and patients alike swear by its efficacy, citing anecdote after anecdote of successful treatment.

In the United States, interest in homeopathic approaches surged after the Civil War but then subsided appreciably after the turn of the twentieth century. In 1900, there were twenty-two homeopathic medical schools in the United States, but by 1918, that number had dropped to six, and now there are none. Interest in homeopathy seems to be rekindling today, however. Homeopathic drug companies report that, in some cases, sales have increased tenfold in the last decade or so. In that time, the sale of homeopathic "cures" has evolved into a $100-million business (currently, these "cures" are not subject to FDA approval). The number of individuals who claim to practice homeopathy has increased, as well, from a nationwide total of 100 in the early 1970s to 2,500 today. Three states—Connecticut, Arizona, and Nevada—now license individuals to practice homeopathy, and in most other states, homeopathy providers may advertise their services as long as they are also board certified as traditional health-care professionals.[1]

This resurgence of interest in homeopathy is important for two reasons. First, homeopathic defections in the patient and practitioner population suggest that at least some are dissatisfied enough with the traditional-care model that they are willing to swim against the tide and try something new, another sign of the decline in trust of traditional care. Second, part of the appeal of homeopathy derives, we suspect, from the close patient-practitioner relationship that the homeopathic philosophy calls for. Homeopaths are encouraged to learn all they can by listening closely to patients, who are allowed to give extended, uninterrupted reports of their symptoms. Practitioners are trained to establish close relationships with their patients, and hour-long consults are not uncommon (Starr, 1982, p. 97). Obviously, this approach varies greatly from that of traditional physicians who are criticized for becoming too emotionally disconnected from their patients.

Patients who are unable to get relief from traditionally trained physicians have given testimony to the value of a wide variety of other alternative approaches to health care, as well. In naturopathy, for example, illness and disease are treated through exercise, diet, and other "natural" means rather than with drugs or surgery. Another alternative, osteopathy (founded by Missouri doctor Andrew Still in the 1890s) takes a very mechanistic approach to medical disorder. Dr. Still encouraged his followers to treat the heart as if it were an engine, the lungs as if they were a fanning machine, and the lobes of the brain as if they were an electric battery (Starr, 1982, p. 108). The body could be repaired, he argued, only by making sure that its parts were in proper relationships with one another. Accordingly, osteopaths emphasize physical manipulation and massage as therapeutic approaches to be used before resorting to drugs or more invasive therapies. Not coincidentally, chiropractic had its beginnings in the same decade as osteopathy, and though the intervening years have produced ups and downs in the field, the chiropractic approach seems to be as popular as ever today.

Acupuncture is yet another increasingly common, nontraditional alternative in health care. This approach was popularized in the United States by *New York Times* writer James Reston, who related his experiences with this ancient Chinese practice that involves inserting needles into the body at specific points and manipulating them to relieve pain and treat illness. More than 2,000 physicians now use acupuncture in conjunction with conventional medicine in the United States (Barasch, 1992).

Some 5,000 other individuals hang hypnotherapy shingles outside their offices. Hypnotherapy is a method of inducing a trancelike state, characterized by the patient's extreme suggestibility, to help the individual relax and control pain or overcome addictions like smoking and overeating. No one thoroughly understands the nature of hypnotherapy's effects, but this alternative, like the others, represents a rejection of traditional medical practice; taken together, these alternatives are now manifest as a multibillion-dollar rival to the traditional care model.

According to a survey reported in the *New England Journal of Medicine*, it is estimated that Americans spent close to $14 billion on alternative medicine in 1990 (Angier, 1993b). Approximately one-third of those surveyed claimed to have engaged in alternative therapies in that year, and one in ten claimed to have visited a practitioner of such therapies. Those under the care of an unorthodox practitioner (most typically, patients were well-educated, middle-income whites between twenty-five and forty-nine years of age) reported making an average of nineteen visits during the course of the year. Multiplied out, that represents a total of 425 million visits—more than the number of trips made by all people to all primary-care physicians (e.g., general practitioners, family doctors, internists, and pediatricians) combined (Angier, 1993b).[2]

The fact that the National Institutes of Health (NIH) opened an Office of Alternative Medicine further testifies to the increasing interest along these lines. According to Dr. Joe Jacobs, the new director of the office, the popularity of alternative medicine demonstrates the "hunger among Americans for a more humane and less invasive type of treatment than ordinarily practiced by standard doctors" (cited in Angier, 1993b). Jacobs believes it is important that "some of these alternative therapies take a holistic and caring view of the patient ... this is hard to achieve in a conventional medical setting, with your feet in stirrups" (cited in Angier, 1993b). Dr. Jules Hirsch of Rockefeller University in New York echoes the sentiment. The interest in alternative medicine, he argues, represents "a cry for new treatments and a criticism of the scientific community for being too cold and too removed from human needs" (cited in Angier, 1993a).

The new office at the NIH is expected to receive requests for funding research in such unorthodox fields as homeopathy, herbal medicine, electromagnetism (to treat arthritis), visualization and guided imagery (to help manage pain), and touch therapy (akin to the traditional laying on of hands). Admittedly, the first-year budget for the Office of Alternative Medicine—$2 million—is minuscule when compared to the total NIH research budget of over $10 billion. Still, the very creation of this office and the growing predisposition of Americans to reject conventional medicine in favor of alternative approaches are harbingers of import to the right-to-die debate. If more Americans are taking health care into their own hands, are they not more likely to take death into their own hands, as well?

The Impact of Organizations

To this point, we have looked at consumerism in health care as manifested in the decline of the physician-patient relationship and the rise of alternative forms of therapy. We now turn to evidence of consumerism as manifested in the activity of groups—primarily interest groups, professional associations, and government committees. The clearest and most explicit expression of health-care consumerism arising from the activity of groups is the Patient Bill of Rights, the end product of a study conducted by the National Welfare Rights Organization (NWRO) in 1970.[3]

The Patient Bill of Rights, a list of twenty-six rights proposals, was presented to the Joint Commission on Accreditation for Hospital Organizations. The Joint Commission is the primary hospital-accreditation agency in the United States, and NWRO was hoping that its rights manifesto would be made a requirement for all hospitals that wished to retain their JCAHO accreditation. After negotiations, the Joint Commission incorporated a number of NWRO rights recommendations into the preamble of its hospital-accreditation manual. Essentially, the new preamble called for hospitals to provide access to care to anyone, regardless of race, color, creed, national origin, or ability to pay. Further, it stated that all patients had the right to be told the truth about their medical condition.

This preamble served as the basis for the American Hospital Association's (AHA) Patient Bill of Rights, issued in 1972. The AHA version reiterated the Joint Commission's preamble and more generally stipulated that all patients had the right to respectful care. Importantly, the AHA proclamation enlarged on the JCAHO manual's treatment of informed consent by stipulating that truth telling must incorporate explanations that "the patient can reasonably be expected to understand" (cited in Rothman, 1991, p. 146). There were also provisions requiring that patient consent be obtained before proceeding with either treatment or experimentation.

In theory, the Joint Commission carries a great deal of weight since it can decertify a hospital, making the institution ineligible for reimbursement under Medicare or Medicaid. Initially, however, the Joint Commission did not exercise its power with regard to patients' rights. Including some of the NWRO positions in the preamble of its accreditation manual really only constituted a statement of a philosophy, not the establishment of hard-and-fast requirements. There were no procedures laid down for enforcement, nor were there any sanctions listed for failure to comply. The AHA document carried even less weight. It provided evidence that change was in the air, but like the Joint Commission preamble, the AHA statement was an expression of philosophy more than a rule of law—an indication of changing attitudes but not necessarily an impetus for changing behaviors. Clearly, however, Joint Commission and AHA attention to these concerns suggested that more rigorous requirements in the area of patients' rights would come into play in the future.

In early 1973, at about the same time the Joint Commission and the AHA were dabbling with patients' rights, Senator Edward Kennedy began holding committee hearings under the operating title "Quality of Health Care: Human Experimentation." Despite the narrow focus suggested by this title, Kennedy's aim was to call all medical practice into question. Although the Kennedy Committee's report was weakened substantially before being made public, it was still strong enough to symbolize the end of the monopoly the medical profession had created for itself in the medical ethics venue (Rothman, 1991, p. 188). The doors to the decision-making process were flung wide open by testimony taken by the Kennedy study group, leading Bernard Barber to predict that the committee would "transform fundamental moral problems [in modern medicine] from a condition of relative professional neglect and occasional journalistic scandal to a condition of continuing public and professional visibility and legitimacy" (cited in Rothman, 1991, p. 188).

The Public Citizen's Health Research Group (PCHRG), one of Ralph Nader's many consumer-oriented organizations, helped to make sure, through the 1970s and beyond, that patients' rights would continue as a high-profile concern on the public-policy agenda (Rothman, 1991, p. 188). The PCHRG stirred the pot by publicizing investigations into medical practices that had gone unscrutinized, by publishing and disseminating its own reports along the same lines, and by testifying before Congress on controversial health-care issues like national health insurance, medical malpractice, unnecessary surgery, and measuring the quality of medical care patients receive.[4]

As much as Americans tend to worship advanced medical technology and those who use it, they seem to be less willing to consider physician-provided treatments as good by definition. And the demographics of U.S. society suggest that this trend will only continue. Baby boomers who cut their teeth during the antiestablishment days of the 1960s are now moving into middle age (the oldest of the lot will turn fifty in 1996). This generation is twice as large as the previous one, and its members will be, we suspect, much more likely to question authority and demand control over their medical care—both in living and in dying—than their parents were.

Those who do make those demands will be relieved to know that the Joint Commission has taken a stronger stand on the issue of patients' rights in recent years, to the point where, instead of being mentioned as a suggestion in the preamble of the certification manual, patient rights have now evolved into a primary and important part of all Joint Commission reviews. According to the 1992 JCAHO standards manual, hospitals are required to have formal procedures in place that protect the right of the patient to make decisions involving health care, in collaboration with his or her physician. This includes the right to refuse medical treatment, to make advanced directives, and to appoint a surrogate decision-maker (all such rights are exercisable to the extent permitted by state law). Further, the Joint Commission requires that, upon admitting a patient, the hospital must make a documented effort to determine if an advance directive exists and to help the individual without one to develop a directive if he or she desires (in the spirit of the Patient Self-Determination Act, which will be described more fully). Any advance directives produced or created as a result must be documented in the patient's record and periodically reviewed, according to commission guidelines.

Thus, the patients' rights movement has produced some tangible results in the twenty years since its humble beginnings. The various rights movements of the 1960s helped to set the stage. Then, as the relationship between physicians and patients began to break down, nontraditional forms of medical care became more prominent. Meanwhile, organizations like the NWRO, the Joint Commission, and the Kennedy Committee were identifying, for the first time, the nature of an appropriate relationship between a caregiver and a patient, with emphasis on the rights of the latter.

All these streams of health-care consumerism ultimately converge in a confluence of activism for patients' rights that is probably nowhere as clearly manifest as
in the women's health movement. This movement illustrates well the trends of
medical decisionmaking in the last few decades. And it may even suggest something about the trajectory of the right-to-die movement in particular.

The Women's Health Movement

Medical consumerism is perhaps most robustly expressed in the area of women's
health care. It may be that the most dramatic changes have taken place in this
arena precisely because this was where the most progress was needed. Indeed, the
history of the interaction between women and their physicians is marked by dom-
inance, deception, half-truths, and even abuse of the former by the latter. The
Hippocratic medical tradition itself reinforced negative conceptions of women,
their predispositions, and their capacities for rational thought.[5] According to that
tradition, a woman's place was deemed to be strictly domestic in nature; she
should not be agitating for her rights in the doctor's office and certainly not practicing medicine.

Women and Medical Training

Male doctors deliberately and systematically excluded women from medical training in the United States at least until recently (The Boston Women's Health Book
Collective, 1984, p. 363). In the nineteenth century, the AMA issued the following
statement in defense of its position that only men should be trained as physicians:
"When a critical case demands independent action, and fearless judgement,
man's success depends on his virile courage, which the normal woman does not
have nor is expected to have" (cited in Kevorkian, 1991, p. 207). In the twentieth
century, the medical establishment built on this and other Hippocratic stereotypes by suggesting that women were unfit to be doctors because menstrual cycles
caused emotional instabilities. Some argued that having women in the classroom
would be an unwholesome distraction for men, and others worried that women
would go on to marry and bear children, proving their training to be a waste (The
Boston Women's Health Book Collective, 1984, p. 570). In addition, many worried
(maybe with good reason) that if women were admitted to the profession, female
patients would prefer physicians of their own gender, especially for childbirth.

Men effectively barred the door to medical school through the 1950s, when only
a trace of females could be found practicing medicine. But numbers grew steadily
through the 1960s as the rights movement began opening all kinds of doors to
those who had previously been discouraged from entering. Today, nearly one in
every eight practicing physicians and more than one in four medical students is

female. This influx of women portends important changes for the doctor-patient relationship (see Chapter 4). Moreover, female physicians serve as strong role models for other women outside the profession who may otherwise have wondered if women really were capable of making medical decisions, either as physicians or as patients.

Women as Patients

The popular media's coverage of issues of particular importance to women has had a galvanizing effect on the women's health-care movement. Headlines about toxic shock syndrome (TSS, a potentially life-threatening malady brought on by the use of superabsorbent tampons), breast cancer (which one in eight women in America today will contract), silicon breast implants and hip implants, and faulty contraceptive devices (like the Dalkon Shield)[6] have, in their way, normalized and popularized health care. Such subjects are now out of the closet and considered something that women can openly discuss and maybe even do something about.

The development and distribution of the birth control pill also had a dramatic effect on women as patients. First approved by the FDA in 1960 and nearly 100 percent effective if properly prescribed and administered, "the pill" was instrumental in empowering women.[7] Availability of the pill drew women into the health-care system earlier and more often than they would have been otherwise, and at the same time, it gave them a degree of control over their bodies that they had not enjoyed in the past. It was now possible for sexually active women to plan pregnancies or avoid them altogether.[8]

Then came *Roe* v. *Wade,* the U.S. Supreme Court's 1973 decision that determined that access to an abortion was constitutionally protected as a "penumbral" privacy right—one of those rights found to exist in the "shadow" of the U.S. Constitution. *Roe* empowered women—even those who chose not to have an abortion or those not needing an abortion—by reinforcing the notion that they could take medical decisionmaking into their own hands. Like the birth control pill, legalized abortion gave women more flexibility, more options, and more control over their own lives, and that emboldened them to expect and even demand more control over their own health care.

Widespread reports of doctors sexually abusing their female patients had an impact, as well, making women leery of male physicians.[9] Even when physicians did not cross the bounds of sexual propriety, their behavior was perceived by many females as imperialistic and autocratic, leading women to regularly complain that their doctors had not listened to them or believed what they said. Too often, women reported, their male medical caretakers were offering tranquilizers and moral advice instead of sound medical care.

Even worse, some physicians systematically withheld knowledge, lied, and treated their female patients without consent. Failing to warn patients of the risks and side effects of treatments, overprescribing drugs, and overcharging in the process are among the indictments of male physicians brought by feminists in recent years. These feminists have urged rejection of the status quo in favor of increasing both patient rights and physician obligations (The Boston Women's Health Book Collective, 1984).

Obstetrics

Some of the most pointed feminist criticisms regarding the treatment of women as patients have been aimed at the way childbirth has become bureaucratized and medicalized in the twentieth century. First, the site of the birth has changed. In 1900, 95 percent of American babies were born at home, commonly with a midwife in attendance. But beginning in the 1920s, many states (with the encouragement of medical doctors) began outlawing the practice of midwifery (Rothman, 1991, p. 135). By 1960, 95 percent of all deliveries were taking place in hospitals, and a centuries-old tradition of domestic childbirth was all but lost.

Even more significant than the change in venue was the change in procedures associated with the delivery of a baby for the entire process had become extraordinarily medicalized. Both baby and mother benefitted greatly during high-risk births. But for many women experiencing an otherwise routine birth, all the added technology turned a natural event into a dehumanizing nightmare. Typically, the woman was forced to lie on her back with her legs spread and feet up in stirrups.[10] Enemas, medical equipment (blood pressure cuffs around the biceps, contraction monitors taped to the abdomen, IVs inserted into the arm), and drugs (analgesia tranquilizers to minimize anxiety, barbiturates to induce sleep, and anesthesia to control pain) were all part of the picture, as well.

Often, if the attending physician did not feel the labor was progressing fast enough, he would break the bag of waters artificially by puncturing the amniotic sac with a small instrument shaped like a crochet hook and inserted through the cervix. Sometimes, electrode sensors would be inserted through the woman's uterus and attached to the baby's body by means of screws or metal clips. The mother's condition might be further monitored by another electrode, introduced into the cervix through a catheter in the vagina. If the delivery was still falling behind schedule, labor might be induced with an injection of Pitocin (The Boston Women's Health Book Collective, 1984, p. 382).

As the baby began to present itself, two more procedures often came into play. First, there was the ever-present possibility of a forceps-assisted delivery. Second, the physician would likely proceed with the most frequently performed obstetric operation in the West: the episiotomy—the only operation regularly effected on the body of a healthy woman without her consent.[11]

This scenario all presumes, of course, that the baby is delivered vaginally. The other option, even more medically intensive, is to deliver the baby through an incision in the mother's abdomen: the cesarean-section delivery. Twenty-five years ago, only 5 percent of babies were born by cesarean section, and a decade before, hardly any were. Today, nearly one in four babies in the United States is born via the ubiquitous cesarean (compared with one in fifteen babies in Japan).[12] The cesarean is increasingly popular among obstetricians at least in part, according to consumer groups, because it allows them to "manage" their "caseload" and maximize efficiency (and profit).[13] This is true despite evidence that suggests that cesareans are more risky for the mother and that many, maybe most, are not even necessary.[14]

In sum, more drugs and technologies are now used in the United States for "normal" births than anywhere else around the world. This reflects, in part, the desire to master, conquer, and control nature that has always been a defining characteristic of the American political culture (Wertz, cited in The Boston Women's Health Book Collective, 1984, p. 362). At the same time, the medicalization of childbirth has tended to restrain and dehumanize the women such procedures are intended to benefit. Today's women are demanding a more humane standard of care, one that adds their feelings and interests into the decision-making mix. Certainly, they want the best care for themselves and their babies. But, because the evidence now coming forth suggests that many interventions and procedures are done solely for the well-being of the physician, women are becoming increasingly suspicious of those who claim to be caring for them.

In an environment of declining trust, women are beginning to demand that their rights and prerogatives be respected, and this sets them up to be more challenging when it comes to making right-to-die decisions, as well. Given their experiences with medicalization in the delivery room, sexual abuse in the examining room, disinformation in the consultation room, and discrimination in medical school, it should come as no surprise that American women are primed to start demanding more control over health-care decisionmaking, both for themselves and for their children. If they are not, perhaps the cases of Angela Carder and Nancy Klein will make them think again.

The Case of Angela Carder. Angela Carder, twenty-seven years of age, had suffered from bone cancer nearly all her life. On two occasions, she had been told by doctors that she had only a few days to live, but Carder, one of the first children to survive Ewing's sarcoma (a cancer of the connective tissue), had proved the experts wrong. By 1984, after being in remission for several years, Carder was married and had hopes of starting a family. With her doctor's blessing, she became pregnant. But in June 1987, when she was twenty-six weeks pregnant, the cancer returned. With an inoperable tumor engulfing her lung, she was admitted to the George Washington University Medical Center in Washington, D.C., where, after examination, doctors determined her condition to be terminal.

Carder had indicated to her doctor at the beginning of her pregnancy that she wanted her own health, not the fetus's, to come first. "She had battled too long to survive to give it all up at this point," according to her mother, Nettie Stoner

(Faludi, 1991, p. 433). Carder's longtime oncologist, who disagreed with the terminal prognosis rendered by the George Washington University physicians, recommended an aggressive treatment of radiation and chemotherapy. However, the
doctors at the hospital, who believed Carder had only days to live, were against
administering this treatment for it would likely endanger the developing fetus.
They decided that if they could prolong Carder's life for several weeks, rather than
save it, they could offer at least some hope for the fetus. So, instead of moving
ahead with a treatment to attack her cancer, doctors administered sedatives, a
strategy used to postpone death. Carder tried to resist the doctors, "thrashing and
twisting on the bed to fend them off." According to her mother, she pleaded, "No,
no, no. Don't do that to me" (Faludi, 1991, p. 435).

At this point, the hospital administration became involved. Aware of a possible
backlash from antiabortion activists for not attempting heroic measures to save
even a severely compromised fetus, they weighed their options. Fearing that if the
fetus was viable, the hospital would be held liable for its death, the administration
recommended that the doctors perform a cesarean section in an attempt to save
the fetus. But in Carder's precarious state, it was highly unlikely that she would
survive this kind of major surgery. She was heavily drugged at this point and virtually unconscious, making it difficult for her to make her own feelings about the
hospital's decision clear. Without waiting for the effects of Carder's sedation to
wear off and without notifying her family, the hospital requested the intervention
of the courts.

Superior Court Judge Emmet Sullivan hastily convened a hearing in a hospital
conference room. Those present included a legal team for the hospital, two city
attorneys, a lawyer representing the fetus, and an attorney appointed by the court
to represent Carder. In the meeting, the medical opinion of each physician in the
obstetrical department was requested, and each doctor called recommended
against the operation. Further questions asked by the judge focused almost solely
around the welfare of the unborn fetus, with the health and welfare of Angela
Carder becoming less and less central. After a brief recess, the judge ruled that
"the court is of the view the fetus should be given an opportunity to live," and
since any delay in performing a surgical delivery increased the risk to the fetus,
the cesarean was to be performed immediately.

Carder's sedatives were just beginning to wear off when Dr. Louis Hamner of
the obstetrical unit arrived to tell her of the decision. When first asked if she
wanted the surgery, Carder indicated yes, but when Hamner returned to her
room a half hour later, Carder clearly and repeatedly said, "I don't want it done, I
don't want it done." According to Hamner, her wishes on the matter were "quite
clear to me" (Faludi, 1991, p. 435). Yet, when he reported this to those still in the
"courtroom," the judge replied, "The court is still not clear what her intent is"
(Faludi, 1991, p. 435). Richard Love, one of the city's lawyers, then argued that
since the court had originally made the decision to operate on the basis that it

would be performed without her consent, her latest indication was immaterial (Faludi, 1991, p. 435). At this point, Carder's court-appointed lawyer called the American Civil Liberties Union (ACLU) Reproductive Freedom Project, and the ACLU attorneys filed an emergency appeal for a stay. Due to the urgency of the matter, a three-judge panel from an appellate court was quickly assembled.

In that hearing, more doubts were raised over Carder's mental capacity to make a coherent decision. The fetus's attorney, Barbara Mishkin, argued that because of Carder's condition, the "right of the fetus to live overrides any interest in the mother's continued very short life." In the end, the three-judge panel upheld the original decision and ordered the hospital to perform the cesarean section. Shortly after, doctors delivered a baby girl who lived only a little over two hours. Carder regained consciousness several hours later and cried when told her child did not survive. Soon after, she slipped into a coma, and two days later, she, too, died. Doctors admitted that the surgery most likely hastened Angela Carder's death.

In April 1990, the Washington, D.C. Court of Appeals issued a decision (*In re A. C.*) affirming the right of a pregnant woman to make her own decisions about health care even if her choices endanger the fetus ("Let the Patient Decide," 1990). Seven months later, in November 1990, the George Washington University Medical Center adopted a new policy that stated that "ethically difficult decisions for treatment of severely ill pregnant women and their fetuses will be made by the woman, her family, and her doctors, not by the courts" (Greenhouse, 1990). Carder's mother issued a statement in response: "It's been a terrible tragedy for us, but positive things have come from it" (Greenhouse, 1990).

Those "positive things" Carder's mother talks about must include the hospital's issuance of a written policy on pregnancy that respects the right of the mother to make decisions and, maybe more importantly, more general changes in attitudes that resulted from the case. Less than one year after the Carder incident, New Jersey passed the first (and, to date, the only) living-will law to give pregnant women the same rights granted in case law by the Washington, D.C. Court of Appeals. We do not have evidence of a causal link between the two events, but it is not hard to imagine that the Carder case helped to set the stage for New Jersey's bold stroke of policy mediation in this area. (For more on New Jersey's law, see Chapter 8.)

The Case of Nancy Klein. Nancy Klein and her family fared a bit better than Carder and her family had when faced with a similar situation, largely because her pregnancy was not as far along when catastrophic illness struck. Still, it took a court fight to settle the matter.

In February 1989, Klein lay in a coma in North Shore University Hospital on Long Island after suffering brain damage in a December 1988 automobile accident. She was seventeen weeks pregnant at the time. Her husband, Martin Klein, sought (with the support of his wife's parents) to be appointed as Nancy's temporary guardian for purposes of authorizing the physicians at the hospital to "inter-rupt the pregnancy ... and to perform such other medical procedures as may be necessary to preserve [Nancy Klein's] life" (538 N.Y.S.2d 274 [A.D.2 Dept. 1989]). Martin Klein was opposed in court by two strangers to the family who sought to prevent the proposed abortion by petitioning for guardianship of the four-month-old fetus.

Both the Supreme Court in Nassau County and the Appellate Division of the New York Supreme Court rejected the strangers' petition, citing *Roe* v. *Wade* and arguing that "a non-viable fetus, i.e., one less than twenty-four weeks old, is not a legally recognized 'person' for the purposes of proceedings such as these." Fur-ther, the court stated, "the State has no compelling interest in the protection of the fetus prior to viability since the mother's constitutional right to privacy, which includes her right to terminate her pregnancy, is paramount at that stage. [There-fore, the] application [of those opposing Klein] is totally without merit." In an emotionally charged summary, the court added that "ultimately, the record con-firms that these absolute strangers to the Klein family, whatever their motivation, have no place in the midst of this family tragedy" (538 N.Y.S.2d 274 [A.D.2 Dept. 1989]). The court also found that, absent any evidence of malicious intent (what the court calls "adverse interest"), case law clearly leads in the direction of grant-ing family members guardianship whenever possible.

The Kleins' victory was a qualified one for the New York courts supported them, it appears, only because the fetus had not reached the magical viability point of twenty-four weeks. Thus, if Angela Carder had been in a New York hos-pital, the fact that she was twenty-six weeks pregnant would apparently have meant that she would have lost in court since her fetus was, in theory, viable. For present purposes, however, it is more important to note that such questions are now being raised in the courts and that both hospitals and states are beginning to make policy in this area. All this activism comes about, at least in part, because of the continued medicalization of health-care in America, which has already pre-cipitated its share of rights activism in the last thirty years.

Women Begin to Regain Control over Their Medical Destiny

According to John Smith, the development of a vital feminism in the United States in the last quarter century has led to some significant changes in women's health care, including everything from "padded stirrups and speculum warmers in the examining room to childbirth education, the resurgence of midwifery, and a wider awareness of 'patients' rights' in general" (Smith, 1992, p. 2). In place of the traditional, profession-dominated medical culture, a therapeutic countercul-ture has emerged in women's health care, in which members of self-help groups coach each other through the travails of infertility, breast cancer, cervical cancer, and sexual abuse. Women also are becoming more comfortable with monitoring their own health status (e.g., by doing breast self-exams and monitoring ovulation for times of peak fertility), all the while taking more responsibility for their own health.

In obstetrics, Lamaze and other "natural" childbirth methods have been advocated since the 1960s. Birthing rooms have become popular accoutrements of the modern American hospital, and now, the infant is allowed to stay with the mother after birth rather than being whisked away to the antiseptic nursery. Some hospitals put a crib in the mother's room to maximize the time mother and child can spend together. There also has been a resurgence in breast-feeding, another development (largely the result of efforts by Le Leche League) that empowers women to take care of themselves and their own.

Women's health issues outside the delivery room are coming to the fore, as well. Smith (1992, p. 14) notes, for example, that a million hysterectomies are conducted in the United States every year, and in nine out of ten cases, there is no medical imperative that the surgery be done. These operations are simply pushed on women, according to Smith (himself an obstetrician-gynecologist), by physicians who favor the aggressive-invasive approach to women's health-care issues.[15] Consequently, approximately three-quarters of all American women have had their uteruses removed by age sixty-five, many unnecessarily. In light of this, Smith and others have recommended that women take control of these decisions themselves. At the very least, they should demand that physicians share decision-making authority with them—and maybe even with other physicians as the second opinion becomes a more realistic option for patients and a requirement of some health-care insurers.

In the end, the women's rights movement—a central and significant part of health-care consumerism (itself a spin-off of the more general civil rights movements ignited in the 1960s)—taught women to reject the "professional autonomy-patient compliance" model that characterized the roles traditionally played when female patients interacted with their physicians. As a result, women of today are well on the way to retrieving some measure of control over their own medical destinies, both in life and, ultimately, in death.

Medical Research
and the Power of the Press

The power of the press was instrumental in converting outrage over women's health issues into something of a coherent mass movement. Headline stories about toxic shock syndrome, the Dalkon Shield, the side effects of birth control pills, and sexual abuse in the examining room encouraged women to demand for themselves more information, more choices, and more accountability in the provision of their health care. And the power of the press was equally important as a force of activism in other health areas, as well.

A Tradition of Influential Exposés

Sometimes, a series of stories and reports, published over time, add up to a significant and annealing force of movement activism. At other times, individual, blockbuster revelations seem to ignite a movement of one kind or another almost entirely on their own.

Upton Sinclair's *The Jungle* was a work of the latter sort. His graphic description of the sausage-making process in the early part of the century was a primary catalyst behind a raft of food-quality regulations that were passed in the years that followed. Rachel Carson's *Silent Spring* is another exposé of this genre, one pointed to by Ralph Nader (1965) as a central, founding treatise of the environmental movement. Nader should know something about such things for his condemning exposé of the Chevrolet Corvair, *Unsafe at Any Speed,* is often credited with launching the consumerism movement.

Nader, Carson, and Sinclair shared the unique quality of being able to stick their fingers in the collective public eye. Their works got people talking—and worried—about their own health and safety. Interest groups formed as agitation became organized and was channeled into various forms of activism that forced government to step into the breach in an effort to protect the rights of the general public. In each case, policy mediation could be traced to an identifiable collection of scathing words distributed for public consumption on the printed page.

It is with this general understanding of how important a single establishment-shaking work can be that we turn back to the field of medicine. Is there anything like the works of Sinclair, Carson, or Nader that has served as a catalyst in the health-care rights movement? One article, in particular, comes as close as any to fitting the bill.

Medical Research and Human Experimentation

The erosion of trust in doctors really began, argues Rothman (1991), with the erosion of trust in medical researchers. And that development only blossomed fully after a stinging indictment of medical research ethics, authored by Harvard Medical School professor Henry Beecher, was published in 1966. The article, entitled "Ethics and Clinical Research," appeared in the *New England Journal of Medicine.*

Medical Research: A Historical Background. Until World War II, medical research was essentially a cottage industry, and human experimentation was limited to individuals and small groups. In those days, it was common for researchers to conduct small-scale trials on friends, neighbors, and family members. For example, Englishman Edward Jenner, an eighteenth-century physician who did ground-breaking research on a vaccination against smallpox, was reported to have experimented on his son and another boy in the neighborhood. Occasionally, partly as an act of good faith and partly out of conviction, these researchers would even use themselves as guinea pigs. In 1767, Dr. John Hunter, the father of modern surgery in the United Kingdom, slit his own penis with a lancet that had been dipped in pus drawn from a patient infected with gonorrhea in an attempt to study the hypothesized relationship between gonorrhea and syphilis (Klawans, 1992, pp. 110–112). A few years later, another European physician, James Simpson, inhaled chloroform during an experiment to develop an anesthetic agent superior to ether; he awoke to find himself lying flat on the floor (Rothman, 1991, p. 21).

The clinical use of humans in experimentation on a large scale did not really come into play until the 1940s. Indeed, the Committee on Medical Research (CMR) projects that were funded during World War II were among the first medical experiments ever conducted in which humans were used in test and control groups to determine, with some degree of statistical confidence, which drugs and procedures were causing what reactions in the client population. Before advances in biochemistry made it possible to isolate and monitor drug doses in trials, it made little sense to conduct large-scale experiments. But rising levels of sophistication in this area, together with the pressing demands of a war (developing treatments for dysentery and malaria, for example, were very high priorities for the military), combined to make such experimentation both possible and necessary.

At that time, attitudes about the ethics of human experimentation were lax, partly because such experiments were so novel, partly because they were considered matters of national security, and partly because so much success seemed to be in the offing. A utilitarian calculus dominated in this environment: Ethical transgressions (if they were even thought of as such) committed in the development of new drugs and therapies through human experimentation were dismissed as inconsequential when compared to the potential benefits of such experiments.

Consequently, all manner of clinical tests were done on large groups of usually unsuspecting subjects without their consent during the 1940s. Orphanages, asylums, and prisons were typically chosen for these trials, as the consideration of ethical dilemmas raised by such experiments were suffused by the expediency of war and the promise of great results. It was almost as if the acquiescence of individuals in these locations was expected as an obligation of citizenship since they were not contributing to the war effort otherwise.

Even after the war years, however, when the national-security argument began to fade and when human experimentation was no longer so novel, researchers continued to play fast and loose with the ethics of their medical experiments on humans. Emboldened by their wartime triumphs over smallpox, typhoid, tetanus, and yellow fever, clinical researchers forged ahead under the old "expedience of war" rules, numb to the ethical objections that could be raised over experimenting on unwitting humans. As Rothman (1991, p. 79) puts it, a "license granted is not easily revoked," and so researchers pressed on in the late 1940s and through the 1950s as if they had an ethical carte blanche.

The 1960s. The era of the laissez-faire laboratory (Rothman, 1991, p. 51) continued into the first years of the 1960s. Early in that decade, Dr. Louis Welt of the University of North Carolina Medical School surveyed eighty university departments regarding their practices and guidelines for human experimentation. Only eight of the sixty-six responding departments had documented their guidelines, and only twenty-four departments (less than half) had or favored the creation of review committees. In another study of fifty-two departments of medicine, only nine had formal procedures for approving research involving human subjects, and only five others indicated that they favored the creation of such procedures. Presumably, the remaining departments were either ambivalent about research protocols or rejected the notion outright. The Welt study concluded that the research community had "a general skepticism toward the development of ethical guidelines, codes, or sets of procedures concerning the conduct of research" (cited in Rothman, 1991, p. 60).

This same rationale seemed to be at work in most major research hospitals during the 1960s, including the flagship institution of the NIH—the Clinical Research Center (CRC). The CRC, a 500-bed, state-of-the-art research hospital in Bethesda, Maryland, was opened by the NIH in 1953. Patients were admitted as research subjects in the formal studies conducted at the institute. But as Rothman (1991, p. 54) states, "The NIH, at least before 1965, never put the matter quite so boldly." Instead, bland and reassuring statements about the importance of patient welfare were offered. The CRC had no formal protocols designed to ensure that the patients' best interests would not be sacrificed to the researchers' own agendas. Indeed, the prospect that the well-being of humanity (the ends) and the well-being of the patient (the means) might often diverge was never officially broached by the research clinicians of the institute.

Not surprisingly, given this environment of ethical neglect, the CRC had no rigorous informed-consent requirements. Instead, the degree to which test procedures, potential benefits and risks, side effects, and possible complications were explained to patients was left entirely up to the discretion of individual researchers. Nor were researchers obliged to consult with their colleagues about the degree to which their experiments comported with ethical standards (as if there were any, beyond the individual conscience of the researcher involved).[16]

Beyond allowing the CRC researchers to create, essentially without oversight, their own experimental protocols, the NIH also allowed those receiving external grants wide discretion. Indeed, grant recipients were not even required to have or report any procedures or guidelines governing the conduct of human-based research at the time of the Beecher article. By 1965, the NIH was the single most important source of research grants for universities and medical schools in the world, supporting over 1,500 projects worth well over $1 billion. Yet, there was no stipulation that these research projects be carried out with even a modicum of sensitivity to the ethical dilemmas that human experimentation posed (Rothman, 1991, p. 59). Then came the Beecher exposé, which shined a glaring light on these researchers and their practices for the first time. And all of a sudden, the gilded age of research no longer seemed so golden.

The Beecher Indictment. Beecher's article cited a series of cases in which human experimentation created, in his opinion, ethical problems of the first order. He wrote of one study in which penicillin was purposely withheld from servicemen so that alternative means of combatting streptococcal infection could be tested. None of the men in this experiment knew this, nor were they aware that their condition could deteriorate into rheumatic fever without treatment by penicillin. In the end, twenty-five men actually did contract this secondary disease.

In another example, live hepatitis viruses were fed to residents of a state institution for the mentally retarded in order to study the progression of the disease under "controlled" conditions. Elsewhere, physicians injected twenty-two elderly patients with cancerous cells to study the body's immunological response. Newborns were the subject of another study. Here, researchers inserted catheters into the bladders of twenty-six babies less than forty-eight hours old, apparently without the consent of the parents, then took a series of X rays to study the function of the bladder as it filled and voided.

The research protocols questioned by Beecher were not unearthed as part of some elaborate, undercover investigation. Instead, the projects he questioned were discussed in published medical research literature, a fact that suggests the researchers thought they were operating well within the realm of standard and acceptable practice when they conducted and reported their work. This becomes even more clear in the unabashed reaction of other medical professionals to Beecher's article. One of his own colleagues at Harvard was moved to write a scathing rebuttal in response to Beecher's suggestion that informed consent be required before human experimentation is conducted. The colleague wrote: "Should informed consent be required? No! For the simple reason that it is not possible. ... Any teaching and research hospital must clearly identify itself as such ... to the patient upon admission. ... The fact that the patient is requesting admission to this hospital represents tacit consent" (cited in Rothman, 1991, p. 91).[17]

Others took a position with less of an edge but still disagreed with Beecher, using the old utilitarian calculus of "the greatest good for the greatest number." It was well understood in the research community that true informed consent would be difficult to extract. In the case of the mentally disabled, questions were raised about whether informed consent was even possible. In the case of the mentally healthy, it was assumed that only those with dire illnesses would subject themselves to experimentation and then only if the procedure offered some hope for alleviating their specific conditions. Mainstream medical researchers claimed that, if the CMR successes of the war years were any guide, a great deal of good could (and had) come from human experimentation. "Even if a few lives were sacrificed along the way, humanity would be better for it in the long run" seems to be a fair representation of the prevailing ethos.

The Beecher article and other stories about the lack of ethical guidelines in human experimentation had a tremendous impact on attitudes in the nonmedical community at the time, but medical researchers just did not seem to get it. They had became experimental junkies in over two decades of experimentation, essentially unencumbered by ethical considerations. But the public was no longer so quick to grant medical researchers the benefit of the doubt. Amid the widespread rejection of the establishment that was expressed in the tumultuous 1960s, Americans began to call medical researchers into question. The Beecher article and others that followed were picked up quickly by the popular press, and they had the effect that might be anticipated—sparking the same kind and degree of outrage that followed the publication of *The Jungle, Silent Spring,* and *Unsafe at Any Speed.*[18]

According to David Rothman (1991, p. 72), "Beecher's article was a devastating indictment of research ethics [that] helped inspire the movement that brought a new set of rules and a new set of players to the medical decision making table." Some of that change was instituted from the top down, as a wounded NIH scrambled to limit the political damage from Beecher's charges by proposing sweeping new regulations on the documentation of informed consent and peer review of ethical protocols. The FDA then got into the act, issuing strict new regulations regarding patient consent in clinical drug trials (Rothman, 1991, p. 93).

Perhaps more important than these top-down reforms was the sea change in attitudes taking place in the United States from the bottom up. The political culture began running counter to the research culture in that decade of social unrest. A loss of trust in discretionary authority in all its manifestations—religion, education, family, and workplace—spilled over to affect the medical community, and things have never been quite the same.[19]

The Funeral Business. It was no coincidence that the 1960s was also the decade during which criticism of the funeral trade began to foment. Two books published in 1963—*The American Way of Death* and *The High Cost of Dying*—were to funeral directors what Beecher's article was to medical researchers. The funeral director, once one of the community's more staid and respected citizens, now became the subject of suspicion and skepticism as potential conflicts of interest were laid bare alongside real-life cases of overcharging and misrepresentation. The situation deteriorated so quickly that the National Funeral Directors Association began a program of damage control, pushing its own enhanced standards of professional conduct on the membership along the way.

Meanwhile, memorial societies began to flourish as the public's disenchantment with funeral directors grew. These new kinds of organizations offered members low-cost body-disposal services by negotiating with mortuaries and crematoriums on a volume basis, thereby effectively cutting out the funeral director altogether. Ultimately, the Federal Trade Commission (FTC) issued its Trade Regulation Rule on Funeral Industry Practices in 1984, based largely on a 1979 study conducted for the FTC. These new federal guidelines set rules regarding pricing, options, and decisions on what was legally required in the disposition of a body.

Informed consent, especially with regard to embalming (which in many states is not required by law) was also a part of what became known in the trade and elsewhere as the "Funeral Rule" (DeSpelder and Strickland, 1992, p. 207). To be sure, the wheels of government turned slowly: Twenty years had passed since *The American Way of Death* and *The High Cost of Dying* were published. But public attitudes and behaviors, as evidenced by the interest in memorial societies, had begun to change almost overnight, as did other attitudes about "business as usual" in the 1960s, those important and formative years of the consumer rights movement.

The 1970s. More research scandals surfaced as the 1960s melted into the 1970s. Things came to something of a head in 1974 when Senator Walter Mondale (D-Minnesota) began conducting a series of congressional hearings under the aegis of a newly formed National Commission for the Protection of Human Subjects of Biomedical and Behavioral Research. Mondale had been trying for years to convene such a committee but did not have the support to do so until the press, on an anonymous tip from a Public Health Service (PHS) researcher, revealed the details of a decades-long study of blacks suffering from secondary syphilis in Macon County, Alabama.

PHS researchers had been traveling to rural Alabama regularly to study the progression of syphilis in the study group there, but they refused to provide any of those afflicted with penicillin, the standard treatment. During the Vietnam War, Health Service officials went so far as to instruct draft boards not to conscript these individuals, fearing they might receive treatment in the service. The PHS defended its actions (or inactions) by arguing that, with the advent of antibiotics, it would never again be possible to study the long-term, untreated effects of syphilis. But the public was outraged, and with support from Senators Hubert Humphrey, Jacob Javits, and Edward Kennedy, Mondale's committee was finally set up, and it began to hold hearings.

The more hearings the committee held, the more scandals were uncovered. There were stories about how diethylstilbestrol (DES, used specifically to prevent miscarriages) and Depo-Provera (used to treat advanced uterine cancer and endometriosis) were approved by the FDA, then prescribed as contraceptives despite evidence to suggest that both were carcinogens. There were stories about Mexican-American women who had gone to a San Antonio, Texas, clinic for contraceptives and unwittingly become part of a study to determine whether side effects of the contraceptive were physiological or psychological. Half the women were given placebos as part of a control group, and several promptly became pregnant (Rothman, 1991, p. 185).

Senators also heard the story of a University of Cincinnati General Hospital study, done in conjunction with the Department of Defense over the course of fifteen years, in which radiation was applied to patients with terminal cancer. The hospital claimed that consent had been granted, but administrators were never able to produce any documentation. Even more troubling, there seemed to be a clear demographic bias in the manner in which the hospital chose those who would be "treated": The test group primarily consisted of indigent African-Americans with only grade-school educations. The committee also took testimony regarding a slew of stories about pharmaceutical companies that relied almost entirely on prisoners—recruited for as little as a dollar a day—for testing new drugs, without the FDA's knowledge (see Mitford, 1973).

These stories all augmented the public's distrust of medical researchers and medical people in general that had begun building in the 1960s. Never again would the doctor be viewed in the same light as every aspect of the medical profession became the subject of suspicion by wary consumers. Medical research abuse had become a flash point for a much larger explosion of interest in the general population regarding health-care rights and wrongs. To be sure, regulatory responses with any bite to them tended to lag well behind the exposés that originally sparked active interest and outrage. But changes did come, largely as a result of the mass agitation provoked by the considerable publicity on professional ethics (or lack thereof) that the scholarly and popular presses provided.

Summary: The Rights Culture and Changing Roles in Health-Care Decisionmaking

The emergence of a rights culture in the United States has caused consumers to question the relationship between patients and their health-care providers. In the process, the patient-physician relationship has been transformed from a monologue into a dialogue, if not yet a partnership. Clearly, the increasingly consumerist American culture is a force of the first order in this transformation. The general public pays more attention to health issues today than ever before, and many people are taking it upon themselves to try new, alternative therapies, partly as a result.

Women in particular have become more aggressive in advancing the right to model treatment decisions and protocols to their own needs and preferences. And they are key to this whole transformation for another reason. Studies show that, overwhelmingly, women rather than men assume responsibility for the health of their offspring. Consequently, as women become more empowered in health-care issues, it is likely that more of an activist orientation will be passed down to the next generation.

The power of the press is a force of activism to be reckoned with, as well, as scandals that foster skepticism within the general population continued to be exposed. No profession, not even the medical profession, can withstand the steady assault of such negative exposure without losing credibility in the process. Power has begun to slip away from physicians, leaving patients in a stronger position to control their own medical destinies as a result. Ultimately, as individuals ask for and get more control over their own health care throughout life, it seems inevitable that they will do the same when it comes time to die. We turn now to a discussion of developments along these lines, in which a specific interest in an agreeable death is beginning to overcome the denial of death that otherwise prevails.

6
Social Activism and the Happy-Death Movement

THERE EXISTS in the United States a collection of interests that coalesce around the idea that death can be a tolerable and maybe even a happy affair. Taken together, groups that advance death with dignity, natural death, and the right to die form what Lofland (1978) calls the "happy-death movement."[1] Whatever the nomenclature, there can be little doubt that, during the last few decades, there has been a rush of activity to construct a new culture of death in the United States (Lofland, 1978, p. 16).

Happy-death activism is suggested by the burgeoning body of academic literature on death. Fears about nuclear technology, concerns about the rights of individuals, and grass-roots organizations also provide robust manifestations of the happy-death movement. Each area will be covered in turn before turning to the topic of assisted suicide, one area where some members of the happy-death movement are blazing a new trail of activism. The chapter concludes with a discussion of this topic, which is just now edging its way onto the public policy agenda.

Ivory-Tower Developments

The academic founding of the happy-death movement can be traced to the 1950s. The first pebble to cast a noticeable ripple may well have been Joseph Fletcher's 1954 publication of *Morals and Medicine*. Fletcher, a Protestant minister and professor of theology and medical ethics, broached the subject of "good death" and patient autonomy when very few writers were dealing squarely with such things.[2] Two years later, Geoffrey Gorer published his seminal work, "The Pornography of Death." This article's title reflects the author's observation that death and pornography seem to have a parallel status in Western cultures: Neither is spoken of explicitly in proper social settings. The Gorer essay was an important piece of thinking that would often be cited and referred to in the work of others who followed.

The third important work of that decade—Herman Feifel's *The Meaning of Death*, published in 1959—is more often described as the founding document of the academic turn toward death. Indeed, this work was so novel that it met with substantial resistance, so much so that thirty years later, Feifel would still be writing about its reception. "What I was up against," he says, "was [a] personal position, bolstered by cultural structuring, that death is a dark symbol not to be stirred—not even touched—an obscenity [borrowing here from Gorer's thrust] to be avoided" (in DeSpelder and Strickland, 1992, pp. 7–8). Despite the chilly reception some gave Feifel's book at first, however, many now look to his volume as the truly seminal work on death and dying of this age. A surge in the publication of works dealing with death and dying seems to bear out this conclusion.

More books were written on death in the 5 years following the release of Feifel's treatise than in the 100 years prior to its publication, and the number of death-related publications expanded from a mere handful to some 400 references in 1964. The next 10 years saw that list grow tenfold, to the point where over 4,000 books and articles on death could be itemized (DeSpelder and Strickland, 1992, p. 9) by the early 1970s. Interest in the subject shows no sign of slackening; another 5,500 new books and journal articles appeared through the 1980s.

The number of college courses on death and dying shows a steady rise, as well, though their appearance and growth have lagged the production of scholarly works. The first courses on the subject began appearing on campuses across the country about a decade after Feifel published *The Meaning of Death*. But growth has been substantial since then, with the number of death-related college courses swelling to over 2,000 by 1987.[3]

Part of this surge in curricular interest can be attributed to Elisabeth Kübler-Ross, who, with her popular *On Death and Dying* (1969), revolutionized understandings and approaches to the subject of death in the clinical setting. The Kübler-Ross thesis—that those who die pass through several distinct emotional stages—has been the subject of a good deal of scholarly and clinical criticism. At the same time, this work put death on the social, cultural, clinical, academic, and political maps for many. Moreover, Kübler-Ross's thesis continues to serve as an academic bench mark, providing others with a context in which to formulate ideas about coping with death.

The year 1969 was also the founding year of the Hastings Institute, a center devoted to discussion and research on biomedical issues, including those associated with the right to die. The Kennedy Institute on Ethics was established the following year at the Georgetown University Medical School for the same purpose. A number of institutes devoted to medical ethics and based on the Hastings and Kennedy Institute models have sprung up since.

More important research on the subject of death took place in the 1970s. Donald Templer (1970) and Avery Weisman (1972) both published important scholarly works that emphasized the American culture of death denial. Ernest Becker advanced the same thesis in 1973 with his often-cited monograph, *The Denial of Death.*[4]

Several academic periodicals focusing on the study of death were launched in the 1970s, as well. Scholarly journals such as *Omega: Journal of Death and Dying* and *Death Studies Journal* gave academics an outlet for publishing their works. Importantly, these journals increased the visibility and legitimacy of scholarly studies about death.

Some academics, especially those with backgrounds in psychology, crossed over into the trade market to sell their death-related works as the 1970s progressed. Some, as David Gutman (1977) noted, focused on "telling us how to compose an aesthetic decomposition—a graceful death." Others, like Raymond Moody's *Life After Life* (1975), went a step further by investigating "near-death experiences" (NDEs)—a phenomenon that some claimed to be evidence of "life" after death. An entirely new subdiscipline of psychology has sprung up in the wake of Moody's work to deal with the emerging body of evidence about the NDE phenomenon. Clinical studies of reincarnation, conducted through hypnotic regression analysis, are also the subject of subdisciplinary attention. Ultimately, this stream of scholarly and quasi-scholarly literature gave rise to a flood of popular, feel-good-about-death articles and books in the 1980s, exposing many to a subject that had been thought of as taboo just twenty-five years before. For the first time in a century, thanks in large part to popular treatments of the subject, a generation of Americans was growing up talking and thinking about death.

Grass-Roots Sentiments

Nuclear Technology

The development of nuclear technology was, of course, one of the most significant scientific achievements of the twentieth century. Nuclear power—used to generate electrical power and, more importantly, to create weapons of mass destruction—is at least partly responsible for Americans' rediscovery of death in the last few decades.

These were the years when the prospect of nuclear war began to hang over the country like a pall of gray smoke. The more the cold war chilled relations among the superpowers and the more weapons of mass destruction were developed and deployed, the more anxiety there was about the prospect of nuclear conflagration. From the eerie bleating of air raid sirens of the 1950s to the residential bomb shelters of the 1960s (stocked with food and, in case things went badly, suicide pills) to the nuclear-freeze movement of the 1980s, the American attempt to reckon with death was evident.

The prospect of death brought on by nuclear power accidents has added to the typical American's appreciation of his or her own mortality. Accidents at Three Mile Island in Pennsylvania and Chernobyl in the former Soviet Union only increased our trepidation. The decade-long struggle to prevent the multibillion-dollar Shoreham nuclear generating plant on Long Island, New York, from becoming operative was another manifestation of the way death was being addressed in public policy. Surely, *The China Syndrome,* a popular movie based on the prospect of a nuclear meltdown, added its own measure of impetus, as well. In a way, nuclear technology—no longer accepted as good by definition—was bringing the concept of death squarely before the public. This brought death out of the closet and made it more likely that Americans would talk and think about the end of life.

Individuals Bring Their Cases to Court

In terms of sources for the growing interest in death-related topics, concern about nuclear technology began to be eclipsed in 1976 by a more focused interest in legal cases involving right-to-die requests. The United States is an extraordinarily litigious society, much more so than its European counterparts[5] and much more so than it was just a few decades ago.[6] And this litigiousness has led to a number of well-publicized, landmark court cases that have, in turn, forced many Americans to confront the issue of the right to die specifically for the first time.

To be sure, only a small percentage of rights cases brought to the courts in the last quarter century have had right-to-die dimensions. But the importance of court cases is not measured by their number but by their impact. Landmark court cases—like media exposés (a la Beecher) and academic milestones (a la Feifel)—adhere to the aphorism *qualis non quantis* ("quality, not quantity"). It is not the number of exposés, milestones, or landmark cases that make the difference so much as their subject matter, their timing, the issues raised, and the resonance those issues have with society as a whole.

It is with this in mind that we turn to the 1976 case of Karen Ann Quinlan. The *Quinlan* case is but one of the many thousands of rights-based cases brought to the bench in the last few decades. But it was Quinlan's predicament, reported in all its detail, that touched a raw nerve: "There but for the grace of God go I" (or for parents, maybe even more poignantly, "There but for the grace of God goes my child"). As such, the *Quinlan* case proved to be a legal turning point, the defining moment of the entire right-to-die debate. Activism has ebbed and flowed ever since, but interest has never dropped below the point where it was prior to 1976. The Quinlan story is the font from which a torrent of popular interest and legal precedents have sprung and will continue to spring, it seems, for the foreseeable future.

Karen Ann Quinlan. It was never entirely clear what had happened to Karen Ann Quinlan when, on April 15, 1975, this seventeen-year-old girl was admitted to St. Clair's Hospital in Denville, New Jersey, after lapsing into a coma. Quinlan had collapsed at a party that night; apparently, a combination of drugs and alcohol taken on an empty stomach had a synergistic and depressing effect on her metabolism, causing her breathing to stop for at least two separate periods of approximately fifteen minutes each. Her condition deteriorated even further after hospitalization, to the point where all examining physicians agreed she had suffered irreversible damage and was now in a persistent vegetative state, without hope of recovery.

After their daughter spent several months in this condition, Karen's parents, Joseph and Julia Quinlan, both practicing Catholics, consulted a Roman Catholic priest, who informed them that they had no moral obligation to continue "extraordinary" means to sustain life when there was no realistic hope for recovery (Worsnop, 1992, p. 155). In this context, "extraordinary means" was taken to refer only to the artificial respirator that enabled Karen to breathe but not the tube that provided her with nutrition and hydration through an incision in her stomach.

Caregivers at the Catholic hospital at first agreed to abide by the family's request to have the respirator removed and even had the parents sign a consent form to that effect. However, the family soon got a call from the primary-care physician, who said his second thoughts and moral concerns made it impossible for him to fulfill their wishes. The hospital backed up the physician's decision, arguing that by any standard, including the Harvard brain-death criteria, Karen was still alive. Given all this, the hospital feared that "pulling the plug" on her respirator would violate the Hippocratic "do-no-harm" principle, thereby exposing the institution (and its employees) to tort liability.

Feeling strongly about their decision, the Quinlans took their case to court. Meanwhile, unbeknownst to the family, medical personnel at the hospital who objected to the Quinlans' position proceeded to wean Karen from her respirator so that if the court decided to allow withdrawal, she would have a chance to breathe on her own. In the end, the New Jersey Supreme Court sided with the Quinlans and ordered the hospital to abide by the parents' wishes that the ventilator be withdrawn, which the hospital did (see Chapter 7 for the legal analysis). By that time, however, Karen had effectively been weaned to the point where she no longer needed a mechanical respirator, essentially rendering the court decision irrelevant.

Still in a hopelessly irreversible coma, Karen Quinlan lived, with artificially provided nutrition and hydration, for another eight years. Her parents wrote, "We understand that, conceivably, all treatment of Karen Ann is extraordinary ... , however, we personally have moral problems with our conscience, with regard to the food and antibiotics" (cited in President's Commission, 1983, p. 192). Adhering to their own moral principles and probably affected by the church's view of artificial nutrition and hydration at the time (that they should be provided in almost every case), the Quinlans never budged on the question of food: Their daughter received ANH throughout her hospitalization. There was some acquiescence on the antibiotics issue, however, for Karen Quinlan finally died in June 1985 from acute pneumonia. Antibiotics that would have fought the pneumonia were not given.

After reviewing the Quinlan story, authors of the President's Commission report on Denial of Life-Sustaining Treatment commented that it was amazing that no similar cases had been brought to court before *Quinlan,* given that these issues had been arising in American hospitals for years.[7] Michael Halberstam, a practicing physician and author of an op-ed piece in the *New York Times,* also expressed amazement, writing that he was surprised the case "is in court at all. Each day, hundreds, perhaps thousands, of similar dilemmas present themselves. ... The decisions are difficult, often agonizing, but they are reached in hospital corridors and in waiting rooms, not courts." The *Quinlan* case, he argued, "represents a failure of the usual—often unspoken, deliberately ambiguous—steps in caring for such a patient" (cited in Rothman, 1991, p. 228).

Apparently, however, given the outburst of right-to-die activism across the states that followed in the wake of publicity about the *Quinlan* case, the unresolved conflicts that were central to the plight of Karen Ann Quinlan were more common than this physician would seem to suggest. Before 1976, right-to-die legislation had been introduced in only five states, and each of the five measures had been defeated. But within one year after the Quinlan story first got national coverage, legislators in thirty-eight states had introduced sixty-seven different pieces of legislation to deal with what they perceived as unresolved or improperly resolved end-of-life treatment conflicts. Eight of these bills were signed into law (in California, Arkansas, Idaho, Nevada, New Mexico, North Carolina, Oregon, and Texas), although the formidable forces of restraint effectively washed the other bills aside for the time. Still, the record of legislative activity—even unsuccessful activity—speaks for itself.

There was evidence of activism outside the statehouses, as well. In the six years prior to *Quinlan,* the Euthanasia Education Council reported having distributed only 750,000 copies of their model living will. But in the eighteen months afterward, they disseminated 1.25 million copies, a nearly tenfold increase in the annual rate of distribution.

The importance of *Quinlan* also is reflected in the amount of interest generated in the scholarly and popular literature of the period. A survey of guides to the medical literature reveals that pre-*Quinlan*, about 6 articles per year were being published on the right to die. But in 1976, the year the *Quinlan* decision was handed down, over 60 scholarly medical articles were published.[8] Legal articles in medical literature were nearly nonexistent before 1975, but the publication rate for scholarly works of a legal nature jumped to an average of 15 per year beginning in 1976. (More recently, the pace has surged to an average of nearly 40 articles per year.) Publication rates in the theological journals also billowed about the time the *Quinlan* decision was delivered, growing from less than 4 right-to-die articles per year to about 22 per year after the New Jersey court issued its landmark decision (two-thirds of these articles were in Catholic journals).

Attention in the mainstream press, as measured by the number of articles appearing on the right to die in the *New York Times*, began its first noticeable rise from a steady state of about 5 articles per year with the publication of 25 articles in 1973. Coverage spiked even more sharply in the *Quinlan* year of 1976, however, when over 100 articles found their way into print.[9]

Quinlan also touched off a spate of court cases. Although court activity prior to *Quinlan* was minimal, there have been over 100 important cases of a right-to-die nature heard in state superior courts in the decade and a half since then. In essence, *Quinlan* stands out as the first right-to-die case of any moment heard by a state superior court in which the court freely injected itself into the sacrosanct doctor-patient relationship as an arbiter of rights and wrongs. The court argued, in ground-breaking fashion, that the *Quinlan* case raised questions that transcended the medical hegemony that had traditionally existed. And in the process, the case personalized the players (even the court referred to Quinlan by her first name in its decision) to the point where medical decisions about life and death began to be considered regular family affairs in legal circles and elsewhere for the first time.[10]

Nancy Cruzan. The case of Nancy Cruzan provides a point of reference for determining how far the right to die had come since the *Quinlan* decision. In addition (and more importantly for our present purposes), the Cruzan story is probably second only to Karen Quinlan's in the degree of media coverage and notoriety it received. As such, it has triggered a secondary wave of activism in the general population, as well as in the courts and the state legislatures.

Early on the morning of January 11, 1983, news reached the Cruzan household that twenty-five-year-old Nancy Cruzan had been involved in an accident. She had lost control of her Nash Rambler on a rural Missouri road late at night and was thrown thirty-five feet beyond her overturned vehicle. Paramedics estimated that Cruzan's brain had been deprived of oxygen for at least fifteen to twenty minutes before they were able to resuscitate her. As a result, although she survived, she was left with irreparable brain damage. Doctors diagnosed her as being in a persistent vegetative state and explained to the family that she could continue to live—with a surgically implanted tube to provide nutrition and hydration—indefinitely, even though her chances of returning to a normal life were virtually nonexistent.

Daily, the once-vibrant Nancy Cruzan became less and less recognizable to members of her family. Her body bloated from tube feeding, and her hands began to curl into gnarled claws from lack of use. Cruzan's spine appeared to round out, and her legs drew up until her body began to assume something of a fetal position. Her sister was moved to say that she "didn't know such life existed" ("The Death of Nancy Cruzan," 1992): It was a life, members of the family came to believe, not worth continuing.

Even though Nancy Cruzan had not left any written instructions about what care she would or would not want under such circumstances, her parents felt very strongly that their daughter would choose not to continue in her present state. Consequently, after five years of tube feeding and physical deterioration and with medical bills of approximately $130,000 per year, her family requested that nourishment and hydration be terminated.

Early in 1988, Judge Charles E. Teel, presiding over the Probate Division courtroom in Jaspar County, Missouri, agreed with the Cruzans and granted their request. But this decision immediately touched off a heated debate over whether the removal of Nancy's feeding tube would simply honor a patient's wishes under "informed consent" or constitute criminal homicide. Appeals of Judge Teel's decision were immediately filed by the state, and, ultimately, the case was moved from the Jaspar County courthouse to Missouri's highest court.

In November 1988, the Missouri Supreme Court refused the Cruzans' petition to make decisions on Nancy's behalf. The court argued that the family's quality-of-life arguments did not carry as much weight as the state's interest in the sanctity of life. Because Nancy's exact wishes were unknown and never would be clear, the court concluded that health-care professionals should stay the course by continuing to maintain her existence.

The family appealed this decision to the U.S. Supreme Court, which, in June 1990, issued a decision that recognized the existence of a right to die, but qualified that finding by arguing that it was entirely appropriate for the states to set "reasonable" standards to guide the exercise of that right (see Chapter 7 for more regarding the legal analysis). The state of Missouri was asking that "clear and convincing evidence" of a patient's wishes be produced before allowing the Cruzans' wishes to be honored. Consequently, since the Cruzans had failed to satisfy the strict evidentiary standard set by Missouri, the U.S. Supreme Court sided with the state and remanded the case back to Missouri.

In November 1990, the Cruzan case was back in the lap of Judge Teel in the Probate Division courtroom in Carthage, Missouri, where more testimony was heard. After learning of Nancy's plight and the decisions of the Supreme Court, several of her friends came forward to testify about conversations they had remembered having with Nancy regarding her preferences in matters such as this. Even her doctor, James Davis, originally against removing Nancy's feeding tube, had begun to acquiesce. When asked by Cruzan's court-appointed guardian if it was in her interest to continue in a PVS, Davis conceded, "No, sir, I think it personally would be a living hell" (cited in Malcolm, 1990b). On December 14, with the weight of this new testimony now hanging in the balance, the Jaspar County Court ruled that there was, indeed, sufficient evidence that Nancy would not wish to be kept alive while hopelessly ill.

The next day, the surgically implanted feeding tube that had sustained Nancy Cruzan for nearly eight years was removed, and her eleven-day journey toward death began; Cruzan would be allowed to die, but no one could aid her in that death. Family members kept the vigil and watched as she slowly died of dehydration. Nancy's lips dried and blistered. Her tongue grew sticky and swollen, and her eye lids dried and began to stick shut. Toward the end, her breathing grew more labored and raspy with every lung-parching breath of dry hospital air she took. Death finally came to Nancy Cruzan, with her family at her side, on the day after Christmas in 1990; she was thirty-three. Earlier, Nancy's parents had issued a statement expressing their hope that "hundreds of thousands of people can rest free knowing that when death beckons, they can meet it face to face with dignity, free from the fear of unwanted and useless medical treatment. [We] think this is quite an accomplishment [for Nancy] ... and [we're] damn proud of her" ("The Death of Nancy Cruzan," 1992).

It is more difficult to gauge the impact of the Cruzan story than the *Quinlan* case. There was extensive newspaper and magazine coverage of the Cruzan situation, and a special, two-hour edition of the PBS program "Frontline" covered the story from beginning to end. But interest in the right to die was already increasing when the Cruzan story first broke, and the litigation spanned several years, making it difficult to sort out the influence of the case itself. Maybe it is enough to note that *Cruzan* got prime-time, front-page coverage almost as a matter of course—a marked contrast to the situation a dozen years earlier when a doctor had told the New Jersey justices that he was surprised the *Quinlan* case was even a matter of public interest.

One can also point to the activities of Missouri's John Danforth, the U.S. senator who introduced, held hearings on, and almost single-handedly pushed through the Patient Self-Determination Act.[11] Danforth, a Protestant minister in addition to being a senator, described the plight of the Cruzan family specifically as the primary reason for his own efforts on this front (Danforth, 1992). That the act is attributable, at least in part, to the *Cruzan* case is important for the PSDA will be playing a prominent role as a source of activism in the right-to-die debate for years to come.[12]

Christine Busalacchi. On May 29, 1987, seventeen-year-old Christine Busalacchi was the victim of a serious car accident. Then a junior in a suburban St. Louis high school, she was left in critical condition as a result. A week later, her father granted consent for doctors to perform a necessary craniotomy, which removed a section of the right frontal lobe of her brain in an effort to save her life. At the same time, a feeding tube was inserted into Busalacchi's stomach to "give her a chance for recovery" ("Another Right-to-Die Case," 1991).

But the damage was more serious than first suspected, and Christine's condition deteriorated to the point where she was no longer able to respond to verbal or visual stimuli ("Another Right-to-Die Case," 1991). In a letter written in October 1990 by Dr. Catalino Daroy, Busalacchi's attending physician, she was described as existing "in generally a persistent vegetative state, although her cognitive function seems to be at a higher level than some other patients classified as such." In another letter several days later, Dr. Daroy wrote, "she does not verbalize and does not follow commands to move her limbs" (cited in "Another Right-to-Die Case," 1991). Sustained on artificial nutrition and hydration at the Midtown Rehabilitation Center in St. Louis, Christine was given a "one-in-a-billion" chance for recovery by some of the doctors.

Christine's father, Peter Busalacchi, considered the prognosis to be hopeless and requested that artificially provided food and fluid be withdrawn from his daughter. After doctors refused, he sought to move her from Missouri to a medical facility in Minnesota, a state that gives family members much greater discretion regarding end-of-life decisionmaking.[13] But administrators at the Missouri institution refused to discharge the patient into her father's custody, and went to court to legitimize their decision.

In December 1990, Judge Scott Sifferman of the Lawrence County Circuit Court issued a ten-day restraining order on behalf of the institution where Christine was being treated, preventing her father from taking actions to move her. Donald Lamkins, the lawyer for the hospital, claimed that, in fact, Christine's prognosis was not as bad as some thought. Further, he accused Mr. Busalacchi of trying to "violate Christine Busalacchi's rights to life under the Missouri and United States' Constitutions" by "terminating her care and treatment" (cited in "Another Right-to-Die Case," 1991).

In January 1991, the case was moved from Lawrence County to the jurisdiction of St. Louis City. At first, Probate Judge Louis Kohn issued another temporary restraining order, but subsequently, he lifted it on January 16, allowing Peter Busalacchi to move Christine if he so desired. The decision was quickly appealed, however, and on January 18, 1991, the Missouri Court of Appeals said that Christine could not be moved until a hospital panel could review the case. In February, the presentation of the Missouri Department of Health's case against Peter Busalacchi began, and a thirteen-minute videotape was released to the local news media, showing an "alert" Christine who was "very much aware of those around her," according to Dr. John R. Bagby, Jr., the state health director ("State Makes Public," 1991). According to Lamkins, this tape provided proof that "Christine was responding well to therapy" ("Missouri Court Rejects," 1991).

At that point, right-to-die issues became intertwined with issues of privacy. Expressing displeasure at the releasing of the tapes without Peter Busalacchi's consent, Robert Trame, one of the lawyers representing him, stated that "they don't have any authority unilaterally to release her medical file." Arthur Caplan, director of the Center for Biomedical Ethics at the University of Minnesota, added that "[it] sounds like a terrible breach of privacy at least in terms of ethics, if not law. The tapes are to document her condition, not to wage their case in the press" ("State Makes Public," 1991). Yet Bagby, the physician who ordered that the tapes be made, claimed his intention was not to use the media as a tool but to update "inaccurate" file clips previously used in television newscasts released by Busalacchi himself, showing Christine in what appeared to be a persistent vegetative state ("State Makes Public," 1991).

In March, as controversy over the tapes subsided, the case turned back to the primary issue of guardianship when the Eastern District Court of Appeals in Missouri issued a 2 to 1 decision rejecting Peter Busalacchi's plea to move Christine. As Judge William H. Crandall, Jr., wrote for the majority, this was "not a right to die case" but one involving a guardian moving a patient out of Missouri. The judge made clear that the court would not tolerate such "forum shopping" in a matter of this great significance ("Missouri Court Rejects," 1991).

In April, the Missouri State Supreme Court agreed to review the case, though the Missouri Health Department continued to maintain that Christine had "recovered from a vegetative state enough that she can be aided by intensive therapy" ("Missouri Justices," 1991). In November 1991, Probate Judge Kohn issued a recommendation to the state supreme court in Peter Busalacchi's favor. He described the situation as a "terrible, terrible dilemma" and concluded that Busalacchi had "the right, the duty, the responsibility to do what's best for this child" ("New Review in Missouri," 1991). The case languished at the state supreme court level until the November 1992 elections when Jay Nixon, a Democrat, was elected to the post of Missouri state attorney general. Nixon's first official act after being sworn in on January 11, 1993, was to ask the state supreme court to dismiss the Busalacchi case. The Missouri court did so without issuing an opinion in the last week of January. That effectively reinstated the trial court decision that had originally affirmed Busalacchi's right to make end-of-life decisions for his daughter (Lewin, 1993).

The story did not end there, however, for three days later, Elizabeth W. McDonald, unrelated to the Busalacchis and a member of a group named Missouri Right to Life, filed a request to be appointed the legal guardian of Christine Busalacchi. With that, Circuit Judge John Kintz issued yet another temporary restraining order that barred Peter Busalacchi from doing what he had intended to do all along: disconnect life-support equipment from his daughter. One week later, however, Judge Kintz dismissed McDonald's petition, arguing that she had no legal standing (reminiscent of New York's *Klein* ruling, discussed in Chapter 5). Within a few weeks of this last decision, Peter Busalacchi directed that life-sustaining treatment be withdrawn from his daughter. Christine, then twenty-three, died of dehydration shortly thereafter.

At one point in the ordeal, Peter Busalacchi, thinking about his daughter and her accident, wondered aloud, "Maybe it would've been best had she died that night" (Gibbs, 1990, p. 62). That certainly would have made for a happier ending to his daughter's life for all parties involved. The statement thus reflects the more general sentiments of an increasing number of Americans regarding the desire for a "happy"—or at least a tolerable—end to life. The *Busalacchi* case is important for other reasons, as well. Although it followed the same sort of tortured legal path as that in *Cruzan* and although both principles had suffered similar fates,[14] the *Busalacchi* case introduced some interesting twists.

First, videotape of the patient was released to the local news media by both parties in the case in an effort to build public support for their respective positions, a move that could not help but widen the audience and increase the level of awareness about the right to die in the general public. Second, the issue of "forum-shopping" was raised, highlighting the disparity in approaches to right-to-die cases in different parts of the country. And third, a popularly elected executive, the Missouri attorney general, took a politically sensitive stand in resolving the *Busalacchi* case in favor of individual rights and happy death, an indication that the happy-death movement may be gaining sympathy among the general population even in conservative Missouri.

Advocacy Groups

The court cases of families requesting the right to die on behalf of their children have precipitated a fair measure of interest in this right. Yet, in a pluralistic society like ours, where it is relatively easy for groups to form and advance their causes, group dynamics have also played an important part in the happy-death movement.

Two kinds of advocacy groups are discussed in this section: those that take a hospice approach to death and those that openly advocate the right to die. Hospice and right-to-die philosophies do not necessarily mix. In a way, they are inimical to each other. Still, the two have one thing in common: They both advocate the acceptance of death. Their differences are really a matter of style and timing.

Hospice and Its Progeny. The hospice philosophy (from the Latin *hospitium*, "hospitality") entails a palliative, nontechnical approach to terminal care that can be traced to Cicely Saunders and her supporters in England during the 1960s. Rooted in the Christian tradition of hospitality toward travelers needing shelter and comfort, Saunders's hospice approach focused on the individuality of the dying person, as opposed to his or her pathology. Saunders emphasized respect for personal needs rather than adherence to institutional routine.

She held that treatment plans should be responsive to the needs, fears, hopes, expectations, and values of the individual, with the family unit serving as the central and natural source of both emotional and physiological support. Her hospice philosophy emphasized caring rather than curing, with medical expertise focused on symptom management and pain relief. Home-based treatments or homelike environments were to be preferred, in which bureaucratic procedures were relaxed and acceptance of death as a natural part of life was encouraged. In this way, the hospice concept is truly reactionary in that it argues for a return to the time, before the middle years of the twentieth century, when care for the terminally ill was provided by family and friends in the home.

The first such program in the United States was set up in 1974 at a site in New Haven, Connecticut. With Elisabeth Kübler-Ross serving as the movement's spiritual leader in the States, the hospice philosophy proliferated rapidly. In 1977, the National Hospice Organization (NHO) was born and shortly thereafter, it began publishing its *Guide to the Nation's Hospices.* By 1983, that guide listed 1,700 organizations serving 100,000 individuals nationwide.

The hospice movement enjoyed a growth spurt of sorts in the 1980s. *The Hospice Journal* began publication in 1983, guaranteeing that those who conducted research and clinical practices in this area would have a scholarly outlet for their work. That same year, hospice care became a potentially reimbursable expense under Medicare, making the hospice option affordable to many who would not otherwise be able to manage such an expense out of pocket. Also, 1983 was the year that the Children's Hospice International, one of the first important hospice-oriented interest groups, got its start as a support network for children, families, and health-care professionals in the United States and abroad. A few years later, in 1986, the Hospice Association of America (HAA) was formed as a lobbying and credentialing organization; it soon began publishing *Hospice Forum,* another symbol and catalyst of academic and professional legitimacy within the happy-death movement.

A number of related organizations to help people cope with death that trace their founding principles to the hospice movement philosophy of caring versus curing also began to pop up in the 1970s and 1980s. Like the hospice movement itself, these related organizations helped to bring death out of the closet and into the light of day, normalizing it and making people more comfortable coping with it in the process. The SHANTI Project of Northern California and the KARA project of Palo Alto, California, have provided volunteer companions for dying patients. Another organization, the Make-A-Wish Foundation, was formed in the early 1980s as a not-for-profit association devoted to granting wishes to children with life-threatening illnesses.

Make-A-Wish got its start in 1980 after an Arizona state police officer kept his promise to Christopher Greicius, a terminally ill boy who wanted a helicopter ride before he died. Not only did the boy get a tour of Phoenix by air, the officers in the unit provided their fan with a helmet, a badge, and an official state policeman's uniform, tailored to fit his small frame. When Christopher died a few weeks later, he was given a full police funeral, with a flag draped over the casket. His grave-stone reads, "Christopher James Greicius, 5-8-72 to 5-3-80, Arizona Trooper." Shortly thereafter, the Christopher Greicius story ran as a feature on "60 Min-utes." Largely due to the publicity garnered from this program, interest surged to the point where there are now over 100 Make-A-Wish chapters nationwide: Over 10,000 wishes have been granted to date. Make-A-Wish, like the hospice move-ment, brings death to light, helps people cope, and breaks down some of the old taboos about death that became such a dominant part of the American culture during the middle third of the twentieth century.

Right-to-Die Advocacy. A number of groups have emerged in the last few de-cades with the expressed intent of providing the grass-roots activism required to advance the right to die as a matter of public policy. This part of the happy-death movement traces its roots back to 1935, the founding year of England's Voluntary Euthanasia Legislation Society.[15] This association—a group of British doctors, Protestant theologians, and prominent intellectuals—was formed to support a bill drafted by an English physician that would have legalized euthanasia in that country. Though the bill was defeated in the House of Lords by a 35 to 14 vote, the British group's advocacy was instrumental as an inspiration to members of the American intelligentsia in New York City, who went on to form the Euthanasia Society of America in 1938.

The American association was no more successful than its British counterpart, however, and interest-group activism ebbed until 1967 when a new organization, Concern for Dying, was formed. Concern for Dying focused on improving the care for and articulating the rights of dying patients. Members also, on occasion, served as family advisers in legal cases and provided *amicus curiae* ("friend of the court") briefs in other related cases. Over the years, Concern for Dying has held education conferences and workshops, provided films and videos for rent, and staffed a speakers' bureau. The organization also supplies living-will forms at the request of individuals or groups (distributing five million copies, to date) and publishes an educational newsletter with information about coping with the problems of caring for terminally ill individuals. Presently, the organization claims to have 250,000 supporters across the nation.

The Foundation of Thanatology, a more clinically based right-to-die advocacy group, was formed in 1967 to improve psychological, social, and medical care for critically ill patients. Two years later, an organization called The Compassionate Friends got its start in England. This self-help group for bereaved parents offers friendship and understanding to other similarly situated individuals in order to promote the positive resolution of grief. It did not take long for the concept to jump the Atlantic, and The Compassionate Friends now claims to have 600 chapters organized in the United States (Kastenbaum and Kastenbaum, 1989, p. 56).

The early 1970s saw the birth of the Euthanasia Education Council (EEC), an organization with goals and tactics very much like those of Concern for Dying. The EEC's day in the sun came shortly after its founding, when it drew up a model living will that was referred to in the syndicated "Dear Abby" advice column. Subsequently, 50,000 readers wrote for copies (Rothman, 1991, p. 239).

A more politically active organization opened for business in 1974 when the Euthanasia Society of America was reactivated and subsequently renamed the Society for the Right to Die.[16] This organization has become one of the most reliable sources of information on issues relating to the right to die in the United States. Unlike the old Euthanasia Society of America, a group that embraced active euthanasia, the new organization limited its advocacy efforts to promoting passive euthanasia—that is, providing terminally ill individuals with the right to be allowed to die. All the while, British branches of Exit—the rejuvenated and renamed chapters of Britain's old Voluntary Euthanasia Legislation Society—were busy advocating the right to die on the eastern side of the Atlantic. The most significant contribution was made by Scotland Exit, which published a thirty-one-page how-to guide to euthanasia in 1979.

The biggest boost for the movement in the United States came with the formation of the Hemlock Society in 1980. Its founder and executive director, Derek Humphry, was the key protagonist. This British-born journalist first became involved in the right to die as a participant in active euthanasia: He helped his first wife, Jean, terminally ill with bone cancer, kill herself in England in 1975. Shortly thereafter, Humphry moved to the United States and started the Hemlock Society in Los Angeles, California, with the help of his second wife, Ann Wickett Humphry.[17]

The Hemlock Society grew steadily through the 1980s and now claims over 57,000 active members in eighty-six local chapters across the States. The goal of these chapters is to "provide a climate of public opinion which is tolerant of the rights of people who are terminally ill to end their own lives in a planned manner" (The National Hemlock Society, 1993). Hemlock issues a quarterly newsletter and has facilitated the publishing of several books that deal with active euthanasia (which Humphry prefers to call "self-deliverance").

The publication list contains three works by Humphry himself. One, *Jean's Way,* traces the story of his wife's euthanasia. It was published by Harper & Row and later was made into a television movie. *Let Me Die Before I Wake,* another of Humphry's books, is a social and legal guidebook to self-deliverance, including exact doses of prescription drugs used in the euthanasia incidents described in the book; over 130,000 copies have been sold. *Final Exit,* the most recent and most popular of the lot, topped the *New York Times* best-seller list for advice books in the summer of 1991, with half a million copies in print at the time and back orders sufficient to warrant a fifth printing. Less than 200 pages long and printed in ex- tra-large type for the benefit of readers with poor eyesight, *Final Exit* is essentially a how-to book on self-deliverance, written specifically with the lay public in mind. It provides tables of suggested drugs, both by trade and generic name, and the recommended lethal dosages.[18]

In the end, the combined effect of all these right-to-die groups and their activi- ties is noteworthy, but it is difficult to say how much real impact they have had. Humphry stands out as the most vocal and well-recognized proponent of the happy-death movement. And *Final Exit* has been the subject of much discussion and brisk sales. Still, it is our reading that these groups and Humphry himself are still viewed as being on the fringe of the happy-death movement, and as such, they do not enjoy widespread credibility in the general population. Individuals who buy *Final Exit*—especially those who take their lives in accordance with its prescriptions—will enlarge the debate in ways that groups like the Hemlock Soci- ety and individuals like Derek Humphry could not hope to do on their own. To date, however, right-to-die organizations have played only a supporting role in a movement that is much less specifically focused than Hemlock and its ilk.

Ebbing Forces of Organized Restraint

Many organizations have taken explicit stands against the right to die, but few have had the impact that the Roman Catholic church has. The National Legal Center for the Medically Dependent and Disabled (NLCMDD) has also played an important role. In addition, various other groups associated with disease research have become sources of policy restraint. Taken together, these groups remain for- midable as forces of restraint, but their influence—especially that of the Catholic church—has been on the wane in recent years.

The Catholic Church. In 1957, Pope Pius XII made a public address before an international group of physicians.[19] In that address, the pope codified the distinc- tion between means of prolonging life for dying patients that were "ordinary" (e.g., according to the pope, food and water, even if artificially provided) and "ex- traordinary" (sometimes referred to as heroic measures—advanced medical tech- nologies that may not provide any long-term benefits to the patient). In his re- marks, the pope advanced the position that extraordinary care might be withdrawn if the patient were in a terminal condition (an important statement of policy in its own right), but he was vehement in his condemnation of the notion that ordinary care might be stopped under the same circumstances.

The ordinary-extraordinary distinction traces back to sixteenth-century Ro- man Catholic moral theology. At the time, the distinction was understood to refer to the potential a medical procedure had for providing some benefit to the patient rather than the nature of a medical procedure itself (Lutz, 1990). According to an author named Banez, writing in 1595, it was reasonable to hold that a human being must act to conserve his or her life by accepting nourishment and medicine and tolerating a level of pain and anguish common to all (Janini, 1958). At the same time, however, one was not bound to endure horrible pain and anguish or undergo extraordinary therapies disproportionate to one's condition. In short, according to the sixteenth-century version of the ordinary-extraordinary distinction, the most sophisticated medical procedures might be deemed ordinary if there is a high level of expectation that it will benefit the patient. At the same time, the simplest procedures can be considered extraordinary—and therefore morally optional—if there is very little indication the patient will benefit from receiving that treatment (Lutz, 1990; President's Commission, 1983).

This is not, however, the way the pope seemed to have read and reported the distinction in his 1957 pronouncement. Instead of adopting the patient-centered, case-based approach common to sixteenth-century understandings, he advanced a treatment-based reading of the ordinary-extraordinary distinction. It was much easier to write in sweeping generalizations, from the pope's perspective: Some treatments can always be considered ordinary, period. But this means taking nothing about the patient's condition into account. Instead, food and water were to be thought of as ordinary treatments, and as such, they should be provided in *almost* every case (even the pope left himself a little leeway here). This position left in its wake a bias in favor of treatment (e.g., always providing food and hydration because that treatment by definition is ordinary) among professionals and patients, Catholics and non-Catholics, alike (Lutz, 1990, p. 31).

In fact, Catholic teachings have always carried a good deal of weight in the United States. For example, the pope's reading of sixteenth-century theology appears time and again in the decisions rendered by state court judges on right-to-die issues through the 1980s. The pope's position also surfaces regularly in the scholarly writings of health-care professionals and medical ethicists (e.g., see Schneiderman and Spragg, 1988). Even the authors of the Presidential Commission on the Denial of Life-Sustaining Treatments saw fit to include the position paper written by the Catholic Conference in the appendix of their report, alongside the statement of the AMA.[20]

Over time, however, the church's position has been mollified, and it has even lost some of its weight in the secular community. Following in the footsteps of the Vatican's 1978 Declaration on Euthanasia, a document that affirms that the dying need not be sustained by "burdensome" life-support systems, the Catholic Conference (Seper, 1980, cited in President's Commission, 1983, pp. 300–307) issued a statement that generally agrees with the basically liberal direction charted by the authors of the Presidential Commission. Although waffling on the nutrition and hydration issue is still in evidence, the language has softened to the point where now it appears the Catholic position is shadowing, rather than leading, opinionmakers in the secular community.[21]

Even when the church leads, it seems to move in a direction that is more tolerant of the right to die than at any time in the recent past. The lobbying effort waged by the Catholic Health Association on behalf of the Patient Self-Determination Act, a bill clearly designed to advance the right-to-die cause, is clear proof of that tendency.[22]

Ultimately, it may be that the Catholic position is simply adapting to the realities of modern medical practice. Artificially provided nutrition and hydration were not even standard medical procedures in 1957 when the pope made his seminal pronouncement on the issue; today, thousands of hopelessly ill individuals are sustained this way for years on end. The church may not be willing to entirely drop its prohibition against withdrawing food and fluids. But whatever resistance remains is becoming increasingly irrelevant for the courts, ethicists, and physicians have broken with the church on that issue. So, too, have some within the church, as the right to die presents just one more in a series of issues (e.g., birth control) on which American Catholic realities do not quite square with Vatican encyclicals. In the end, interest in a happy death has grown as the forces of restraint associated with the Catholic church have ebbed in recent years.

The NLCMDD. The National Legal Center for the Medically Dependent and Disabled has its most profound impact in the legal community. The NLCMDD publishes a respected bimonthly legal journal called *Issues in Law and Medicine*, which is dedicated to clarifying the legal standing and rights of medically dependent and disabled individuals. As such, this journal (which is cosponsored by the Legal Services Corporation) has a decidedly prolife, anti-right-to-die cast to it. The NLCMDD also publishes a litigation manual of over 600 pages, laying out the legal precedents for those who are handling the cases of medically dependent and disabled individuals; the clear intent is to advance the right-to-life position. In addition, the NLCMDD has, on occasion, petitioned state courts as a third-party litigant in right-to-die cases, such as the one involving Sue Ann Lawrence and argued in an Indiana court in 1991.

Since childhood, Sue Ann Lawrence had been a victim of debilitating disorders precipitated by a tumor in her brain. As she got older, her condition progressively worsened. After a 1987 fall from a wheelchair, Lawrence lapsed into a persistent vegetative state. Her father, an Indianapolis dentist, explained that his family had coped "very well" with his daughter's handicaps for more than thirty-two years but that Sue Ann now had no consciousness, no hope of recovery, and "no potential for life, even compromised life" (cited in Lewin, 1991). The Lawrences came to believe that continued existence in this state would not be in the best interest of their daughter. So, after Sue Ann had been in a PVS for a year, the family unanimously decided to request that life support be withdrawn (Lewin, 1991). In May

1991, the Hamilton County Court approved the request by Lawrence's parents to withhold feedings.

This action was quickly challenged by the NLCMDD, which argued that withdrawing artificially provided nutrition and hydration would constitute discrimination against the disabled and that such a course of action would constitute a violation of basic human rights. This was all in accordance with the standard NLCMDD modus operandi, which involved categorizing the PVS patient as disabled, then applying law regarding the rights of the disabled to shield the individual from the actions of others that would lead to his or her demise. The Lawrences agreed to resume feedings until the Indiana Supreme Court could issue a ruling in the matter. Before the case had been decided, however, Sue Ann Lawrence died, on July 18, 1991, at the age of forty-two. At the family's request, Indiana's highest court continued to examine the case.

James Bopp, president of the NLCMDD and, at the same time, general counsel to the Right to Life Committee, argued the standard case before the court. But in September 1991, the Indiana Supreme Court ruled that the family had authority, without judicial intervention, to halt artificial feedings. In the plain language of the majority opinion, Chief Justice Randall T. Shepard wrote, "The law of the state permits the family to decide in consultation with their physicians, that tube feeding of a loved one in a persistent vegetative state should be ended" ("Indiana Court Backs," 1991).

The Lawrences won but not without a fight, and fights can have a chilling effect on those who do not have the stomach to see a long, public, and possibly ugly legal battle waged over what is already a heartrending situation. In that way, the actions of the NLCMDD may have caused some ripples of restraint, and therefore, its efforts in the Lawrence case may not have been in vain. Yet, the impact of groups like the NLCMDD cannot help but ebb as courts all across the country converge on the consensus opinion that individuals and families acting in good faith have the right to forgo life-sustaining treatments.

Other Groups. In addition to the Catholic church and the NLCMDD, we should also note the existence of the many disease lobbies that are organized to support research and treatments for those suffering from various afflictions. Groups associated with cancer, Alzheimer's disease, heart and kidney disease, and a raft of other infirmities push hard for research and treatment funds. Generally speaking, they are not particularly interested in seeing the right-to-die cause advanced since the importance of finding a cure is potentially lessened if those afflicted are granted the right to end their own lives.

The medical lobby is also important as a force of restraint. The American Hospital Association, the American Medical Association, and many of the specialized professional associations all have powerful voices in the debate, voices that typically advance a positive treatment bias when it comes to the right to die. Anesthesiologists, for example, with support from their national professional association, usually decide unilaterally not to honor DNR orders in the operating room. For their part, the AMA and AHA were active in opposing (albeit unsuccessfully), the passage of the Patient Self-Determination Act. More recently, however, the AMA and other professional associations are beginning to change course. Increasingly, attention to informed consent and inclusion of patients in the decision-making matrix is being advocated in professional medical circles.

Senior-citizen groups also add a potentially important voice of restraint. The American Association of Retired Persons (AARP) and other such organizations that claim to represent the interests of seniors have, in the past, pushed hard for more and better care for the elderly, while either opposing or ignoring the right to die. But change seems to be in the air with these groups, as well. Recently, AARP has added the right to die to its issues docket as a cause worth pursuing. And it now puts out a glossy, sixty-four-page publication called *Tomorrow's Choices* in which members are urged to take end-of-life issues—including the right to die—into their own hands by executing legal documents that clearly state their intentions and wishes.

The National Legal Center for the Medically Dependent and Disabled and various right-to-life groups across the country may prove to be the last line of defense; as they continue in their steadfast opposition to the right to die, organized resistance from other quarters seems to be on the wane. The erosion of Catholic resistance and influence is most notable, but, as mentioned, other natural enemies of the right to die seem to be having second thoughts of their own. It seems as if whatever group resistance remains is being slowly but inexorably overwhelmed by the forces of activism, leaving many opportunities for the happy-death movement to spread and flourish.

Assisted Suicide

Interest in assisted suicide—possibly the most dramatic manifestation of the happy-death movement—is the last stop in our survey of policy forces of activism that seem to be percolating from the grass roots up.[23] As previously noted, the Dutch seem to be much more comfortable with the concept of assisted suicide than Americans. Approximately 10 percent of doctors in the Netherlands admit to engaging in euthanasia sometime in their careers, and the populace seems to be in general agreement with the standing policy (Humphry and Wickett, 1986, p. 180).

Those who advocate or practice euthanasia do not enjoy the same level of acceptance in the United States, and nowhere in this country is assisted suicide openly tolerated. (It is patently illegal in only thirty-two states; see Figure 6.1.) But change does seem to be in the offing. The recent assisted-suicide ballot initiatives in Washington (1991) and California (1992) are evidence of that. Even though

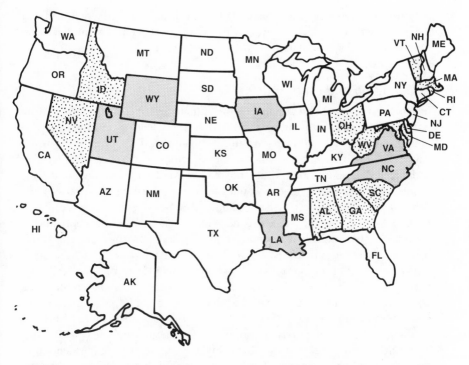

States with statutes that explicitly criminalize assisted suicide: (32 states: Alaska, Arizona, Arkansas, California, Colorado, Connecticut, Delaware, Florida, Hawaii, Illinois, Indiana, Kansas, Maine, Michigan, Minnesota, Mississippi, Missouri, Montana, Nebraska, New Hampshire, New Jersey, New Mexico, New York, North Dakota, Oklahoma, Oregon, Pennsylvania, South Dakota, Tennessee, Texas, Washington, and Wisconsin).

Jurisdictions that criminalize assisted suicide through the common law of crimes (the District of Columbia and 12 states: Alabama, Georgia, Idaho, Kentucky, Maryland, Massachusetts, Nevada, Ohio, Rhode Island, South Carolina, Vermont, and West Virginia).

States in which the law is unclear concerning the legality of assisted suicide (6 states: Iowa[a], Louisiana[b], North Carolina[c], Utah[c], Virginia[a] and Wyoming[c]).

[a]Case law exists that may or may not be applicable to assisted suicide.
[b]State constitution stipulates that "no law shall subject any person to euthanasia."
[c]State has abolished the common law of crimes and therefore does not explicitly prohibit assisted suicide.

FIGURE 6.1 Assisted-suicide laws in the United States. Source: © Choice in Dying, 1993. Reprinted by permission.

both initiatives were rejected, the level of support they received, combined with the related activities of two noteworthy practitioners, suggests that interest in and support for the happy-death movement is on the rise.

Washington and California

In 1991, citizen groups in support of the euthanasia concept circumvented the state legislature in Washington State by successfully placing an assisted-suicide initiative on the ballot: Proposition 119. If it had passed, Proposition 119 would have changed the current law, which carries penalties of up to five years in prison and a fine of up to $10,000 (though no one has ever been prosecuted under this statute). The proposed initiative would have made it legal for physicians to help patients die if they were certified as having six months or less to live. According to the proposition, only the written requests of conscious and competent patients, witnessed by two individuals with no familial connection to the patient and no financial stake in the patient's estate, would be considered valid.

The vote on Proposition 119—what noted bioethicist Arthur Caplan called the most important biomedical event in the United States ("Washington State Voters," 1991)—attracted a great deal of media attention, and divided the religious and medical communities across the state and the nation. Organized labor, the Washington Democratic Party, groups of AIDS advocates, and the Gray Panthers all sided with proponents of 119. Surprisingly, a number of religious denominations also came out in support: The General Assembly of the Church of Christ— the first major religious denomination to accept suicide for the hopelessly ill (Rosenblatt, 1992, p. 347)—endorsed Proposition 119, as did other mainline-to-liberal Protestant churches, including the General Synod of the United Church of Christ (representing 1.6 million members) and the Pacific Northwest Conference of the United Methodist church (Rosenthal, 1991).[24]

Those arrayed against the proposition included the American Medical Association (although some physicians were quite vocal in support of the initiative), antiabortion groups, the Roman Catholic church, and the Southern Baptist Convention. Some antiproposition activists raised the specter of Washington becoming the nation's "fly-and-die" state if Proposition 119 were to pass. Others argued that there were not enough safeguards built into the act. Most importantly, detractors noted the lack of a cooling-off period for those who said they wanted to die and the lack of a requirement for a witness to be present at the time of death. Some were distressed by the fact that the initiative did not spell out any family notification requirements, and others were bothered by the fact that Proposition 119 did not require the individual requesting assisted suicide to undergo a psychological exam.

Then, just a few weeks before the vote, Jack Kevorkian, the retired Michigan pathologist that some have come to know as "Dr. Death," assisted in the double suicide of two patients, in direct contravention of a court order. The cavalier and unrepentant nature of Kevorkian's actions seemed to bolster antiproposition sentiment in the state. Ultimately, even though polls were giving the initiative solid support six weeks before the vote (61 percent in favor, 27 percent opposed, with 12 percent undecided) Proposition 119 went down to defeat on election day by a margin of eight points: 54 percent to 46 percent.

Even in defeat, however, Proposition 119 is both evidence for and a source of activism. The nationwide news coverage of the measure put assisted suicide in the public mind, a first and crucial step toward policy mediation. Pat Nugent, a seventy-one-year-old cancer patient and activist for the Washington proposition, described the impact of Proposition 119 in simple terms: "Grandma's been talking to Grandpa and Grandpa's been talking to the kids and the grandkids. It's been a dinner table topic now like never before" (cited in Gross, 1991).

In 1992, California had its turn in the limelight of this issue with another ballot initiative: Proposition 161. The initiative was coauthored by Robert Risely, whose wife, Darlena, died in his arms after losing a battle with ovarian cancer. On several occasions, Risely had discussed with her what he could or should do to help her die if the pain became unbearable (Reinhold, 1992). In the end, Risely had decided that a law ought to be passed that would guarantee an individual's right to choose death when in a condition like the one his wife had to endure. The requisite number of signatures were gathered, and the California Death with Dignity Act was made an official part of the general-election ballot for 1992.

A now familiar patchwork of groups arrayed themselves on either side of the debate as the vote neared. Much of the support came from grass-roots organizations of individuals who felt as though they had some personal stake in the outcome. In the meantime, the right-to-life groups, most physicians' groups, and the Catholic church once again stood in opposition. The Catholic church went so far as to take up collections to pay for some of the radio and television spots that were part of a $1.4-million advertising campaign waged to fight the initiative. Meanwhile, in a clear manifestation of the deep ambivalence and profound sensitivity of the subject matter, none of the four candidates running for the two U.S. Senate seats open that year chose to take a stand on the issue. In the end, the California initiative failed by the same margin as its sister initiative did in Washington State, with the same, apparently damning criticisms being raised.

These criticisms (e.g., no requirements for cooling-off periods, death witnesses, family notification, or psychological examinations), though substantial, would seem to be relatively easy to address. If, in fact, it was these criticisms that meant the difference between victory and defeat for the two assisted-suicide propositions voted on to date, it is likely that a reformed ballot question, modified to address these perceived flaws, would be relatively easy to fashion and pass. Clearly, general support for assisted suicide in the United States continues to be strong. According to one Gallup poll, conducted in January 1991, 58 percent of those surveyed reported that they supported the right to end life when faced with an incurable disease. That percentage jumped to 66 percent if the dying individual was suffering great pain without hope of relief. And fully 65 percent said yes when asked: "When a person has a disease that cannot be cured, do you think doctors should be allowed by law to end the patient's life by some painless means if the patient and his family request it?" (Worsnop, 1992, p. 157).

Given all this, it will be interesting to see how well the next state—probably Oregon in 1994—does with an assisted-suicide question once again on the ballot. Together, the relatively noncontroversial nature of criticisms leveled at the Washington and California initiatives, the apparently enduring support that Americans have for assisted suicide as a general principle, and the panoply of activism forces currently at work in the nation seem to indicate that physician-assisted suicide will be a legal option in a growing number of states in the not-too-distant future.

Medical Practitioners

There are some in the United States who must observe all this public handwringing about assisted suicide with a sense of bemusement—the doctors who either have assisted patients in dying at some point in their careers or at least have first-hand knowledge of such events occurring in their midst. Indeed, even though thirty-two states have laws that explicitly forbid assisted suicide, it goes on anyway and in every state.

The percentage of physicians who engage in assisted suicide or active euthanasia is difficult to gauge, given the illegal nature of such practices in most places and the professional intolerance of such acts generally. Estimates vary substantially from study to study, but clearly, the number of physicians who have engaged in assisted suicide or active euthanasia (through either passive acquiescence or active participation) is greater than zero—and probably much greater (Rosenblatt, 1992, pp. 18–19, 349; Quill, 1993, p. 22). Indeed, Dr. Alister Brass, writing as the senior editor of the *Journal of the American Medical Association*, declared that euthanasia was practiced by physicians to a "wide extent"—and that was in 1970, nearly twenty-five years ago (cited in Schoenfeld, 1978, p. 52). As Sidney Wanzer and his colleagues (1989, p. 848) note:

> Some physicians, believing it to be the last act in a continuum of care provided for the hopelessly ill patient, do assist [in the suicides of] patients who request it, either by prescribing sleeping pills with knowledge of their intended use or by discussing the required doses and methods of administration with the patient. The frequency with which such actions are undertaken is unknown, but they are certainly not rare.

The case of Dr. Timothy Quill can probably be taken as prototypical, except for one minor detail: Quill wrote about the experience in a public forum and signed his name. Most would not even contemplate such a move.

Dr. Timothy Quill. In March 1991, Dr. Timothy Quill, a forty-one-year-old internist and respected faculty member at the University of Rochester Medical School in upstate New York, publicly revealed his complicity in the suicide of a terminally ill patient. In a letter published in the *New England Journal of Medicine* (the same journal that published Henry Beecher's indictment of medical research ethics twenty-six years before), Quill gave a detailed account of the case of a patient identified only by the pseudonym "Diane."

Quill described Diane as a fighter, someone who had come from an abusive home and struggled successfully to overcome bouts with alcoholism, depression, and vaginal cancer before showing up at his office with complaints of fatigue. These symptoms turned out to be early signs of Diane's next and last challenge: acute myelomonocytic leukemia.

This form of cancer could be treated with chemotherapy and full-body radiation, followed by a bone-marrow transplant. But the success rates for treatment were low (only about 25 percent of those undergoing treatment survived), and treatments themselves would be drawn out and painful. At the same time, the consequences of the "no-treatment" alternative were clear: death in days, weeks, or, at most, a few months (Quill, 1991, pp. 691–692).

After discussing her situation with her husband and college-age son, Diane returned to Dr. Quill and informed him of her desire to forgo treatment. At that time, she expressed her clear preference to live what life she had left outside the hospital, with her family. According to Quill (1991, p. 692), "It became clear that she was convinced she would die during the period of treatment and would suffer unspeakably in the process (from hospitalization, from lack of control over her body, from the side effects of chemotherapy, and from pain and anguish)." In assuring himself of the soundness of her decision-making faculties, Quill requested that Diane repeat her understanding of the process of the treatment she was refusing. After "clarifying a few misunderstandings," Quill concluded that she "had a remarkable grasp of the options and implications."

Quill left the door open for a change of heart on Diane's part while home hospice care was arranged. With every day that passed, however, she seemed more resolved to stick with her decision to refuse treatment, and concern turned more toward making her remaining time as fulfilling and comfortable as possible. Soon, Diane came to Dr. Quill to express a desire that she be allowed to die when her disease advanced to the point where she could no longer maintain her dignity. After assuring himself that she was mentally alert and only after discussing the situation fully with Diane's family, Quill referred her to the Hemlock Society for further information.

A week later, Diane phoned Quill with a request for barbiturates, an essential ingredient in a Hemlock Society suicide, and he asked Diane to come to his office to talk things over. After further discussion, Quill decided to help, reporting that he felt his assistance in the matter would set Diane "free to get the most out of the time she had left." He made sure she knew how to use the barbiturates for sleep and also that she knew the amount needed to commit suicide. He then wrote the prescription "with an uneasy feeling about the boundaries I was exploring: spiritual, legal, professional, and personal" (Quill, 1991, p. 693).

Diane survived for several months more before the pain of the spreading cancer became uncontrollable without the heavy sedation that would lead to the dependency and humiliation she had hoped to avoid. Diane met one more time with Quill, as she had promised she would, so they could say their good-byes. Two days later, on May 19, 1990, Quill received a call from Diane's husband with the news that Diane had died peacefully on the couch that afternoon, after asking to be left alone for an hour. Diane was forty-five.

In March 1991, after Quill disclosed the details of Diane's case, Howard R. Relin, the Monroe County district attorney, announced he would discuss details of the case with the medical examiner and then make a decision about convening a grand jury. The charge Relin was considering was second-degree manslaughter—the intentional assisting of another in the commission of suicide—carrying a penalty of five to fifteen years in New York (Altman, 1991b). At first, Relin decided not to convene the grand jury since there was no physical evidence of the crime. But in June, an anonymous tip to the district attorney's office led investigators to the body of Patricia Diane Trumbill, forty-five, of Pittsford, New York.

After her death, Trumbill's cadaver had been kept at the Monroe Community College for dissection. Autopsy findings revealed that there was a fatal dose of barbiturates in the body and that Trumbill was, indeed, the patient Quill had described. With this new development and because of his belief in the need for a referendum of sorts in this controversial case of medical ethics, Relin took the case to a grand jury. But in July 1991, the grand jury declined to indict Quill on charges suggested by the district attorney.

A few months later, a three-judge panel from the New York State Health Department announced a unanimous decision that "no charge of misconduct was warranted." According to the panel, since Quill himself had not participated directly in the taking of a life, his prescribing of barbiturates was not inappropriate "because he could not know with certainty what use a patient might make of the drugs he has prescribed" (cited in Foderaro, 1991). At the same time, in a seemingly contradictory pronouncement, the State Medical Society of New York reaffirmed its policy, stating, "The use of euthanasia is not in the province of the physician" (cited in Altman, 1991b).

The AMA was more confrontational in asserting its qualms about Dr. Quill's conduct, claiming that his actions did not fall within the standards of suggested practice. Dr. John Ring, president of the AMA, said, "I have reservations about supplying a patient with medication and instructions as to what the lethal dose is. I think the AMA is pretty clear that for a physician to assist a patient in a suicide is not ethical. We certainly sympathize with Dr. Quill, and more so with the patient. This is a terrible, terrible dilemma" (cited in Roan, 1991).

For his part, Quill defended his decision to publicly admit his role in the case and expressed his hope that "a deeper appreciation of the suffering of dying people is achieved as a result of this process" (cited in Glaberson, 1991). Quill had focused much of his previous work on efforts to increase patient autonomy in medical treatment, and following the publication of his letter, he reported that he had learned from the many accounts relayed to him by others that his story was just the "tip of the iceberg": Many other doctors, it turns out, had faced similar situations and taken similar actions (Altman, 1991a, 1991b).

Later, in an interview following the dismissal of his case, Dr. Quill expressed his belief that it was time to drag the whole right-to-die issue out of the closet, arguing that "the debate needs to go on and be broadened" (cited in Altman, 1991b). The activities of Dr. Jack Kevorkian—a better-known and more aggressive practitioner of assisted suicide—seem tailor-made to do just that.

Dr. Jack Kevorkian. Jack Kevorkian is a licensed medical doctor trained in clinical pathology, although he does not maintain an active practice in the traditional sense. Instead, he has turned his efforts toward advancing acceptance of the practice of assisted suicide.[25] Now in his sixties, he is known popularly as "the suicide doctor" or "Dr. Death." Both titles flow from his complicity in a string of assisted suicides beginning in June 1990, when he used a machine that he fashioned out of readily available materials to assist in the suicide of Janet Adkins, a Portland, Oregon, woman suffering from Alzheimer's disease.

Kevorkian connected Adkins to an intravenous line that fed a harmless saline solution into her arm as she lay in the back of his rusty 1968 Volkswagen van, which was parked in a public campsite north of Detroit. When she was ready, Adkins pressed a button on Kevorkian's contraption (he prefers to call it a "mercitron"). Immediately, the line carrying the innocuous flow of saline was shut off, and another line attached to a bottle of thiopental automatically opened up. This drug, the barbiturate used in executions, caused Adkins to lose consciousness after just a few seconds. A bit later, an automatic timer shunted the deadly contents of a third bottle, filled with potassium chloride, into the IV tube in her arm. Janet Adkins's heart stopped beating about six minutes later (Worsnop, 1992, p. 158). Kevorkian (1991, p. 230) reported that Adkins's last words were, "Thank you, thank you," to which he replied, "Have a nice trip."

In a suicide note released after the incident, Adkins—a former English teacher, mother of three, and a member of the Hemlock Society even prior to her illness—stated that her decision was made "in a normal state of mind and is fully considered. I have Alzheimer's disease and I do not want to let it progress any further. I do not want to put my family or myself through the agony of this terrible disease" (cited in Lewin, 1990).

Shortly thereafter, Richard Thompson, the Oakland County prosecutor, filed a charge of criminal homicide against Kevorkian, a charge that eventually was thrown out on two grounds. First, the judge found there was a lack of evidence of Kevorkian's complicity as a perpetrator of homicide. Second, since Michigan had, at the time, no law that specifically proscribed assisting in a suicide, Kevorkian's actions raised no legal questions on that score. The judge did issue a court order prohibiting Kevorkian from any further use of his suicide machines, though it was unclear what legal weight such an order would carry.

Of the decision, Dr. Marcia Angell, executive director of the *New England Journal of Medicine* (cited in Lewin, 1990), writes:

> I think the whole episode, which certainly had its bizarre aspects, underscored a very real problem, that we now have technical capacity to maintain life past where it has any meaning or pleasure for the person living it. I'm very pleased about the ruling, because whatever you thought of what Dr. Kevorkian did, it certainly wasn't murder. And we in medicine have got to come to better grips with the fact that increasing numbers of our patients will be seeking our assistance in ending their lives.

These sentiments represent something of a minority position, however, for mainstream medical, ethical, and legal opinions have tended to run against the Michigan physician. In the general public, there seems to be some ambiguity: Public-opinion polls indicate that many disapprove of the man, personally, even though they may support what he does.

After seventeen months of inactivity, Kevorkian decided to begin challenging the medical and legal establishments again. His next two "patients" were Sherry Miller, a forty-three-year-old victim of multiple sclerosis and Marjorie Wantz, a fifty-eight-year-old woman suffering from chronic, uncontrolled pelvic pain. Miller and Wantz agreed to commit suicide on the same day, October 23, 1991, two weeks before the vote on Washington's Proposition 119.

Wantz was a veteran of some of the best pain clinics in the country. (According to her husband, Marjorie's screams of pain could regularly be heard by the neighbors). She had turned first to the advice Derek Humphry provided in his *Final Exit,* but she failed in an attempt to take her own life. She then turned to Kevorkian, who, after considerable consultations, decided that she would be an appropriate candidate for his services. He fitted her with a breathing mask that was attached to a canister of carbon monoxide, which Wantz activated with the push of a button. Meanwhile, Miller chose to use a mercitron similar to the one used by Janet Adkins. Both Miller and Wantz committed their final acts in a rented cabin in the Bald Mountain Recreation Area, a state park about forty miles north of Detroit. Technically speaking, neither woman was terminally ill.

Once again, the Oakland County prosecutor tried to bring murder charges. But once again, he was unable to produce sufficient evidence that Kevorkian did anything more than assist in the suicides of these two individuals. Consequently, the judge threw out the charges of murder. Oakland County Circuit Judge David Breck even seemed sympathetic to Kevorkian's position, writing that "for those patients, whether terminal or not, who have unmanageable pain, physician-assisted suicide remains an alternative" (cited in Anderson, 1992).

Kevorkian's case number four involved another woman with multiple sclerosis. On May 15, 1992, Susan Williams, fifty-two years of age, blind, and wheelchair-bound for the last twelve years of her life, was assisted by Kevorkian in her Detroit home. She, like Marjorie Wantz, chose the canister of carbon monoxide as a means of "self-deliverance." In a letter that was released after her death, Williams wrote that "the quality of my life is just existing, not living ... I pray Dr. Kevorkian will be exonerated of any wrongdoing in this case. I am so thankful he was able to help me" (cited in "Michigan Doctor," 1992).

Kevorkian's fifth patient was a fifty-two-year-old woman with terminal lung and brain cancer who, like Wantz and Williams, chose the increasingly popular carbon-monoxide option. A sixth patient, yet another woman, was helped to commit suicide in the company of four friends shortly thereafter. When Kevorkian was asked why all his patients to that point were women, he commented that "women are just far more realistic about facing death, and [they] have got the guts to do it " (Kevorkian, 1992).

Meanwhile, several bills had been introduced in the Michigan State Senate that would proscribe the practice of assisted suicide entirely. In each case, however, passage was held up in the house, which was controlled by the Democrats. The house appeared to be more sensitive than the senate to polls in Michigan that consistently showed that nearly two-thirds of the state's residents supported laws permitting physicians to help individuals commit suicide. Two and a half years later, after Jack Kevorkian had decided to take matters into his own hands in six assisted suicides, a bill was passed in both houses of the legislature that made assisted suicide an illegal act, punishable by up to four years in prison and a $2,000 fine. The law was to take effect on April 1, 1993, and sunset (expire automatically unless the legislature acted to renew it) after a special commission set up to study the issue published its recommendations in July 1994.

On December 15, 1992, just hours before Republican Governor John Engler signed the bill into law, Kevorkian assisted in suicides number seven and eight. Marguerite Tate, seventy, and Marcella Lawrence, sixty-seven, both used the carbon-monoxide option in Tate's Auburn Hills home. Tate had amyotrophic lateral sclerosis (ALS), and Lawrence suffered from heart disease, emphysema, and arthritis in the back. Appearing at a news conference held to protest the passage of the new Michigan law a few days earlier, Lawrence had stated: "The pain I have, I wish they [the legislators] could have for just one night. ... If I were up on the thirteenth floor right now, I would jump" (cited in "Doctor Assists 2 More," 1992).

One month later, Jack Miller, fifty-three, a former tree trimmer who suffered from bone cancer and emphysema, became Kevorkian's ninth client, the first male to take part in a Kevorkian-assisted suicide. Then, on February 4, 1993, Stanley Ball and Mary Biernat became the principals in Kevorkian's third case involving a double assisted suicide. The eighty-two-year-old Ball, a retired agricultural extension agent who was still swimming and skiing in his seventies, had contracted cancer of the pancreas; the condition blinded him and left him in constant pain. Biernat, a seventy-three-year-old woman with breast cancer spreading in her chest, was driven to Ball's home by her children. Both patients opted for the carbon-monoxide device. Four days later, Elaine Goldbaum, a forty-seven-year-old woman suffering with multiple sclerosis, became the twelfth individual to be assisted by Kevorkian.

Interestingly but maybe not surprisingly, public concern with Kevorkian's activities, as reflected by the reactions of the news media, slackened substantially over time. According to David Margolick (1993), "As the death toll mounts, the bizarre has become almost banal. The local police come and go more quickly. Local television stations no longer broadcast news conferences live, and succeeding suicides make only the inside pages of the Detroit papers." For better or worse, it seems that Kevorkian's activities were becoming commonplace and almost acceptable in an ad hoc, de facto sort of way.

Hugh Gale, seventy, became Kevorkian's next (and, ultimately, most problematic) client on February 15, 1993. The thirteenth individual but only the third man to successfully avail himself of Kevorkian's services, Gale suffered from emphysema and heart disease. Patient number fourteen, forty-four-year-old Jonathan Grenz, and patient number fifteen, forty-one-year-old Martha Ruwart, became the fourth pair of Kevorkian's patients to participate in a double assisted suicide shortly thereafter, on February 18, 1993. Grenz had cancer of the neck, lungs, and chest, and Ruwart had cancer of the ovaries.

Agitated by Kevorkian's increased rate of activity, the Michigan legislature amended its original assisted-suicide prohibition so that it would take effect immediately. On the day that Governor Engler signed the amendment, law enforcement authorities converged on Kevorkian's Royal Oak apartment in search of evidence that Hugh Gale, patient number thirteen, was a less-than-willing participant. Also on that day, a right-to-life advocate produced documentation to that effect after rummaging through a Kevorkian associate's garbage can and finding what appeared to be records indicating that Gale panicked and tried to back out of the suicide. This led Oakland County prosecutors to think in terms of building a case of attempted homicide against Kevorkian.

Apparently, Gale did panic after about forty-five seconds of breathing the carbon monoxide fed into his lungs via a mask over his mouth and nose. According to the document retrieved by the right-to-life advocate, "The patient became flushed, agitated, breathing deeply, saying 'Take it off!'" ("Suicide Tried," 1993).

Then, according to the retrieved record, the patient calmed down after about twenty minutes and requested that the assisted suicide continue. Whether a second request was made to discontinue the suicide is a matter of some dispute, however. Kevorkian, his associates, and members of Gale's family who attended the assisted suicide corroborated the original request to discontinue the assisted suicide but argued that the process then proceeded without incident. But the retrieved record led right-to-life advocates to claim that a second request to terminate the suicide went unheeded. Without any more evidence along these lines, however, the prosecutor's office decided to drop the notion of bringing homicide charges.

Kevorkian challenged the new law by assisting in his sixteenth suicide on May 16. He was arrested for violating the new ban, but before the week was out, Judge Cynthia Williams of the Wayne County Circuit Court found the Michigan law to be unconstitutional on procedural grounds. She then granted a temporary injunction to allow parties on both sides of the issue the chance to explore, with appeals to higher state courts, whether the law violated the Michigan constitution on substantive grounds as well. (Although Judge Williams refused to rule on the substantive question, her sentiments on the issue became clear when she stated that: "This court cannot envisage a more fundamental right than the right of self-determination. Without that right none of the others ... can have meaning or effect," ["Judge Strikes," 1993]). In June, however, the Michigan Court of Appeals stayed the injunction put in place by Judge Williams, effectively reinstating the law banning assisted suicide pending a more complete review of the statute.

With the implications of this most recent ruling still unclear Kevorkian resumed his crusade on August 4 when he assisted in the death of thirty-year-old Thomas Hyde. Hyde, suffering from Lou Gehrig's disease, was the youngest of Kevorkian's seventeen assisted suicide patients to date. Once again, the Wayne County prosecutor charged Kevorkian with violating Michigan law, but after a preliminary hearing the defendant was released on his own recognizance pending commencement of a criminal trial. Kevorkian used this period of freedom to assist in the suicide on September 9 of another individual: Donald O'Keefe, a seventy-three-year-old man suffering from bone cancer. Shortly thereafter the prosecutor in Wayne County filed his third charge of assisted suicide against Kevorkian, although he expressed his misgivings about the law at the same time. Even the judge scheduled to handle this third case—Kevorkian's eighteenth assisted suicide—sympathized with the doctor, calling him "very courageous" and arguing that "it would be difficult for many of us to say there isn't some right to say how we can leave here" ("Kevorkian at Suicide Scene," 1993).

Kevorkian remained free on bond pending the start of the Hyde and O'Keefe trials. This allowed him to assist in another suicide, his nineteenth. Merian Frederick, a seventy-two-year-old woman with Lou Gehrig's disease, was no longer able to speak and was fed through a tube in her stomach. Frederick was, however, able to express her desire that Kevorkian help to end her life, which he did on October 22. The death was attended by Frederick's son and her Unitarian church minister. This time Kevorkian's actions fell within the jurisdiction of Oakland County, where the county prosecutor—Richard Thompson, a long-time foe of Kevorkian and the man who attempted to bring homicide charges against the doctor prior to passage of Michigan's assisted suicide law—filed charges under the new law and demanded that Kevorkian be jailed. As he had promised, the doctor refused to accept solid food, taking in only water, fruit juice, and vitamins. After three days of high-profile media coverage, however, an opponent of Kevorkian's position bailed him out of jail in the hopes of diverting media attention away from Kevorkian's cause.

The tack did not work very well, however, for on November 22, while free on bail, Kevorkian struck in Oakland County again by assisting in the suicide of Ali A. Khalili, a sixty-one-year-old physician and a pioneer in rehabilitative medicine, who was suffering from the advanced stages of bone cancer. Khalili, an assistant professor of rehabilitative medicine at Northwestern University and former chairman of the Department of Rehabilitation at Grant Hospital in Chicago, was said to be in tremendous pain despite being on a pump that injected him with constant small doses of morphine. Once again Kevorkian was jailed on charges of violating Michigan's law banning assisted suicide. He then resumed his hunger strike.

On December 13, 1993, Judge Richard C. Kaufman of the neighboring Wayne County Circuit Court did what his Wayne County colleague Judge Cynthia Williams seemed inclined to do in May: He struck down Michigan's assisted suicide law on substantive grounds. In his decision Judge Kaufman argued that "when a person's quality of life is significantly impaired by a medical condition and the medical condition is extremely unlikely to improve" that person has a "constitutionally protected right to commit suicide," so long as the decision to take one's life is a reasonable one made of the suffering person's own free will ("Suicide Law Struck Down," 1993). The next day Judge Kaufman ruled that, at the very least, charges against Kevorkian in the Wayne County case of Donald O'Keefe should be dropped. Using the Supreme Court's 1990 ruling in the case of Nancy Cruzan and also referring to *Roe* v. *Wade*, the judge reasoned that "it is hard to imagine a state action that would have a greater intrusive effect upon a person's quest to make decisions based upon their personal moral beliefs than the state's blanket proscription on assistance of rational suicide." Ultimately, the Wayne County judge argued, the right to suicide was "implicit in the concept of ordered liberty" ("Suicide Law Struck Down," 1993).

At first authorities in Oakland County argued that the Wayne County judge's ruling had no bearing on the two cases (Frederick and Khalili) pending in the Oakland County jurisdiction. Subsequently, however, an Oakland County judge lowered Kevorkian's bond from $50,000 to $100. A supporter of Kevorkian's, who vowed to commit suicide if the doctor died in jail, posted that bond, and Kevorkian was freed after promising not to help anyone else commit suicide "for the time being" (Prodis, 1993). Kevorkian was also required to wear an electronic monitoring device. Clearly weakened from his latest hunger strike, which lasted seventeen days, Kevorkian was driven directly to Sinai Hospital in Detroit for treatment. The entire situation is now under review within Michigan's appellate court system. Meanwhile, Compassion in Dying—a newly formed group based in Seattle and inspired, at least in part, by Kevorkian's machinations—has begun assisting terminally ill patients end their lives in Washington state. It is the first such organization in the United States to provide comfort and technical assistance for those wishing assistance in the planning and execution of a suicide (Belkin, 1993).

All told, Kevorkian has assisted in the deaths of twenty patients: four instances of double suicide and twelve singular acts. Though Kevorkian's early patients were predominately women—the first eight patients were female, as were ten of the first twelve—the gender ratio began to even out over time; in all, twelve women and eight men have availed themselves of Kevorkian's services. Thomas Hyde was the youngest to die, at age thirty, and Stanley Ball was the oldest patient, at age eighty-two. Cancer was the most common affliction in the group, being the primary diagnosis in ten of the twenty cases. We also should note that though many of Kevorkian's patients were in great pain and suffered extensive physical disability, most were not, technically speaking, terminally ill. Indeed, Janet Adkins—Kevorkian's first assisted suicide—suffered from the early stages of Alzheimer's disease and may well have lived for many years had Kevorkian not intervened. Likewise, although Marjorie Wantz complained of being in great pain, an autopsy revealed no life-threatening physiological problems of any kind (see Table 6.1).

Point-Counterpoint

Perhaps more than any other topic debated within the happy-death movement, assisted suicide highlights the ethical issues that are so often brought into play when the right to die is in question. The first and foremost issue has to do with the appropriate role of the physician. The "slippery slope" is also a central concern to many—that is, many fear that allowing assisted suicide in particular cases will inexorably lead society down the slippery slope toward the abusive and illegitimate use of this procedure. And the sanctity of life lies at the heart of the debate, a notion that is often pitted against the right to self-determination.

Role of the Physician. Many who argue against assisted suicide on ethical grounds do so by invoking the Hippocratic oath. How can one participate in an assisted suicide without violating the "do-no-harm" pledge? Very few medical students are required to take this oath upon graduating from medical school now,

TABLE 6.1 Jack Kevorkian and Assisted Suicide

Patient's Name (Age)	Date of Suicide	Patient's Condition	Comments[a]
1. Janet Adkins (54)	6/4/90	Alzheimer's	• first suicide and a member of the Hemlock Society • homicide charges filed and dismissed • judge barred Kevorkian from using "mercitron" • Michigan suspended Kevorkian's medical license
	17-month layoff		
2. Sherry Miller (43)	10/23/91	multiple sclerosis	• first double suicide • homicide charges filed and dismissed
3. Marjorie Wantz (58)	"	uncontrolled pain in the pelvis	• tried and failed at a Hemlock suicide first • autopsy revealed no clinical cause of pain
4. Susan Williams (52)	5/15/92	multiple sclerosis	• blind and wheelchair-bound for 12 years
5. Lois F. Hawes (52)	9/26/92	lung and brain cancer	• technically, first patient considered "terminally ill"
6. Catherine Andreyev (46)	11/23/92	breast cancer	• considered acutely ill
7. Marguerite Tate (70)	12/15/92	amyotrophic lateral sclerosis (ALS)	• second double suicide • both patients considered acutely ill
8. Marcella Lawrence (67)	"	heart disease, emphysema, and arthritis	• on same day, Governor Engler signed bill making assisted suicide illegal in Michigan (effective 4/1/93)
9. Jack Miller (53)	1/20/93	bone cancer and emphysema	• first male patient
10. Stanley Ball (82)	2/4/93	pancreatic cancer	• third double suicide • Ball was blind, in constant pain, and the oldest suicide
11. Mary Biernat (73)	"	breast cancer	
12. Elaine Goldbaum (47)	2/8/93	multiple sclerosis	
13. Hugh Gale (70)	2/15/93	heart disease and emphysema	• Gale had second thoughts, aborted suicide attempt at least once before going ahead as planned

14. Jonathan Grenz (44)	2/18/93	neck, lung, and chest cancer	• fourth double suicide • Governor Engler signed a new bill making assisted suicide illegal immediately
15. Martha Ruwart (41)	"	ovarian cancer	
16. Ronald Mansur (54)	5/16/93	bone and lung cancer	• Kevorkian arrested under new law • judge struck down law on 5/20 • law reinstated on appeal
17. Thomas Hyde (30)	8/4/93	ALS	• youngest suicide • Kevorkian arrested; released on bond to await trial
18. Donald O'Keefe (73)	9/9/93	bone cancer	• Kevorkian arrested again and released on bond
19. Merian Ruth Frederick (72)	10/22/93	ALS	• patient unable to talk; fed through a stomach tube • Kevorkian jailed on 11/5 for assisted suicides of Hyde and O'Keefe and began hunger strike • an opponent of Kevorkian bailed Kevorkian out of jail, against Kevorkian's will, on 11/8
20. Dr. Ali Khalili (61)	11/22/93	bone cancer	• Khalili was prominent pioneer in rehabilitative medicine, assistant professor of rehabilitative medicine, Northwestern University, and former chair of the Department of Rehabilitation, Grant Hospital, Chicago • Kevorkian rearrested on 11/30 for death of Frederick. Bail set at $50,000, and Kevorkian began another hunger strike (taking in only water, juice, and vitamins)

NOTE: Legal update—On December 14, 1993, Wayne County Circuit Judge Richard C. Kaufman—ruling on the case of Donald O'Keefe—struck down Michigan's ban on assisted suicide as unconstitutional, and charges against Kevorkian in that case were dropped. Kevorkian remained in an Oakland County jail for the death of Merian Frederick, however, pending an appellate court ruling on the Wayne County judge's decision. Charges regarding the death of Ali Khalili—another Oakland County case—were also pending.

[a]Kevorkian's first two patients (Adkins and Miller) committed suicide using what Kevorkian calls a "mercitron" (with which patient activates the flow of toxic chemicals through an intravenous line attached to his or her arm). Kevorkian's medical license in Michigan was suspended in November 1991, making the purchase of the chemicals difficult. Since then, he has used carbon monoxide, which flows from a canister, through plastic tubing, and into a mask placed securely over the patient's face. As with the mercitron, the patient is responsible for initiating the flow of the lethal agent.

but most continue to use the oath in rationalizing the aggressive approach to therapy that most practitioners take.

There are some who doubt the validity of the Hippocratic oath, however, suggesting that it does not reflect the thinking of Hippocrates at all. Instead, critics of the oath's validity hold that it is a contrivance created by the Pythagoreans, a small, secretive sect of Greeks who, the critics contend, concocted the Hippocratic oath well after its namesake had died.[26] If this reading of history is accurate, then prevailing medical ethics are grounded in a pledge that really only reflects the thinking of an isolated and religiously extreme group of believers, who also forbade surgery as an unholy enterprise: "I will not use the knife, not even on sufferers from stone" (see Edelstein, 1943, p. 28).

Given its proscriptions, the oath was not accepted by many premoderns. Indeed, for centuries, ancient physicians practiced surgery, administered abortive remedies, and assisted patients in committing suicide (Edelstein, 1943, p. 63), all things the oath appears to forbid. Only at the end of antiquity, with the emergence of Christianity and religious control of the healing arts, did those practicing medicine begin to conform to the oath's principles, and that is when the oath began to take on the significance that is currently—and, according to all the evidence, falsely—attributed to it (Edelstein, 1943).

A better source for the Hippocratic philosophy, according to Stanley Joel Reiser (cited in Knowles, 1977a, pp. 50–51) is the group of texts written by different men and passed down by Hippocrates' disciples as a collective work known as *Corpus Hippocratum*. Here, one finds a different sort of philosophy than that suggested by the Hippocratic oath. How far should the physician extend medical techniques to fight nature? *Corpus Hippocratum* seems to advocate restraint. According to "The Art," one of the works in *Corpus Hippocratum*, the physician's responsibility is to do away with the suffering of the sick, to lessen the violence of their disease, and to "refuse to treat those who are overmastered by their disease, realizing that in such cases medicine is powerless" (cited in Reiser, 1977, p. 51; see also President's Commission, 1983, pp. 15–16).

In the end, for those who rely on Hippocrates for answers to the ethical dilemmas posed by end-of-life medical decisions, one can only advise caution. Generally, it must be remembered, the Hippocratic school embraced a holistic approach to medicine. Thus, it is quite possible and even probable that Hippocrates would have rejected the degree to which medicine has embraced the narrowly focused, specialized approaches that are characterized today by the technological imperative (which is often rationalized using the "do-no-harm" principle), almost to the exclusion of the softer side of human experience (Bronzino, Smith, and Wade, 1990, p. 546).

Jack Kevorkian criticizes modern medicine on these grounds, claiming that medicine should be just as concerned with alleviating suffering as it is with prolonging life (Kevorkian, 1991, p. 159; see also DeSpelder and Strickland, 1992, p. 358).[27] Otherwise, he warns, there will be a proliferation of botched and degrading, "back-alley" assisted suicides.[28] Even when clandestine suicides succeed, they do not provide the dying individual with the opportunity to leave this world with much dignity. Instead, those who would take their own lives are forced to scurry around behind closed doors, usually alone lest family members, friends, or physicians become implicated in the act. And, of course, organs that might be donated are wasted when assisted suicides take place secretly. For those who advocate assisted suicide, mottos like "do no harm" hardly have currency in modern medicine, if they ever did.

The Slippery Slope. A second important case made against assisted suicide on ethical grounds involves the "wedge" or "slippery-slope" argument. According to this line of thought, advanced by the NLCMDD and others, legitimizing mercy killing in any context permits entry of a "wedge" that would inevitably lead to a complete breakdown in application, with euthanasia performed as a matter of convenience, without thought to the rights of the physically disabled, the old, the mentally infirm, and others. This would lead us down the "slippery slope": One step onto the assisted-suicide ramp would cause society to slide downward uncontrollably, to the point where euthanasia would be administered without consent in some cases and where potential candidates would feel pressured (and maybe even obliged) to choose the euthanasia option rather than burden family and friends by prolonging the inevitable.

The same argument has been made for years in other rights contexts: Minor restrictions on gun ownership would eventually lead down the slippery slope to the entire loss of the right to bear arms; legal restrictions on abortion will take us down the slippery slope to a complete gutting of *Roe* v. *Wade* protections; setting restrictions in the arts and entertainment fields leads down the slippery slope toward onerous censorship. It is a powerful argument that is sometimes phrased in terms of opening up either Pandora's box or the proverbial can of worms. A. A. Brill uses another metaphor in the context of euthanasia when he notes, "The lust for killing can only be held in leash with the greatest effort, and like the proverbial sleeping dog, it is best not to disturb it" (cited in Schoenfeld, 1978, pp. 54–55).

Some counter these analogies with rhetorical parallels of their own, suggesting that critics of assisted suicide are crying wolf; like Chicken Little, they worry needlessly about how the sky is falling. Those concerned about assisted suicide are said to see a tempest in a teapot, making a mountain out of a mole hill in the process. Ultimately, in this particular battle of aphorisms and parables, just one thing is clear: Only time will tell which side sees the situation more accurately. The only problem, contend those who advance the slippery-slope argument, is that once we start down that road, it may be too late to turn back, regardless of how badly things turn out.

Sanctity of Life Versus Individual Autonomy. The sanctity of life is a central concern of the religious and spiritual community. Those who argue along the sanctity-of-life line often identify God as the author of all life, claiming it would violate the most fundamental of religious tenets to tamper with the life He has created. This is not to say, however, that this argument is irrelevant within the secular world. Indeed, the sanctity-of-life principle is widely understood to operate in the public sector as a rationale for all kinds of policies, including prohibitions on late-term abortions.

Often pitted in direct conflict with the sanctity-of-life ethic is the principle of self-determination: Individuals should be allowed to choose for themselves. The sanctity-of-life principle is deductive in nature in that those who support it believe the principle should apply regardless of the situation. In contrast, the principle of self-determination is driven more by context and is thus more inductive in nature, demanding that individuals be allowed to make decisions, case by case, as they see fit. Often, constitutional protections are invoked in assisted-suicide issues by those who advocate self-determination.

Ultimately, the ethical positions intersect when it comes to human dignity. Both camps argue that human dignity is a consideration of supreme importance; they differ only on the means used to achieve that end. Is the dignity of human life greater when individuals are kept alive regardless of their preferences or situations? Or is it enhanced most when individuals are allowed to choose (knowing they will not always choose wisely)? There are no clear answers, but the policy debate increasingly favors the right to self-determination, on constitutional and political-culture grounds, sanctity-of-life arguments to the contrary notwithstanding (see Chapter 7 for more along these lines).

Other Practical Issues. In addition to the ethical debate, a number of practical issues have fueled the debate about assisted suicide. Some argue that making assisted suicide an option will take the wind out of the research sails, weakening the incentive to find cures and treatments for painful diseases along the way. Typically, this argument is advanced by those lobbying for research funds for a specific disease. Daniel Callahan (1990, especially Chapter 2) counters the argument by noting that medical advances simply create "needs, endless needs" and that we may now be at or near the point of diminishing returns when it comes to investing in research. Thus he contends, our research dollars would be more humanely spent caring for individuals rather than trying to cure every infirmity that exists.

Others have raised concerns about the potential erosion of patient confidence if physicians have the assisted-suicide option at their disposal in troublesome cases or with troublesome patients. In light of this criticism, Kevorkian proposes that only retired physicians should be allowed to administer euthanasia, either on a salaried or a pro bono basis. This, he believes, would eliminate any concerns about professional or financial conflicts of interest for patients and physicians alike.

Daniel C. Maguire (1974, p. 182) and J. B. Wilson (1975, p. 111) raise another issue. They argue that medical professionals are uniquely ill suited to handle assisted suicide because of their marked aversion to death in the first place. This would make it difficult for them to help their patients come to grips with the notion. As Maguire points out (in Schoenfeld 1978, p. 53), not only do medical schools usually avoid formal consideration of mercy killing, the prejudice against euthanasia may already be well crystallized before prospective doctors even enter medical training.

This is something of an oblique attack that does not criticize the concept of assisted suicide outright; it only argues against the capacity of physicians to be involved. But Kevorkian counters that physicians *must* be involved. They are the ones with the expertise in diagnosis and prognosis, the ones who can prescribe drugs and understand their effects, and the ones who can take action when things go wrong. And they are still among the most trusted and trustworthy individuals in society today. For all these reasons, Kevorkian says, physicians can and must undertake the responsibility that is naturally theirs to bear.

America of Two Minds

There is a history of euthanasia in American medicine. As Andrew Malcolm (1990a) notes, "It was common procedure years ago for a doctor, on his own, to administer extra morphine to a dying patient. The objective was to relieve the pain. But the inevitable side effect was that the patient's breathing also slowed and death came much sooner." And, as the response to Quill's article suggests, euthanasia is practiced in the medical community today. Indeed, as Schoenfeld (1978, p. 50) states, "Surveys among physicians reveal a considerable incidence of mercy killing, particularly when pain-ridden and terminally ill cancer patients are involved." Despite all the training and professional pressures that militate against assisted suicide, one recent survey reported that 60 percent of the physicians interviewed favored legalized euthanasia (Rogers, 1992).

When polled anonymously, physicians still exhibit considerable tolerance for the practice of assisted suicide. But few (Quill and Kevorkian are exceptions) are willing to risk going public. Moreover, the same poll that revealed 60 percent support for assisted suicide in theory also found that less than half of those favoring legalized euthanasia would actually be willing to perform it (Rogers, 1992). Meanwhile, the professional associations continue in their opposition to assisted suicide. As we have noted, the AMA lobbied hard against the initiatives in Washington and California, and though it sympathized with Quill's situation, it denounced his actions. Moreover, although the professional community commiserates with Quill, it almost uniformly denounces Kevorkian, despite the many similarities between their actions.[29] Apparently, the medical community is of two minds on the issue.

That is all to be expected, given the ambiguous sentiments of the American people on the subject. Nearly 80 percent of Americans support the use of living wills, but only 10 percent execute them. And even though 65 percent of the people surveyed say they supported the assisted-suicide initiative a few weeks before the Washington vote, only 45 percent had the stomach to go to the polls and vote for it.

The legal system seems to be of two minds, as well. In spite of the prosecutors' best efforts, both Quill and Kevorkian have walked away from their actions legally unscathed. Nor were the fates of these two physicians exceptional. According to Wilson (1975, p. 149), "Prosecutors and grand juries tend not to indict those who kill ... to relieve suffering or to prevent unconscious existence when there is no hope of recovery." And even when indictments are handed down, juries tend to vote for acquittal; if they convict, punishments tend to be mild and are often alleviated by pardons (Schoenfeld, 1978, p. 50).

In fact, between 1920 and 1985, criminal charges associated with a mercy killing were filed in only fifty-six cases. Only ten of the individuals involved were found guilty of criminal homicide and imprisoned; twenty were granted suspended sentences or probation, and fifteen were granted outright acquittals (often on the grounds of temporary insanity). In six cases, the charges were dismissed, and five others were not even brought to trial (Humphry and Wickett, 1986, p. 219). Even more important than the generally lenient disposition of these fifty-six cases, however, is the fact that thousands of other physicians who must have participated in acts of euthanasia over the years were never charged in the first place.

Obviously, positions on assisted suicide are in flux. Quietly tolerated in the past, the issue is now out in the open. The public, the legal community, and the physicians—all of two minds on the subject—are struggling to cope with the activism that is slowly overwhelming right-to-die restraint on the assisted-suicide question. The current ambiguities might be defended as good public policy on the ground that such ambiguity "permits mercy killing where needed, and yet avoids the unsettling effect upon the populace—'the unwanted repercussion on the delicate forces which restrain killing'" (J. Wilson, cited in Schoenfeld, 1978, p. 50). We suspect, however, that Americans will slowly begin to reject the clandestine, restricted, quasi-legal status that assisted suicide now has. Over the years, Americans have made the demanding of specific, legally protected rights something of a political cause célèbre (voting rights, abortion rights, rights not to be discriminated against because of age, gender, ethnicity, religion, disability, and so on). As restraint slowly gives way to activism, we believe that, for better or worse, the right to assistance in dying will be added to the list.

Summary: Society Begins to Embrace the Happy-Death Concept

Has there been a fundamental reconstruction of our cultural stance toward death as a result of the happy-death movement? After all is said and done, Charmaz

(1980, p. 12) is not so sure, arguing that the social structures of our institutions, families, hospitals, and legal systems remain essentially intact. Of course, she states, there are trends and drift, but fundamentally, denial maintains its grip on a culture more concerned with consumption and rejuvenation than with expiration. Writing twelve years after Charmaz made that assessment, we would offer a different conclusion for the social structures of our hospitals and legal structures *have* undergone dramatic changes in the interim.

In that time, the U.S. Supreme Court has reaffirmed what the state courts have been affirming for a decade or more: The right to die does exist. Forty-six states and the District of Columbia have passed living-will laws. The federal government has also gotten into the act, with the Patient Self-Determination Act designed to ensure that everyone admitted to a hospital for any reason will be apprised of their rights under state law.

Ethics committees were still largely an abstraction when Charmaz put pen to paper, and DNR orders were just beginning to be taken seriously. Today, nearly every hospital in the country has an ethics committee, and all honor an explicit DNR protocol. Meanwhile, assisted suicide has become the subject of a great deal of debate nationwide. State initiatives in Washington and California, the rise of Derek Humphry's *Final Exit* to best-seller status, the machinations of Jack Kevorkian in Michigan, the revealing confession by Timothy Quill in the *New England Journal of Medicine,* with a sequel that lays out a six-part criterion for the legitimate use of euthanasia (see Brody, 1993b) all guarantee that the issue will have staying power. Thus, it is clear that our cultural stance toward death has begun to change in the last dozen years or so. And it is equally clear, given such developments, that there will be no turning back.

In a way, we are all unwittingly part of the happy-death movement, a movement that cuts across lines of age, race, class, gender, ethnicity, and religion. We are all aging in the inexorable march toward death that life is from its inception. Furthermore, most people would likely agree with Norman Cousins's belief that "death is not the ultimate tragedy of life. The ultimate tragedy is depersonalization—dying in an alien and sterile area, separated from the spiritual nourishment that comes from being able to reach out to a loving hand, separated from the desire to experience the things that make life worth living, separated from hope" (cited in DeSpelder and Strickland, 1992, p. 576). In the end, it is presumed that most of us would prefer a happy death—one that is comfortable rather than painful, expeditious rather than protracted, humane and dignified rather than depersonalizing and humiliating. Anyone who hopes for that kind of death is a potential participant in the happy-death movement, creating a vast reservoir of activism just waiting to be mobilized.

Death with dignity—a happy death—was considered the norm for the first thirty years of this century. Then, a number of social and technological changes conspired to alter the way Americans conceive of death. Today, the notion of death with dignity will continue to motivate activism as long as it is not the norm. And death with dignity will not be the norm, writes Morgan (1989, p. 95), until mankind's ethical standards expand to encompass changes in the technology and sociology of death that were visited on this culture in the middle third of the twentieth century. All indications are that, today, America is ripe for just such an ethical expansion.

7

Policy Mediation in the State Courts: Consensus on the Cutting Edge

To THIS POINT, we have discussed the forces of policy restraint, the forces of top-down activism associated with a profound transformation in the medical profession, and the forces of bottom-up activism associated with important social changes.[1] With that framework in place, it is time to consider the forces of mediation that do not set the policy agenda so much as they shape policy outcomes in the areas where activism succeeds in overwhelming restraint. Activism and restraint set the stage for policymaking by mediators—the individuals and institutions that then go on to forge policy results.

Policy mediation takes place in a number of different venues. The courts make policy all the time in the form of case law. Courts interpret statutory law in light of the state and federal constitutions, taking case-law precedents from past decisions across the nation into account. Statutory law is the work of the legislatures. Legislators introduce bills, hold hearings, and pass legislation that is sent to the executive, who either signs the bill into law or rejects it. The executive branch of government can make policy as well, in the form of executive orders issued by the executive or regulations formulated and promulgated by executive-branch agencies. Sometimes, policy mediation is relegated to private entities. In that case, policy takes the form of institutionally based guidelines that affect the way the public is treated in areas that are associated, in theory, with some measure of public-sector responsibility.

With regard to the right to die, the governors have stayed out of the policy mediation business for the most part, although various state departments of health have had some passing interest in certain aspects of this issue; for example, the New York State Department of Health became involved in the case of Timothy Quill, and the Missouri Department of Health argued cases against the Busalacchi and Cruzan families in state court. Private entities have been more involved, particularly in terms of formulating policies on the execution of DNR orders. These exceptions aside, however, the real epicenters of right-to-die policy mediation have been the state courts and, to a lesser degree, the state legislatures. Chapter 7 provides a survey of the state courts' role in this mediation, and Chapter 8 discusses the role played by the state legislatures.

We find that the state courts and legislatures have been engaged for some years in a game of legal tennis. For the most part, the courts have been serving all along. The legislatures have occasionally returned serve with weak shots, but more often, they have been aced. In short, state-court judges are the political actors who have taken the lead in applying policy alternatives to the right-to-die problems on the agenda, and the legislatures, when pressured to act, have dragged their collective feet if they have done anything at all.

Legal Foundations for a Right to Die

In the decade and a half since 1976, the year the New Jersey Supreme Court decided the landmark case of Karen Ann Quinlan, the state courts have played the central role in legitimizing the right of dying patients to refuse medical treatments. Though the establishment of right-to-die precedents has proceeded incrementally across the States, several common premises have emerged in the case law.

First, the state courts have leaned almost exclusively on two legal pillars in building a case for the right-to-die premise: (1) a common-law recognition of human autonomy and self-determination, as manifest in the informed-consent doctrine, and (2) constitutionally grounded rights to both liberty and privacy. Second, the courts have struggled to establish enduring criteria for surrogate decisionmaking when the principal is incompetent in right-to-die cases, although judges have exhibited a general tendency to be lenient in recommending that decisions be placed in the hands of others (typically, those of the families and health-care professionals) whenever possible. Third, the courts have come to accept the notion that artificial nutrition and hydration is a medical procedure that a patient—or the surrogate making decisions for an incompetent patient—may choose to forgo in exercising the established right to die. And fourth, the right to die applies to both those who are terminally ill and those who are in a persistent vegetative state.

Common-Law Grounds

There is a long-standing common-law tradition in American jurisprudence that recognizes and protects human autonomy and self-determination, based on eighteenth-century English common law. This principle, the basis for what is commonly referred to as informed consent, is regularly applied in cases where petitioners are requesting that medical procedures be withheld.

Case law that draws on this principle of informed consent traces back at least 100 years to the seminal U.S. Supreme Court ruling of 1891, in which the court held that a plaintiff could not be ordered to submit to a surgical exam against his or her will (*Union Pacific Railroad* v. *Botsford*). In addressing the issue of bodily control, the court stated: "No right is held more sacred, or is more carefully guarded by the common law, than the right of every individual to the possession and control of his own person, free from all restraint or interference by others, unless by clear and unquestionable authority of law."

Justice Benjamin Cardozo reaffirmed this premise twenty-three years later when writing an opinion in *Schloendorff* v. *Society of N.Y. Hospital* (1914). In a much-quoted statement from that decision, Cardozo writes that "every human being of adult years and sound mind has the right to determine what shall be done with his body." In effect, Cardozo used this case to expand the liberty concept that preserved the individual's right to resist invasive therapies against his or her will by incorporating a positive obligation on the part of medical personnel to inform patients of their alternatives. Thereafter, the tort doctrine of informed consent would be thought to oblige health-care professionals to explain, in good faith, proposed medical procedures and associated risks to prospective patients, then obtain consent, if possible, before proceeding. Moreover, in Cardozo's words, "a surgeon who performs an operation without his patient's consent commits an assault, for which he is liable in damages."

Although Cardozo may not have been thinking along right-to-die lines when he charted this informed-consent doctrine, no one today questions the applicability of his doctrine in right-to-die cases. The motivations of patients exercising informed consent may vary: A patient in George Washington's predicament, where the ministrations of health professionals only serve to hasten death, may refuse treatment just as right-to-die patients may refuse treatments out of fear that medical interventions will keep them alive. Regardless of the motivation, however, common law is thought to protect both kinds of patients equally.

Constitutional Grounds

As we have noted, the doctrine of informed consent is well established in American tort law as a common-law basis for decisionmaking. But common law falls short of offering the sort of enduring protection that typically accompanies rights grounded in the U.S. Constitution. For this reason, although most all courts begin their inquiries into right-to-die cases by calling on informed consent, many look to the Constitution for further guidance. Some courts argue that they have found this guidance in two places: in the penumbral privacy-rights protections embedded in the Bill of Rights and in the liberty protections of the Fourteenth Amendment.

The liberty interest found in the Fourteenth Amendment's due process clause is actually something of a constitutional rationale for the common-law informed-consent doctrine. That is, the Fourteenth Amendment's guarantee of "life, liberty, and property" is considered in this context to codify the common-law right of informed consent, which prohibits others from invading one's body—for purposes of surgery or otherwise—against one's will. The privacy interest is much less explicit in the Constitution. For this, one must look to court cases, beginning with the 1965 *Griswold* v. *Connecticut* decision in which the Supreme Court struck down state legislation that prohibited the use of contraceptives and the dispensing of birth control information among married couples (Kelly and Harbison, 1976).

Writing for the majority in *Griswold*, Justice William Douglas advanced the idea that "specific guarantees in the Bill of Rights have penumbras formed by emanations from these guarantees that give [those guarantees] life and substance" and provide "zones of privacy" for the individual. Douglas found that these penumbras were cast by the guarantees of the First, Fourth, and Fifth Amendments as "protection against all governmental invasions of the sanctity of a man's home" (cited in Kelly and Harbison, 1976, p. 963).

The right to privacy established in *Griswold* was further extended in the 1973 landmark abortion case, *Roe* v. *Wade,* which struck down a Texas law that made abortion a criminal offense. In reaching its decision in this case, the court relied on a series of privacy-rights cases that constitutionally protected decisions concerning procreation, marriage, and family life.[2] For state courts considering right-to-die cases, it was a small and inevitable step to include death, the next logical (and chronologically the ultimate) zone of private life, under the privacy-rights blanket (Borst, 1985, p. 906).[3] This, in essence, is how the New Jersey Supreme Court approached the case of Karen Ann Quinlan.

The Supreme Court View

Fourteen years after *Quinlan* was decided in New Jersey, the U.S. Supreme Court heard its first case ever dealing explicitly with the right to die: *Cruzan* v. *Director, Missouri Department of Health* (1990). Although the Cruzan family technically lost that case, the Supreme Court did affirm that there was, indeed, a long-standing common-law tradition of informed consent that could be appropriately applied in right-to-die cases. More importantly, the Court agreed that there were constitutionally protected rights at stake—specifically, the liberty interest supported by the Fourteenth Amendment.

At the same time, while the majority decision is clear and forceful in its elaboration of liberty interests, there is a conspicuous absence of discussion regarding privacy rights. This is the case, we suspect, because privacy rights are what the

Roe v. *Wade* abortion decision rests on. Conservative justices have chafed at the penumbral, evanescent nature of privacy rights, thinking the whole concept to be an ideological fabrication of liberal justices. Thus, William Rehnquist and the conservative wing of the court were not about to find privacy rights in the Constitution that would support the right to die for this would only lend legitimacy to the rationale that undergirds the *Roe* decision—a decision that conservative justices would just as soon overturn, given the opportunity.

Despite the fact that many state courts have alluded to the privacy-rights argument in defense of the right to die, Chief Justice William Rehnquist—author of the majority opinion—buried his only reference to the privacy question in a footnote, pointing out that "although many state courts have held that a right to refuse treatment is encompassed by a generalized right of privacy, we have never so held. We believe this issue is more properly analyzed in terms of the Fourteenth Amendment liberty interest."[4]

Even then, the court hedged its bets by arguing that although there was a constitutional basis for the right to die, this right was not absolute. In explaining the majority's opinion on this score, Chief Justice Rehnquist contended that it was reasonable for states to counterbalance constitutional liberty interests against relevant state interests in preserving life, preventing suicide, protecting innocent third parties, and maintaining the integrity of the medical profession. Accordingly, "determining that a person has a 'liberty interest' under the Due Process Clause [of the 14th Amendment] does not end the inquiry; 'whether respondent's constitutional rights have been violated must be determined by balancing his liberty interests against relevant state interests'" (*Youngberg* v. *Romero*, 1982).

Given this restrictive reading of the Constitution, it is conceivable that the constitutionally protected right to die could be turned on its head. That is, in cases where the principal is incompetent, the Fourteenth Amendment's due process clause could be relied on to protect the state's interest in preserving life as much as it might be relied on to protect an individual's right to decide, on behalf of another, to forgo life-sustaining treatment. In other words, not only must an individual's Fourteenth Amendment rights be balanced by the state's interest in preserving life, the state itself may find some protection of its prerogatives in the Constitution's due process provisions.

For example, Missouri's *Cruzan* decision required that guardians of an incompetent patient produce clear and convincing evidence (in accordance with due process) of a patient's wish to have life-sustaining procedures withdrawn. According to Rehnquist's opinion, this was a perfectly acceptable qualification to the right to die, given that this evidentiary standard had been found appropriate in other kinds of Fourteenth Amendment cases where the state had an interest in protecting the rights of an individual (e.g., cases involving deportation, denaturalization, civil commitments, contracts, and wills). If clear and convincing evidence of intent was required in other, more pedestrian civil cases, Rehnquist argued, the same evidentiary standard surely would be appropriate in cases of greater moment, such as those involving life and death.[5]

There may be no denying an individual's right to refuse life-sustaining treatment under the due process clause of the Fourteenth Amendment, including (according to the Supreme Court) the right to withdraw food and fluids. However, when the principal is incompetent to make the decision, questions arise as to what evidence of a patient's wishes will qualify as valid. Under the liberty-rights rationale grounded in the due process clause, the Supreme Court argued that plaintiffs might reasonably be required to produce clear and convincing evidence sufficient to overwhelm the state's interest in preserving life. Otherwise, the state's interests would be allowed to prevail.

Incompetent Patients and Surrogate Decisionmakers

No court, including the U.S. Supreme Court, has left much doubt about the firm common-law and constitutional basis of the right to die. This makes the right straightforward for those who are competent enough to make their wishes known. And doctors (some more than others) have become increasingly receptive to this notion that patients might refuse treatment at the end of their lives, consistent with the principle of informed consent.

The rub comes when individuals get into right-to-die situations but are unable by reason of incompetency to make those critical life-or-death decisions for themselves. What meaning can informed consent have when patients can no longer communicate their wishes or even understand information about their condition? Can third parties give informed consent in the name of an incompetent principal? That is, can third parties exercise a principal's liberty interest? These, it turns out, are the questions that have tried judges' souls.

Decision Criteria

The fact is that the overwhelming majority of the 100 or so right-to-die cases that have ended up in state courts since *Quinlan* have involved the disposition of incompetent patients—individuals who left no clear instructions as to their wishes before they became incapable of making informed decisions for themselves. Indeed, nearly 85 percent of all right-to-die cases heard in the state courts from 1976 through 1992 involved surrogates who were trying to make decisions for patients whose ability to decide was somehow—and in most cases, severely—impaired. The federal courts have heard six right-to-die cases in that same time frame, five of which involved incompetent patients and surrogate decisionmakers (National Center for State Courts, 1992, pp. 155–172). Court consensus was relatively easy to achieve on the basic issue of the right to die; the only controversy that remains re-garding that basic right concerns what parts of the Constitution apply in such cases. But the issue of incompetency has proved to be a much harder nut to crack.

The "Substituted-Judgment" Standard. The New Jersey Supreme Court took a relatively liberal position on the question of incompetency. With *In re Quinlan* (1976), it was argued that the constitutionally protected right to die could be exer-cised by a family on behalf of an incompetent patient as long as the family could establish that its decision was consistent with the decision the incompetent prin-cipal would make if able to do so. This knowledge might include understandings about the principal's religious beliefs, general attitudes regarding medical care, and other substantial (albeit indirect) evidence of that person's frame of mind with regard to right-to-die issues.

As the *Quinlan* court put it: "We have no doubt in these unhappy circum-stances, that if Karen were herself miraculously lucid for an interval (not altering the existing prognosis of the condition to which she would soon return) and per-ceptive of her irreversible condition, she could effectively decide upon discontinu-ance of the life-support apparatus, even if it meant the prospect of natural death." This reasoning would become known as the "substituted-judgment" standard, which holds that a third party's best guess about the wishes of the incompetent patient could be substituted for that which was impossible to obtain: the ex-pressed wishes of the patient.

The term *substituted judgment* actually originates with the Massachusetts case *In re Spring* (1980). In this case, the court decided that a seventy-eight-year-old incompetent individual with end-stage kidney disease could forgo hemodialysis, based on what was known about the individual's general preferences in such mat-ters. No written or specific oral instructions would be required as long as the principal's predisposition toward the withdrawal of life support could be reason-ably demonstrated by a third party.

The "Best-Interests" Standard. In another important Massachusetts case, *Su-perintendent of Belchertown State School* v. *Saikewicz* (1977), the court seemed to expand coverage of the constitutionally protected right to die beyond those who were currently incompetent to those who had never been legally competent. Jo-seph Saikewicz, the principal in this case, had been mentally retarded since birth. But the Massachusetts court hearing the case presumed that those who knew him could reasonably determine what his wishes might be, even though he himself had never been legally competent to make such decisions on his own behalf.

Extending the *Quinlan* rationale to *Saikewicz* was something of a stretch for the substituted-judgment standard, however, leading the *Saikewicz* court to intro-duce the notion that other factors might be considered, including age (Saikewicz was sixty-seven), the pain associated with continued therapy, the chances for therapeutic success, the suffering associated with the continuation of life, and the inability to cooperate with therapy when in a degraded mental state. This move to the consideration of other factors broadened the realm of possibilities for those seeking to establish the right to die, and in the process, it laid the groundwork for what would become a second kind of test: the *"best-interests" standard*, a term that was actually not coined until the New Jersey court heard the case of Claire Conroy five years later.

Claire Conroy was an eighty-four-year-old nursing-home patient who had lapsed into a condition similar to that of Karen Ann Quinlan without leaving any clear instructions regarding further medical treatment (Humphry and Wickett, 1986, p. 257). The *Conroy* (1985) court, when petitioned by a nephew interested in removing life support from the patient in question, argued that even though there was not enough evidence for a substituted judgment to be made, a patient's right to die might be secured using a second standard. This alternative standard, based on the best interests of the incompetent patient as balanced against the interests of the state in preserving life, codified what the *Saikewicz* court had only alluded to.

The *Conroy* solution involved weighing the net benefits derived from treatment as compared with the burdens imposed by treatment (e.g., the degree of the treatment's invasiveness, the degree of humiliation, and the extent of uncontrollable discomfort or pain). Also to be considered, according to the court, were the net benefits to the sustained individual of continued existence with treatment, as balanced against the burdens that treatment would impose on the individual (e.g., the degree of dependency and, again, the extent of the uncontrollable discomfort or pain).

This cost-benefit formulation was intended to serve as a guide to what, if any, actions would serve the best interests of the patient. The *Conroy* court argued that, by taking such evidence into account, the decisionmaker could choose to withdraw treatment if clearly satisfied "that the burdens of the patient's continued life with the treatment outweigh the benefits of that life for him"—for example, if "the pain and suffering of continued life markedly outweigh any physical pleasure, emotional enjoyment, or intellectual satisfaction that the patient may still be able to derive from [that] life."

The state courts that have made decisions following *Saikewicz* and *Conroy* have generally agreed with the expansion of rights using the best-interests standard. But there has been a notable exception to this trend, first enunciated by the New York court with its *Eichner* and *Storar* decisions in the early 1980s and echoed by the Missouri court with its important *Cruzan* decision later in the decade.

The "Subjective-Decision" Standard. *In re Eichner* (1980) was a New York case, decided in 1981, involving the disposition of Brother Fox, a man who had suffered a cardiac arrest while undergoing hernia surgery. Fox was left in a persistent vegetative state as a result.

Father Philip Eichner brought the case to court, seeking appointment as Brother Fox's guardian for purposes of withdrawing life support. The court found in favor of Eichner, but it rejected an open-ended reading of the *Saikewicz* court in the area of incompetence by suggesting that an incompetent could exercise a right to die *only* as long as there was "clear and convincing" evidence of the patient's earlier wishes. As it turns out, Brother Fox had expressed his desire— while competent, in previous discussions on the matter—that he not be kept alive by extraordinary measures. Satisfied with that evidence, the court granted Father Eichner's petition to have life support withdrawn from Brother Fox.

In the other right-to-die case heard by the New York court that year, however, the "clear and convincing" test proved to be more detrimental to the petitioner's case. *In re Storar* (1981) involved the case of John Storar, a man who (like Saikewicz in Massachusetts) had been profoundly retarded since birth. Storar had become terminally ill with bladder cancer, and his mother was asking that necessary blood transfusions be stopped. The court denied the mother's request, arguing that since the patient was—and always had been—mentally retarded (i.e., incompetent in the eyes of the court), he could not possibly have made competent indications as to his desires should a right-to-die scenario ever develop. In the court's words, it was "unrealistic to attempt to determine whether [a lifelong incompetent] person would want to continue life-prolonging treatment if that person were competent." By holding that the *Storar* case failed the substituted-judgment standard sketched in *Quinlan* and by rejecting the move toward the best-interests standard advanced in *Saikewicz*, New York's *Eichner* and *Storar* decisions really introduced a third kind of decision-making criteria: the "subjective-decision" standard.

The New York court argued that life support must be provided unless clear and convincing evidence was produced, demonstrating that a patient, while competent, had made a "subjective decision" regarding his or her wishes should he or she become seriously ill and incompetent at some future time. Ultimately, the decisions of the New York court and, later, the Missouri court (with *Cruzan* following roughly in the footsteps of *Eichner* and *Storar*) stand as important exceptions to the stream of state-court decisions to come—decisions that would more closely follow the evolutionary path charted by court cases using the substituted-judgment standard (e.g., *Quinlan* and *Spring*) or the best-interests standard (e.g., *Saikewicz* and *Conroy*).

Emergence of a Loose Consensus. New York's subjective-decision test remains an important, precedent-setting exception to the rule. Other state courts have generally seemed willing to find that individual interests, however derived and expressed through family members or advocates, more than outweigh the interests of the state in preserving life (even when lacking clear and convincing evidence of the patient's wishes). This liberal course in decisionmaking is what Thomas Mayo describes as the more mainstream current of jurisprudence. He writes: "State courts that have considered the question have been, on the whole, quite yielding. They generally recognize a qualified right to refuse life-sustaining medical treatment that may be exercised by competent patients and by guardians or others on behalf of incompetent patients" (Mayo, 1990, pp. 103–155). New Jersey's second landmark case in this area, *In re Conroy,* did much to solidify this emerging consensus.

At the same time, however, it would be incorrect to assume that much has been settled in the area of surrogate decisionmaking. First, controversy continues over which standard or standards do the best job of resolving disputes in right-to-die cases involving incompetent patients: substituted-judgment, best-interests, or both (or even neither, as with New York and Missouri's adherence to the subjective-decision standard). And even when a standard is agreed upon, the inquiry has only begun. For example, if operating under the substituted-judgment standard, what should be done when close family members disagree about what the incompetent patient would want if that person were somehow able to make the choice? Under the best-interests standard, who is to weigh the degree of pain and discomfort, the value of continued life, the degree of humiliation felt by an incompetent patient, as compared with the state's interest in preserving life? And if both standards are to apply, how will decisions be made when different conclusions are drawn by using the different approaches?

The courts may have agreed in principle to defer to surrogate decisionmakers, but the matter of surrogate decisionmaking is hardly settled. Moreover, controversy over who should do the deciding persists. Indeed, deciding exactly who the decisionmaker(s) should be continues to be one of the larger sticking points in the entire right-to-die debate.

Who Should Decide?

At this point, the only thing we can say about the "who" question is that the courts have charted a meandering course that has taken some interesting twists. "In short," according to Norman Cantor (1987, p. 106), "the development of a definitive and comprehensive legal approach to decision-making authority on behalf of terminally ill incompetent patients has not yet occurred." The courts have understandably beseeched their respective state legislatures—both in written decisions and in public pronouncements—to take the lead in codifying surrogate decision-making rules. The response from the legislatures has been slow in coming, however (when it has come at all), leaving the courts to struggle with the implementation side of the policy equation.

Still, there is a general trend in court decisions toward devolution of responsibility away from the bench and toward those with a personal and professional interest. For example, the *Quinlan* court introduced the notion that hospital ethics committees, made up of physicians, social workers, ethicists, attorneys, and theologians, be formed to review and approve all right-to-die decisions.

The *Saikewicz* court in Massachusetts stepped in at this point to issue a notable exception to the *Quinlan* philosophy of letting private parties make decisions. Indeed, *Saikewicz* moved in exactly the opposite direction in arguing for a stronger judicial role, stating that "we take a dim view of any attempt to shift the ultimate decision-making responsibility away from the duly established courts of proper jurisdiction to any committee, panel, or group, ad hoc or permanent." This judicially centered approach held that, no matter who was involved in the decision-making process at the lower levels, all parties should repair to the courts for the final decision.

The Washington court returned to the path blazed by the New Jersey court with its *In re Welfare of Colyer* decision of 1983, while at the same time adding its own peculiar twist. This court took a more medically oriented approach than its New Jersey counterpart by suggesting that a prognosis board, two physicians specializing in the patient's condition along with the attending physician, be used to guide the decision-making process.

The following year, this same court explicitly rejected the *Saikewicz* approach in its *Hamlin* decision, a case involving Joseph Hamlin, a man who was blind, severely retarded since birth (reminiscent of Saikewicz and Storar), and without any immediate family members. Hamlin's case ended up in court after he was diagnosed as being in a persistent vegetative state. The court argued that a suitable guardian, chosen on behalf of an incompetent patient, should be allowed to proceed with decisionmaking without any further intervention on the part of the judiciary (*In re Guardianship of Hamlin*, 1984). On this score, the Washington state judges were quite explicit, arguing that the court "need not always be involved in the actual substantive decision [to terminate treatment], even for lifetime incompetents" (cited in Robertson, 1985, p. 868).

Ultimately, with the weight of these two Washington cases added to the precedent established in *Quinlan*, the judicial trend advocated in the courts would be one where the judiciary's role would diminish and the part played by family, guardians, and health-care professionals would expand. Instead of taking the path outlined by the Massachusetts court in *Saikewicz* (that courts should play a central decision-making role)[6] or following in the footsteps of the New York court's *Storar* and *Eichner* decisions (that lifetime incompetents cannot have the right to die exercised on their behalf because they could not possibly satisfy the "clear and convincing" test), the courts have generally preferred to entrust the decisionmaking to private parties, acting as referee only in cases where consensus among such parties fails to emerge.

The Decision-making Maze

Ironically, what the courts have done with their surrogate decisions is simply to ratify the private-professional decision-making cooperative that has existed ad hoc for years, even before *Quinlan*. It is more and more common for physicians and family members to make decisions for incompetent patients, quietly and privately in waiting rooms and at bedsides in American hospitals. The courts really only added a sense of legitimacy to these arrangements by discussing them openly and in a favorable light, while setting a few guidelines along the way.

At the same time, it should be noted that the issue of what criteria these interested parties should apply—the criteria the courts would presumably apply when a guardian's decision is challenged legally—has proved to be much more difficult to resolve for judges across the States. Perhaps it is not surprising that the state legislatures have had even less success in this realm.

Artificially Provided Food and Fluids

Although the state courts may have labored with the surrogate decision-making issue, most seem to have become relatively comfortable with what for many is still a very contentious issue: the right to withdraw artificially provided food and fluids. The central role that food plays in our culture makes the nutrition and hydration issue especially controversial outside the courtroom (Callahan, 1990). For the most part, however, the state courts are clearly moving toward sanctioning the withholding or withdrawal of ANH for patients who otherwise qualify under the emerging set of right-to-die rules.

The ground-breaking case in this area was *Barber v. Superior Court* (1983). In that case, the family of the plaintiff, Clarence Herbert, had asked that tube feeding be discontinued, and the attending physicians consented. Herbert died six days later. Shortly thereafter, his two attending physicians were charged by the Los Angeles district attorney with murder. Sustaining the lower courts, the California Court of Appeals ruled that the administration of ANH could be categorized as medical treatment exactly as the use of mechanical supports was since ANH was "more similar to other medical procedures than to typical human ways of providing nutrition and hydration."

To expand on the explanation, the court went on to argue that the distinction between ANH and other medical procedures "seems to be based more on an emotional symbolism of providing food and water to those incapable of providing for themselves rather than on any rational difference." Furthermore, "medical nutrition and hydration may not always provide net benefits to patients."

Importantly, the court rejected the distinction between extraordinary and ordinary treatment enunciated by the Catholic church and often bandied about by ethicists, physicians, and lawyers, as well as judges. Catholic teachings since the 1957 encyclical of Pope Pius XII had held that food and fluids were ordinary treatments that could not morally be withheld or withdrawn from seriously ill patients, a position that has carried great, albeit diminishing, weight in religious and secular circles alike. But beginning with the Herbert case, courts began to conceive of ordinary treatments as those that offer reasonable hope of benefit to the patient without incurring excessive cost or subjecting the patient to excessive discomfort. Extraordinary treatments, then, would be taken to mean everything of a medical nature that offers little hope of benefit to the patient, while incurring excessive costs or producing excessive discomfort (Meisel, 1989, p. 83).

In other words, though the Catholic church had determined artificially provided food and fluids to be ordinary by definition, the courts now began to depart from that understanding. Instead, the Herbert case marked the beginning of a judicial tendency to take a more flexible approach that would allow for a determination that, in some cases, ANH could be withdrawn. This would be determined, according to California's *Barber* decision, using a "benefits versus burdens of treatment" test (i.e., the best-interests standard) under which the removal of ANH might be an entirely appropriate course of action if the burdens of treatment were perceived to outweigh the benefits.

A 1984 Massachusetts case, *In re Hier*, was the next to deal with the ANH issue in an explicit and important way. Mary Hier was a ninety-two-year-old woman who had lived in a psychiatric hospital for fifty-seven years (Humphry and Wickett, 1986, p. 255.) Unable to take food orally, she was fed through a gastronomy tube, which she continually pulled out. In this case, the Massachusetts court reaffirmed what the California court had established in the *Barber* decision: that artificially provided nutrition and hydration is a medical procedure that could be withheld or withdrawn like any other, even for incompetents. The court cited a three-part rationale in coming to its decision: (1) the burden and intrusiveness of the proposed surgery (to reimplant the feeding tube), (2) the patient's earlier objections to treatment (even though she was legally incompetent when she made them), and (3) the decreased benefits of treatment because of the patient's lack of cooperation (Collins, 1987, p. 273).[7]

New Jersey's *In re Conroy* (1985) followed close on the heels of the California and Massachusetts precedents. In this case, Claire Conroy's nephew (and legal guardian) had petitioned the superior court to have his aunt's nasogastric tubes removed. The court agreed, but Conroy's court-appointed lawyer objected to the decision and filed an appeal. In their appellate decision, the New Jersey court equated artificial feeding through tubes with artificial breathing through the use of a respirator. Then, in an attempt to remove some of the emotionalism from the issue, the court ruled that "naso-gastric tubes, gastrotomies, and intravenous infusions ... are medical procedures with inherent risks and possible side effects, instituted by skilled health care providers to compensate for impaired physical functioning." The court went on to explain that "once one enters the realm of complex high-technology medical care it is hard to shed the 'emotional symbolism' of food. However, artificial feeding such as nasogastric tubes, gastrotomies and intravenous feedings are significantly different from spoon feeding. They are medical procedures … and can be seen as the equivalent to artificial breathing" (*In re Conroy*, 1985, p. 1236).

Lastly, there is the Florida case of *Corbett* v. *D'Alessandro* (1986), which is important for its role in explicitly rejecting right-to-die limitations imposed by statutory law. Florida's natural-death law at the time specifically excluded "sustenance"—the legislature's term for food and fluids—from the category of procedures that could be withdrawn under right-to-die rules. Though this law gave pause to the lower courts, the Appeals Court ruled that the individual's prerogative to have a nasogastric tube removed was a constitutional right that could not be infringed upon by legislation.

Interestingly, given the courts' clear and generally unwavering trend toward allowing the withdrawal of food and fluids, many states passed living-will legislation throughout the 1980s that expressly forbade the withdrawal of ANH. The courts had been asking, both publicly and in their judicial decisions, that the legislatures provide statutory guidance in the right-to-die area. But this invitation to the legislatures was neither an open nor unqualified one. Indeed, as the Florida court's decision illustrates, judicial mediators would not hesitate to reject those provisions of state law that were found to violate some essential aspect of what the courts considered to be constitutionally protected rights—in this case, a right to withdraw food and fluids from individuals who are either terminally ill or in a persistent vegetative state.

Who Qualifies to Exercise the Right to Die?

This all brings us to the last critical issue: Who qualifies to exercise the right to die? There are really four possible classes of individuals to consider. First, there are the terminally ill individuals—those with life-threatening illnesses who have a finite amount of time left (six months or less is one generally accepted standard). Second, there are those in a PVS. These are individuals who, even though their eyes may be open, have no consciousness of their surroundings. People in a PVS are not terminally ill in the traditional sense, however, for theoretically they can exist for years and even decades with the appropriate life-support assistance. The third class consists of individuals who suffer from chronic, irreversible medical afflictions. These afflictions are not terminal either per se. Yet, even though death is not imminent for these individuals, their conditions are painful or debilitating enough to lead some to think life is not worth living. The fourth class involves everyone else. Let us consider the classes in reverse order.

No one makes the case in court (or anywhere else) that suicide should be granted as an individual right in the absence of a serious medical condition. Suicide has been and continues to be taboo in Western civilization, and we see no evidence of that changing. Consequently, the fourth class of individuals is eliminated a priori from qualifying under right-to-die rules.

The third class of individuals, those with chronically painful or seriously debilitating medical conditions, prompt significant controversy. Because some of these individuals will not necessarily die if medical procedures are withheld or withdrawn, they actually need assistance in dying. And that opens up the entire assisted-suicide debate. Generally, the courts have been tolerant. Aside from slapping a restraining order on Jack Kevorkian, which did not seem to be having much effect, the Michigan courts have more or less buckled under on the question of assisted suicide. The same could be said regarding Timothy Quill's case—lots of handwringing went on, but Quill was left unscathed by the judiciary. There is also the landmark California case involving Elizabeth Bouvia to consider.

Elizabeth Bouvia was twenty-eight in 1986 when she asked that medical personnel withdraw food and fluids from her so that she could die. A quadriplegic with severe cerebral palsy and intense arthritic pain, she was almost entirely dependent on others for her care. Over time, Bouvia came to believe that her condition made life not worth living. When the hospital refused her request to have food and fluids withdrawn, she took her case to the California courts, which ultimately found in her favor. One of the majority opinions put the matter quite bluntly: "The right to die is an integral part of our own destinies so long as the rights of others are not affected. That right should, in my opinion, include the ability to enlist assistance from others, including the medical profession, in making death as painless and quick as possible" (*Bouvia* v. *Super. Ct. of Los Angeles County*, 1986).

By and large, however, today's judiciaries are not engaged in euthanasia cases of this sort. Instead, the courts have been dealing primarily with the first two classes of individuals in this schema: the terminally ill and those in a persistent vegetative state (or irreversible coma).[8] Here, we can report overwhelming consensus: Those who find themselves in either of these conditions has the right to die, period. The courts, as has been noted, run into trouble when the individuals in question are rendered incompetent before having a chance to leave clear instructions on what they would want done. But the central point is that there seems to be little if any dissention.[9] Both those who are terminally ill and those who are in a persistent vegetative state qualify, in theory, to exercise an inherent, constitutionally protected right to die.

Case Law in Perspective

Although the courts continue to grapple with issues and standards of surrogate decisionmaking for incompetent patients, there is a general agreement on the three other central issues addressed in the right-to-die policy context. First, there is not much question about the right to die in the state courts. That right usually functions as a bottom-line foundation, below which the state courts are unwilling to go. New York's "clear and convincing" test can and has proved to be an important qualification to the right to die, as in the cases of *Storar* and, in Missouri, *Cruzan*. Still, most state case law supports the concept of a right to die. And the only Supreme Court decision on the right to die, *Cruzan* v. *Missouri*, suggests that the state courts are on firm ground here.

Second, when it comes to ANH, it seems clear that this is a medical therapy that can be either withheld or withdrawn pursuant to the right to die. And third, all patients who are either terminally ill or in a persistent vegetative state qualify for right-to-die status. Even conservative courts grant that much, as long as clear and convincing evidence can be produced as to the patient's wishes. The sole exception here seems to be for lifelong incompetents. In subjective-decision states like New York and Missouri, these individuals apparently must forgo any constitutionally protected right to die in favor of the state's due process interests in preserving life.

All this consensus begs the question: Why is there such widespread agreement? Theories of federalism suggest that the states have the capacity to operate independently of each other and that, absent rulings from the Supreme Court, the state courts are on their own to formulate decisions in cases that come before them. Of course, the courts do not operate in a vacuum: They are guided by constitutions, statutory laws, common laws, political culture, and judicial precedents within their own states. But if this were all there was to state-court decisionmaking, we would have to conclude that consensus was the serendipitous result of the various state courts stumbling, independent of each other, to the same policy conclusions.

Actually, this is not as improbable as it might sound at first blush. Indeed, the fifty states operate within political cultures in which similarities among laws, common-law traditions, and constitutional frameworks are the rule rather than the exception. In addition, there is a good deal of commonality to the cases that end up in the state courts.[10] Incompetence is one common theme. The overwhelming majority of patients were either clearly incompetent (80 out of 108 patients) or marginally incompetent (another 6 patients) at the time their cases were heard. Combining these two categories reveals that in 4 cases out of 5, the patient's ability to make decisions for himself or herself was impaired to one degree or another.[11] Usually, family members were allowed to serve as decisionmakers in such situations (court-appointed guardians were involved in only 11 of 80 cases involving incompetents).

Artificial nutrition and hydration provides another common thread of contention running through the body of case law: ANH was an issue in 43 percent of the cases (46 out of 108 cases).[12] Old age was also a common characteristic of principals involved in right-to-die cases. There is a small bulge in the age distribution at the beginning of life (9 cases involved infants) but a much larger bulge at the end of life. Although those over seventy years of age make up only 10 percent of the general population, nearly one-third of all right-to-die cases heard to date (34 out of 108) have involved patients seventy years or older. Indeed, more right-to-die patients are in their seventies (19, not counting the 17 cases in which the exact age of the patient is not reported) than in any other ten-year age bracket.

But a close look at right-to-die decisions suggests that more than a combination of serendipity and common denominators is at work here. Not only have the state courts tended to agree in principle on such decisions, they have also borrowed language from each other and cited each other's decisions extensively in the process. Despite their capacity for acting independently, state courts have not reinvented the wheel every time they have been confronted with the right to die. Instead, there has been a good deal of interstate borrowing. Indeed, there is a stream of policy literature that deals with this very phenomenon of "policy diffusion." Observers of the process argue that the courts "interact as part of a larger network of parallel organizations, using each other's decisions in different ways as part of their own policy process" (Glick, 1990, p. 94).

Policy Diffusion

Policy diffusion is a communications process in which judicial opinions of one court are picked up and used in the formulation of the decisions of another court in a different state. Often, lawyers are the messengers, making judges aware of innovative opinions in other states through their oral arguments and legal briefs. And, of course, court clerks do their own interstate reviews of decisions when helping judges draft decisions of their own. The proliferation of interest groups willing to file amicus curiae briefs (these are unsolicited, "friend of the court" advisories, filed by interested third parties) and the proliferation of computerized legal data bases have combined in recent years to facilitate the diffusion process. There may be no sound constitutional reason for state courts to give out-of-state court decisions any weight in their own deliberations, but it is clear that these rulings have an important impact on in-state decisionmaking nonetheless.

The 1976 case of Karen Ann Quinlan is a quintessential example of diffusion at work. The *Quinlan* decision was cited as a legal precedent in no less than 80 percent of all rulings rendered by superior state courts since the New Jersey case was heard. This is not to suggest that all the courts that have cited *Quinlan* agreed with that decision without qualification. Indeed, both the Massachusetts and New York courts made important qualifications to *Quinlan* in their own opinions.[13]

The New York court decision enjoyed some diffusion of its own: The Missouri court adopted New York's "clear and convincing" test, as did the court in Maine. Still, we should not let these admittedly important exceptions cloud the larger picture. State courts around the country, including those in New York and Missouri, have used *Quinlan* almost as if that were a precedent in the body of case law in their own state. And New Jersey's 1985 *In re Conroy* decision, legitimizing the withdrawal of food and fluids from terminally ill and hopelessly vegetative patients, was used the same way—again, just as if it were an in-state precedent upon which to build. Obviously, then, state courts borrow from each other, but we are still left to wonder why this is so.

One of the more durable explanations for borrowing holds that some trendsetting, activist courts are traditionally considered beacons of jurisprudence. As Glick (1992, p. 141) puts it, a "small subset of states with large and diverse populations and complex economies and government structures are much more likely to generate model litigation than simpler, homogeneous states." These trendsetters are looked to, it is argued, with some regularity by courts in other states. The state courts in California, New Jersey, New York, and Massachusetts are among those most often mentioned in this light.

It should come as no surprise to those familiar with the "beacons of jurisprudence" explanation of policy diffusion that twelve of the seventeen important right-to-die cases discussed in some detail in this chapter come from the courts of these four states.[14] Nor would it be a surprise that, within this group, New Jersey's three decisions have stood out as landmarks among landmarks, for the New Jersey court has been a jurisprudential leader in the specific area of individual liberties for two decades (Sullivan, 1990).[15] "Intrinsically," argues John Sexton, dean of the New York University Law School, New Jersey "is just one of fifty voices among the state courts. ... But time and time again other state courts and the Federal Court in constitutional and common law matters tend to follow the reasoning of the New Jersey Supreme Court" (Sullivan, 1990).

Still, two important questions about trendsetting might legitimately be raised. First, how does a state become a trendsetter? Part of the answer to this question may relate to the fact that controversial issues are more likely to arise and get dumped in the laps of justices who preside in states with heterogeneous populations, concentrated in densely packed cities and suburbs. The four beacon states cited here—California, New York, Massachusetts, and New Jersey—would certainly qualify on this score. Political subculture (Elazar, 1984, pp. 134–142) may be in play here, as well. Citizens in states with "individualistic" political subcultures might be predisposed to bringing their rights-based claims to the courts for mediation. According to Elazar, the populations of all four states noted here as trendsetters have dimensions of individualism to their political subcultures, with New Jersey the most individualistic of all. In addition, the judges in these states (who are products of this individualist political subculture themselves) may be more likely to take an activist role in setting precedents.

The second question the theory of trendsetting courts begs has to do with the following: Why do other states follow trendsetters' leads? The answer to this question may have something to do with the absence of prominent intrastate precedents. With newly emerging issues like those swirling around the right to die, diffusion may become something of a necessity. The absence of federal-court leadership is important to note here, as well. In such an environment, it becomes "increasingly important," according to Stewart Pollock (1985, p. 992), "for the courts to communicate with each other about significant decisions affecting fundamental rights. Horizontal federalism, a federalism in which states look to each other for guidance, may be the hallmark of the rest of the century."

There is one other possible explanation: It could be that trendsetters and followers alike are actually following a third source of guidance. This may well be the case with right-to-die issues for the dearth of precedents, both legislative and judicial, and the technicality of the subject matter have forced courts to look elsewhere for guidance. Apparently, the President's Commission report is one place the courts have looked with some regularity. That landmark document was cited in approximately 70 percent of all right-to-die court cases decided in the five years following its 1983 release. The position paper released by the American Medical Association in 1982, stating that it would be ethical for physicians to withhold or withdraw life-support systems (including ANH) from hopelessly ill individuals (including those in a PVS), was also heavily cited by courts in the years following its release (Glick, 1992, pp. 139–140).

Whatever the merits of this alternative explanation and regardless of whether the courts continue to adhere to Pollock's advice, it is enough for our purposes to note that state courts for the most part have followed each other's leads on the right to die. Naturally, then, they have also ended up in roughly the same places.

Summary: Case Law Versus Statutory Law

Overall, despite some twists and turns on the incompetency question, the courts have come to a consensus on the major right-to-die issues. But the same degree of general consensus in this area cannot be attributed to the state legislatures. Indeed, it was not until 1985 that a majority of the states even had living-will laws on the books to codify the right to die. And today, even though all but four states have such laws in force (the four holdouts are Massachusetts, Michigan, Nebraska, and New York), not much of a controversial nature has been resolved by that body of statutory law.

State judges, such as members of the New Jersey Supreme Court in its *Conroy* decision, have all but begged the legislatures to be more responsive in dealing with the right to die. But the legislatures, with a only few notable exceptions, have resisted the call. And even if state-court decisions have stimulated legislatures to address the right to die (Glick, 1992, p. 158), the substance of most laws that have been passed leave many important questions unanswered. Treatment of incompetent patients, artificial nutrition and hydration, and a number of other important matters have been dodged by many states, leaving one to wonder what exactly the legislatures have accomplished to date. We will answer that question in the next chapter, in order to shed some light on where the right-to-die debate is headed. We will also explore other problems that may lie on the horizon for those who wonder whether the right to die, for themselves and for their family, will be protected or even continue to exist under statutory law.

8

Policy Mediation and the State Legislatures: Common Ground, Divergence, and Liberal Trends

STATE-COURT JUDGES, if they can be believed, do not like making right-to-die policy.[1] Many, former Chief Justice Warren Burger among them, would go further and argue that the courts have no business making policy. As Justice Burger put it more than two decades ago, "In a democratic society legislatures, not courts, are constituted to respond to the will and consequently the moral values of the people" (cited in Kevorkian, 1991, p. 182).

In this spirit, state judges have for years been extolling, cajoling, and even begging the state legislatures to step into the breach and establish statutory rules and procedures for right-to-die cases. But the fifty state legislatures have been reluctant to respond. With only a few notable exceptions, the states have been led by the courts, codifying parts of what the courts have decreed, trying to put the brakes on or even attempting to reverse other court initiatives, and leaving for further litigation many of the more controversial issues faced by the courts in the last decade and a half. We turn first to a survey of the right-to-die legislation that has passed to date, before moving on to explain how this curious body of statutory law came into existence.

Statutory Overview

The state legislatures make right-to-die policy primarily by passing two kinds of legislation: durable power of attorney for health-care provisions and living-will laws.[2] Power of attorney provisions are important but restricted in their scope.

187

The laws themselves are usually brief and straightforward: Typically, the only details covered are those involving the legal and medical mechanics of declaring incompetency. As such, durable power of attorney for health-care provisions usually do little more than shunt the decision-making dilemma from a principal to a
surrogate, an individual who is sometimes referred to as a "health-care proxy."

By contrast, living-will legislation is more robust, which is why we spend more
time focusing on it. Consequently, it is through a survey of such legislation (with
reference to power of attorney laws as appropriate) that we will be able to assess
the progress the states have made in coming to grips with right-to-die issues that
the courts have been dealing with now for a decade and a half.

Common Ground

The California legislature led all others by passing the first living-will law in 1976,
the same year the *Quinlan* decision was handed down.[3] But California was not
alone for long, as seven more states passed laws the following year. After this ini-
tial surge, however, legislative activity slowed. The only three states to pass laws in
 the next four years were Kansas and Washington (1979) and Alabama (1981),
bringing the total number of states codifying the right to die to ten (see Table 8.1).

By 1992, thirty-seven of the remaining forty-one jurisdictions (the District of
Columbia included) added living-will laws to their state codes. All this legislative
activity is a bit deceiving, however, for only a few of the bills passed or being considered deal in a substantive way with the controversial issues that the courts have
been handling in the same time frame. Indeed, the state legislatures, for the most
part, have been codifying only the rudiments of the right to make advance directives regarding health-care decisions of the seriously and terminally ill. Thus,
many of these laws have a great deal in common regarding the mechanics associated with executing advance directives.

For one thing, living-will laws in most states are relatively brief and to the
point; in most cases, they run only a few pages. Other commonalities can be
lumped into six categories: (1) the rationale for existence of the law, (2) the kinds
of conditions covered, (3) the procedures for executing advance directives, (4) the
release of liability for health-care professionals, (5) health-care and life insurance
restrictions, and (6) the nature of the rights explicitly conveyed.

Rationale

Most living-will or natural-death acts establish an explicit rationale that addresses
the way in which the rush of medical technology has the potential to impinge on
dignity and autonomy of patients in terminal conditions. The statutes—borrowing from the text of state-court decisions—tend to make the argument that medi-

TABLE 8.1 Living-Will Legislation by Year of Passage (with selected court cases in parentheses)[a]

Year	State(s)
1976	California (*Quinlan*)
1977	Arkansas, Idaho, Nevada, New Mexico, North Carolina, Oregon, Texas
1978	No living-will laws passed
1979	Kansas, Washington
1980	(*Saikewicz, Spring*)
1981	Alabama (*Eichner, Storar*)
1982	Delaware, Washington, D.C., Vermont (*Bouvia*)
1983	Illinois, Virginia (*Colyer, Barber*)
1984	Florida, Georgia, Louisiana, Mississippi, West Virginia, Wisconsin, Wyoming (*Hier*)
1985[b]	Arizona, Colorado, Connecticut, Indiana, Iowa, Maine, Maryland, Missouri, Montana, New Hampshire, Oklahoma, Tennessee, Utah (*Conroy, Hamlin*)
1986	Alaska, Hawaii, South Carolina (*D'Alessandro*)
1987	No living-will laws passed
1988	No living-will laws passed
1989[c]	Minnesota, North Dakota (*Klein, Couture*)
1990	Kentucky (*Cruzan, Carder*)
1991	New Jersey, Ohio, Rhode Island, South Dakota (*Wanglie, Busalacchi*)
1992	Pennsylvania (*Donaldson, Busalacchi*, pending)

[a]States without living-will legislation (as of January 1, 1993) are: Nebraska (L. 671, on General File); Michigan (H. 4931, in the Judiciary Committee); New York (S. 2712, in the Health Committee); Massachusetts (no legislation pending; H. 2129 died in Senate).

[b]The Uniform Rights of the Terminally Ill Act (URTIA) was adopted by the National Commissioners on Uniform State Laws in 1985.

[c]A completely revised version of the URTIA was adopted by the National Commissioners on Uniform State Laws in 1989.

cal procedures today do not always provide something medically necessary to the patient. Consequently, the heath-care codes must be restructured to reflect that reality.[4]

Conditions Covered

All state laws currently in effect cover those who have been clinically diagnosed as terminal (but only thirteen states include the persistent vegetative state as a quali-fying condition). Although the clinical definition of *terminal* varies widely from state to state, it almost always refers to a condition in which life-supporting or life-sustaining procedures only serve to "prolong the dying process" or "postpone the moment of death." Most laws specifically exclude procedures designed to pro-vide comfort, care, and alleviation of pain from the kinds of therapies that may be withdrawn under living-will rules. In addition, the terminal prognosis typically must be certified in writing by an attending physician and a second physician, both of whom are physically present to examine the patient (a variation of the prognosis board proposed by the Washington court decision *In re Welfare of Colyer*).

Explicit distinctions are then usually drawn between what the law intends to sanction (allowing terminal patients to die) and those actions that the law is not meant to condone (mercy killing and euthanasia).[5] To drive home the point even further, the typical statute points out that a death covered under living-will provi-sions does not constitute a suicide or homicide. Similarly, actions taken pursuant to the act are not generally allowed to be considered or listed as the official cause of death.

It is clear from reading the statutes that a great deal of thought (and anxiety) went into considering what kinds of deaths were being sanctioned across the states. In general, the legislatures seemed to be quite deliberate in attempting to distinguish the very limited types of actions that they intended to sanction as part of a "natural death" from every other kind of "arranged death" (e.g., active eutha-nasia or assisted suicide), which would continue to be deemed medically unpro-fessional, morally reprehensible, and legally punishable under criminal law in most states.

Execution of the Living Will

The majority of living-will laws also converge in the more legally technical area associated with executing an advance directive. Typically, living wills need only be executed once as long as they are completed with all the same care as an estate will would be.[6]

In most cases, living-will forms can be obtained and completed without the as-sistance of an attorney. Several state laws require the dissemination of information on these wills as part of a program to inform the public of their legal rights to refuse medical care when in a right-to-die situation. A recent amendment to Maine's living-will law mandates that the appropriate forms be made available in local department of motor vehicle offices. Nevada law mandates that health-care facilities inform patients of their rights and make forms available on admittance, and Wisconsin law charges its Department of Health and Social Services with responsibility for distributing forms and information.[7]

Almost always, the declarant must be of majority age: eighteen years in most states, although Oklahoma uses twenty-one as the cutoff and Kansas prefers not to stipulate any particular age as a measure of legal competency. The document must usually be witnessed by two individuals, neither of whom have financial responsibility for the declarant or a financial stake in the disposition of the declarant's estate. In addition, falsification, destruction, or purposeful withholding of a living will or coercion associated with the execution of it is expressly prohibited and punishable under criminal law in most states.

Some states publish a model living will as part of their statutes, and most claim to honor any directive that is properly executed within the state or elsewhere, as long as the document adheres—generally and in spirit—to the principles and guidelines set down by the legislating state. Living wills generally enjoy severability in the states, as well; that is, if parts of any will are found to be invalid, the offending sections are legally severable from the whole so that defects in portions of the will in no way impair the validity of what remains.

In addition, descriptive personal statements—communicated orally, in writing, or otherwise—by the patient in a qualifying condition (i.e., terminally ill and of majority age) are also considered to be valid under living-will provisions in most states. The revocation of a living will also can be made by the personal statement—however communicated—of the qualified patient. Moreover, revocations usually can be made regardless of the patient's level of competency. Indeed, the Hawaii legislature recently considered and rejected an amendment to their living-will law that would have made revocation of a directive contingent on the competency of the patient.

Liability for Health-Care Professionals

Many have raised the issue of potential liability for health-care professionals who are involved in implementing an advance directive. Here again, most states seem to be in agreement. Generally speaking, living-will legislation explicitly protects health-care professionals by releasing them from legal liability for wrongful death when a good-faith effort has been made to comply with a declarant's wishes.[8]

On the one hand, if medical personnel choose to take part in allowing an individual to die, state laws will shield them from professional sanction as long as they participate in good faith and in accordance with a valid advance directive.[9] On the other hand, if caregivers find that, for moral or professional reasons, they cannot participate in the implementation of an advance directive, they generally are charged only with the responsibility of transferring the care of their patient to another provider who, presumably, would be more inclined to act in accordance with the patient's wishes.

Insurance Provisions

The issuance of insurance is yet another area in which the states have seen fit to promulgate, as a group, similar regulations regarding advance directives. Most states explicitly prohibit health insurers from requiring that a living will be made out as a qualification for health-care coverage.[10] Likewise, the states tend to expressly prohibit life insurers from disallowing benefits to the estates of patients who had a living will in force at the time of death. Many life insurance policies are voided in the case of a suicide, and the living-will statutes usually go to some length to explain that dying under living-will rules does not constitute such an act.

The Nature of the Rights Explicitly Conveyed

Lastly, most of the state laws end with a series of rights disclaimers. Two of the more prominent disclaimers address the unassuming and unrestrictive nature of the respective living-will statutes. In the first instance, state law generally makes it clear that no presumptions should be made regarding those who fail to execute a living will. That is to say, the failure of an individual to execute a living will should not be considered as presumptive evidence of his or her desire to be sustained on life-support equipment without limitation. Individuals, therefore, do not cede their right to have life support withdrawn simply because they failed to complete a legal directive to that effect.

In the second instance, states typically add the disclaimer that rights expressed within the laws are cumulative. That is, rights codified by the legislature add to the rights an individual enjoys outside the statute (in common law, in the case law, or as a matter of constitutional law). In other words, codification is not meant to infringe on, impair, or otherwise circumscribe the unstated rights and liberties of individuals under state jurisdiction. The message of these last two qualifications is clear: State statutes should be considered a place to start when divining what rights an individual has regarding the withholding and withdrawing of life-sustaining procedures, but the statutes are no place to end such an inquiry.

To What End?

We find this minimalist interpretation of statutory law entirely appropriate. The states agree on the fundamentals, but the more contentious issues—the specific definition of the word *terminal,* coverage of those in a persistent vegetative state, the artificial nutrition and hydration question—have been sidestepped by the majority of states.

The courts have moved a good way down the road toward building a consensus around the granting and protecting of rights to die for the terminally ill, but the legislatures have only been able to agree on rudiments. One need only take a look at the tremendous diversity in state laws that overlay the fundamental agreements we have just sketched to appreciate how really trifling all this legislative activity has been to date.[11]

Statutory Specifics

Arthur Berger (1990, p. 141) notes that when it comes to the right to die, legislatures can "muddy the waters" by drafting statutes that limit case-law rights and may even undermine patient autonomy in the process. That is, patients may have been better off had the legislature not acted at all. But the states have acted and in a variety of ways. A review of the diversity in living-will provisions across the states will put the limitations of current legislation into perspective.

Diversity Across the States

The diversity among existing statutes can be categorized into four general areas: (1) qualifying conditions under which rights to die may be exercised, (2) provisions for surrogate decisionmakers in cases of patient incompetence, (3) the treatment of artificial nutrition and hydration, and (4) consideration of women who are pregnant at the time they otherwise qualify under right-to-die rules. The first three areas roughly parallel categories of central consideration in the case law: existence of the right to die, incompetence, and ANH considerations. The fourth area—pregnancy—is one almost wholly untouched by the courts to date (with the exceptions represented by *In re Klein* and *In re Carder,* discussed in Chapter 5), and the only area where the legislatures have taken the lead in attempting to mediate potential right-to-die disputes.

Qualifying Conditions. Though all forty-seven jurisdictions with living-will statutes (forty-six states plus D.C.) target the terminally ill, the clinical definition of what passes for terminal varies in some important ways across the states. In addition to this definitional variation, there is also the question of individuals in a persistent vegetative state: Some states cover those in a PVS under their living-will statutes, but others do not (see Figure 8.1).

Under definitional distinctions, the state laws can be grouped into three categories of linguistic construction: conservative, liberal, and neutral. We use the

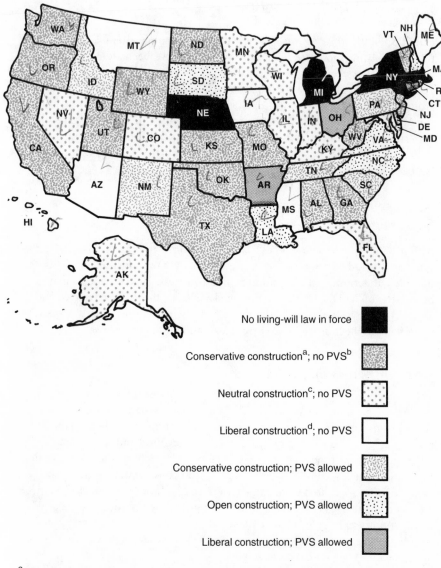

No living-will law in force

Conservative construction[a]; no PVS[b]

Neutral construction[c]; no PVS

Liberal construction[d]; no PVS

Conservative construction; PVS allowed

Open construction; PVS allowed

Liberal construction; PVS allowed

[a]Conservative construction: law allows the withdrawal of life-sustaining treatment only in cases in which death is imminent, regardless of whether life-sustaining treatment is maintained or withdrawn.

[b]PVS: a persistent vegetative state in which the patient has lost, permanently and irreversibly, all sensory perception of his or her surrounding environment—32 of the 33 states categorized as "no PVS" give no guidance regarding comatose states, and North Dakota alone specifically excludes patients in that condition.

[c]Neutral construction: language regarding qualifying conditions is simple and left open to interpretation.

[d]Liberal construction: law allows the withdrawal of life-sustaining treatment when such therapies are the only thing prolonging the life of a terminally ill individual; this is the Uniform Law Commissioners' recommendation (1989).

FIGURE 8.1 Qualifying conditions of living-will provisions regarding the terminal condition and persistent vegetative state (as of August 1, 1989).

word *conservative* here to refer to a restrictive reading of the concept *terminal;* *liberal* indicates a more expansive reading, and *neutral* implies that the term is not well enough defined to fit into either category.[12]

The twenty-one jurisdictions using the conservative definitional construction for the terminal condition require that death be imminent "whether or not" or "regardless of whether" life-sustaining treatment is continued (Figure 8.1). This definition is classified as conservative in construction because, if literally adhered to, laws employing this language provide little if any added decision-making authority to the individual. Strictly speaking, if death is imminent, regardless of whether or not life-sustaining procedures are employed, there is little point in having a statute permitting the withdrawal of such procedures (see Uniform Rights of the Terminally Ill Act, 1989, p. 5). That is, what good is a living-will statute granting an individual the right to die if death is imminent anyway?

Nine states use a more liberal construction. Their statutes consider individuals to be terminal if death would be imminent without the application of life-sustaining procedures (Figure 8.1). In other words, the individual must be seriously ill with an affliction that has shortened life expectancy substantially (some states use six months as a bench mark), but death need not be imminent, as long as life-sustaining procedures are maintained. This reading of the concept "terminal" comports with the model living-will legislation passed by the Uniform Commissioners in 1989, and it is the definition that the courts have embraced.

The remaining sixteen states use simple, neutral language to describe the "terminal" concept, thereby avoiding the "regardless of" versus "without" debate altogether (Figure 8.1). Instead, the word *terminal* is left open to interpretation. Consequently, no one knows ahead of time what kinds of situations would or would not be covered under the given statute.

In addition to these three definitional constructions, there is the important question of the persistent vegetative state. The question is important because there are approximately 14,000 cases of PVS in the United States today, and a substantial proportion of court cases involve individuals in this condition (approximately three out of four).

Although the clear consensus in the courts is to cover the PVS condition under right-to-die rules, the consensus of the states is to do just the opposite: Thirty-three states and the District of Columbia disqualify individuals in a persistent vegetative state from being covered under their living-will statutes. The remaining thirteen states with related laws on the books have complied with the Uniform Commissioners' 1989 model living-will law by including PVS patients in their coverage (Figure 8.1).

Inexplicably, some states that take the relatively bold and liberal step of adding permanent unconsciousness as a qualifying condition under the law use the conservative construction of what counts as terminal (among them is South Carolina, where all patients must be treated for at least six hours before treatments can be withheld). Likewise (but maybe less remarkably), not all states using the relatively liberal construction of the word *terminal* have taken the next logical step to expand the concept and include individuals in persistent vegetative states (Figure 8.1). At least several states have adopted each of the six permutations derived by combining the three constructions of the "terminal" concept with the two possible alternatives on PVS (to cover or to exclude).

The only thing that does seem clear, then, is that there is not much clarity in the institutional minds of the legislatures across the states when it comes to the codification of qualifying conditions. In this area, the state legislatures have dragged their feet in response to the state courts because no courts—not even the conservative Missouri and New York courts—have expressly prohibited the withdrawal of life support from those in a persistent vegetative state the way thirty-three states and D.C. have. Neither have the courts seen fit to adopt a conservative definition of the word *terminal* the way twenty-one state legislatures have. Apparently, the legislatures, bowing to the forces of restraint, have tried to put the brakes on court-made policy.

Health-Care Proxies. Health-care proxies are surrogate decisionmakers that have the legal power to make right-to-die decisions on behalf of incompetent principals. At this writing, only Alaska, Nebraska, and Oklahoma have no provisions to legally designate proxies or surrogates. Alaska's durable power of attorney law expressly prohibits proxies from making decisions on the "termination of life sustaining procedures" (Alaska Statutory Form Power of Attorney Act [1988]). In Oklahoma, an attorney general's opinion states that the Durable Power for Attorney Law in that state *cannot* serve as the basis of authority for health-care proxy decisionmaking (Society for the Right to Die, 1991). Nebraska simply has no law that deals with medical proxies.

The remaining states are hardly in agreement, however, for there is a good deal of variety associated with the designation mechanisms, designation types, and proxy restrictions that apply (see Figure 8.2). The mechanisms come in two varieties. First, proxy designations can be made through the execution of a durable power of attorney. Otherwise, provisions for designating a health-care proxy can be "built in" to the living-will law itself. Some states provide individuals with both alternatives (Florida, Indiana, Louisiana, Maine, Texas, Virginia, Wyoming).

There are also two different types of designation. Prospective designations are those made by the principal before becoming incompetent, and they identify by name the person or persons to whom decision-making authority would devolve should the principal become incompetent. The other type, ad hoc designations, identify a list of potential proxies to whom decision-making power would automatically flow in the absence of a specifically designated proxy.

Forty-four jurisdictions have durable power of attorney laws or living-will statutes that explicitly give declarants the ability to designate a surrogate decision-

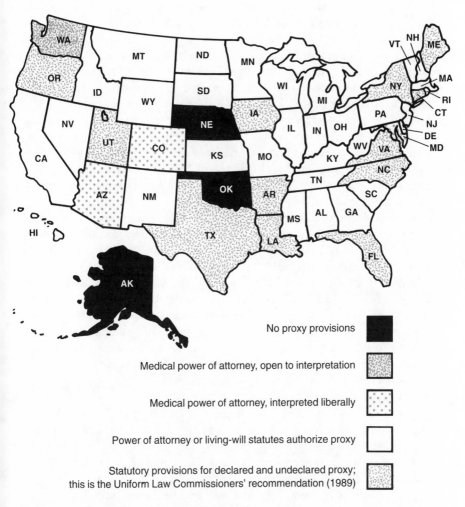

FIGURE 8.2 Provisions regarding the appointment of proxy decisionmakers for living wills and durable powers of attorney (as of August 1, 1991).

maker, by name (Society for the Right to Die, 1991). Three other states (Arizona, Colorado, and Maryland) have medical power of attorney laws that, through court decisions, opinions issued by attorneys general, or other statutes, have been interpreted as giving third parties the right to make decisions involving the withholding or withdrawal of life support (Society for the Right to Die, 1991). One other state, Washington, has a law on the durable power of attorney for health care that does not explicitly deal with the right-to-die scenario. In this case, the status of the law in right-to-die cases is a matter of some legal dispute.

Taken together, these forty-seven jurisdictions clearly reflect the consensus of courts across the states in at least acknowledging the possibility that a surrogate could make decisions for the principal. Meanwhile, the remaining three states continue to swim against the tide in this regard. However, consensus breaks down in the state laws—just as it did (but to a much lesser degree) in the state courts—when it comes to identifying decisionmakers.

For example, in Alabama and Hawaii, individuals can only declare physicians as proxies. In contrast, the laws in both California and Ohio expressly prohibit health-care professionals from acting as surrogate decisionmakers. Regulations regarding the witnessing of health-care proxy designations vary, as well. In five jurisdictions (California, North Dakota, South Carolina, Washington, and the District of Columbia), there are special provisions for patients who have been institutionalized. In these instances, at least one of the witnesses must be a patient advocate (e.g., an ombudsman from the department of health, aging, or social welfare). In a sixth jurisdiction, Georgia, a physician must be one of the two individuals witnessing an institutionalized patient's advance directive.

In several other states, the attending physician takes on the role of superproxy. In these states (California, Connecticut, Indiana, North Dakota, and Nevada), the relevant statutes do not require the physician to abide by a medically and legally sound advance directive. Rather, these laws only require that the physician give "great weight" to the declarant's wishes. Provisions in these states effectively give attending physicians veto power over the declarant and his or her legally designated proxies, thereby establishing a whole new class of de facto proxies.

Eleven of the forty-two jurisdictions with laws providing for declared proxies also give guidance in their living-will legislation regarding the designation of ad hoc proxies when a terminally ill patient is incompetent and no proxy has been previously designated. Typically, these states issue a prioritized list of individuals to whom decision-making authority devolves when a patient who has not specifically designated a surrogate becomes incompetent. The list varies from state to state, with some interesting twists.

Most states roughly adhere to the Uniform Commissioners' prescription, laid out in the 1989 version of their Uniform Rights of the Terminally Ill Act (URTIA). Here, decision-making authority devolves to the first available classification of individuals in the following list (National Conference of Commissioners on Uniform State Laws, 1989, pp. 12–13):[13]

1. the [adult] spouse of the individual;
2. an adult child, or, if there is more than one adult child, a majority of the adult children who are reasonably available;
3. the parents of the individual;
4. an adult sibling, or, if there is more than one adult sibling, a majority of the adult siblings who are reasonably available; or
5. the nearest adult relative of the individual, by blood or adoption, who is reasonably available for consultation.

Iowa adopts the URTIA standard in toto. In a minor variation, Florida and Louisiana adopt the same standard but place the legal guardian ahead of the adult spouse as the decisionmaker with top priority. In a further revision, Arkansas and New York add guardian at the top of the list, then go on to substitute in loco parentis individuals and the majority of adult heirs, in that order, for the fifth classification of the Uniform Commissioners' version. In a similar vein, Texas and Virginia list guardian, spouse, adult children, parents, and next of kin as the appropriate priority for decisionmakers.

In another interesting twist worthy of note, Utah lists guardian, then spouse, then reverses the following two classifications, putting parents ahead of adult children in order of priority. North Carolina law adds still more variation to the URTIA theme by listing spouse, then guardian, the majority of first-degree relatives, and the attending physician as those with ordered priority for decisionmaking. And in a radical and rather loosely constructed departure from the Uniform Commissioners' standard, Connecticut law authorizes the attending physician to "gather whatever information he/she can regarding intentions of the principal" in order to determine what course of action to take in right-to-die situations where no proxy has been designated for an incompetent patient (Connecticut Gen. Stat., 1992).

More important than these minor variations on the URTIA theme, however, is the fact that a number of important questions go unaddressed altogether. For example, what happens if a group of individuals within a decision-making class cannot reach consensus (e.g., adult children)? Should the majority rule? Should any one individual in the class have veto power over the rest? Should split decisions go to those who favor the preservation of life? These are all possible resolutions, but neither the Uniform Commissioners nor the state legislatures provide any clues on which direction to take in this matter.[14]

Even more importantly, not one state has broached the subject of decision-making criteria. The state courts have labored in this vineyard since the New Jersey court handed down the *Quinlan* decision in 1976. Since that time the courts have wrestled mightily with the subject, codifying several loose standards (the substituted-judgment, best-interests, and subjective-judgment standards) along the way. Yet, the state legislatures have ducked the matter entirely. The surrogacy issue is only partly about who should play the role of decisionmaker for the real crux of the matter has to do with *how* the surrogate should make the decision. In this regard, the entire body of statutory law passed to date is essentially no help at all.

Artificial Nutrition and Hydration. The withholding or withdrawing of artificial nutrition and hydration is one of the most controversial issues raised by the debate over the right to die. As noted in Chapter 7, consensus has emerged in the courts: ANH is generally considered to qualify as a medical procedure that might potentially be withheld or withdrawn in right-to-die situations. Even generally conservative Chief Justice of the Supreme Court William Rehnquist argued, in the *Cruzan* decision, that "we assume that the United States Constitution would grant a competent person a constitutionally protected right to refuse lifesaving nutrition and hydration" (*Cruzan v. Director, Missouri Department of Health*, 1990). The socially conservative Catholic church has also moderated its stand in recent years by acknowledging the propriety of withdrawing food and fluids in "exceptional" cases (see Chapter 6; also Catholic Bishops, 1991, p. 22). At the same time, most state legislatures have been more cautious in their approach.

The most common tack has been to avoid the issue altogether: Twenty of forty-seven jurisdictions with living-will laws in force make no mention whatsoever of artificial nutrition and hydration, despite its central importance to the debate (see Figure 8.3). When ANH is mentioned, a fair number of states either limit (Colorado, Florida, Illinois, Kentucky, North Dakota, Ohio, and South Dakota) or equivocate (Arkansas and Indiana) about the right to withdraw or withhold artificially administered food and fluids. Only thirteen states have codified what is now the mainstream case-law position in which ANH qualifies as a procedure that a patient or surrogate decisionmaker might choose to forgo in a right-to-die situation (Figure 8.3).

In the seven other states that mention but limit the right to withdraw ANH, circumstances in which ANH is allowed vary in the degree of restriction. In Kentucky and North Dakota, the law allows for the withdrawal of ANH only if it can be established that continued provision will be painful or excessively burdensome to the patient. Colorado and North Dakota laws make the distinction between artificial feeding (naso- or gastrointubation), which can be withheld or withdrawn, and the more conventional methods of obtaining nutrition and hydration (eating and drinking through the mouth, even if artificially assisted): The latter does not qualify as something that can be withheld or withdrawn in either state. Tennessee and Illinois laws allow for the withholding and withdrawal of ANH as long as lack of nutrition and hydration is not considered to be the official cause of death. And,

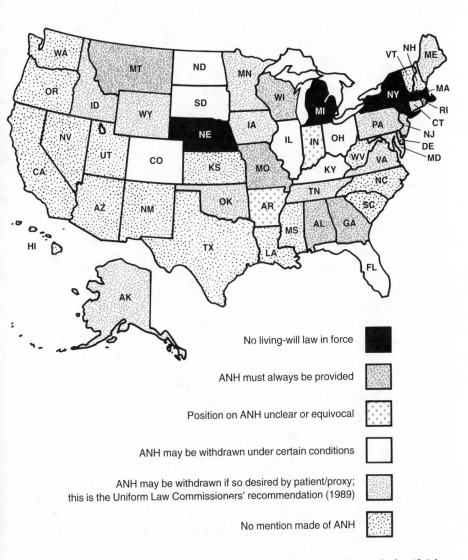

FIGURE 8.3 Living-will provisions regarding the withholding or withdrawal of artificial nutrition and hydration (as of August 1, 1991).

in more liberal language, Florida allows for the withdrawal of ANH if its sole purpose is to artificially postpone an otherwise imminent death.

Meanwhile, in a move that seems designed to flout the mainstream case-law position, five states (Alabama, Georgia, Missouri, Montana, and Wisconsin) have passed or amended their laws to explicitly prohibit the withholding or withdrawal of ANH. Missouri is especially interesting in this regard, given that it was the venue of Nancy Cruzan's case, in which, with guidance by the U.S. Supreme Court, ANH was allowed to be withdrawn after seven years of legal battles.

Thus, it seems that only a small proportion of the state legislatures have been able to reach the same conclusion that the state courts have with regard to artificial nutrition and hydration. Again, forces of restraint have apparently had more impact on the legislators, and judges have enjoyed more freedom in responding to the considerable forces of activism that have welled up in American society in the last several decades.

The Impact of Pregnancy on the Right to Die. The right of pregnant women to make right-to-die decisions is one area in which the states seem to be ahead of the courts when it comes to establishing rules. For the most part, the lack of direction offered by the state courts in this area might be attributed to a lack of opportunity: In the 106 cases involving the right to die that were cited by the National Center for State Courts (National Center for State Courts, 1992, pp. 155–172) from 1976 through 1992, only three involved a pregnancy, and only two (*In re Klein* [1989] and *In re A. C.* [1990]) involved a decision by the court. This makes the activism of state legislatures even more interesting. Despite the lack of court-sponsored impetus and despite the relative rarity of right-to-die cases involving pregnancy, the clear majority of states—thirty-five of forty-six states with living-will laws in force—have proceeded to address the issue of pregnancy in their right-to-die legislation. Almost all of these states—thirty-four of thirty-five—have gone on record to foreclose the right of women to control medical decision-making in right-to-die situations when they also happen to be pregnant (see Figure 8.4).

Many states (twenty in all) disqualify pregnant patients, without exception, from exercising the right to die. In these states, pregnancy automatically voids the validity of an advance directive, written or otherwise. The remaining states that mention pregnancy pull back from a blanket prohibition but leave substantial obstacles in the way nonetheless.

Six states (Arkansas, Arizona, Idaho, Illinois, Minnesota, and Ohio) qualify their pregnancy exclusion by stipulating that the advance directives of pregnant women will be voided if the continued development and live birth of the fetus is "possible." In more liberal language, five other states (Alaska, Colorado, Iowa, Montana, and Rhode Island) void advance directives only when the continued development and live birth of the fetus is "probable." This is also the position ad-

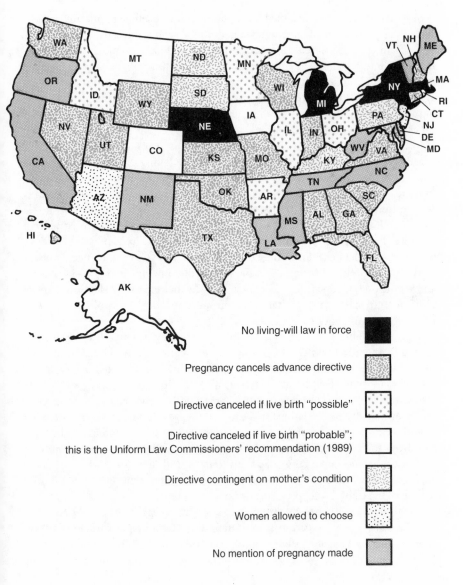

FIGURE 8.4 Living-will provisions regarding pregnancy (as of August 1, 1991).

vanced by the Uniform Commissioners in the 1989 version of the model living-will bill (Section 6[c]).

Several other states have added more specific tests, disallowing the advance directives of pregnant women except when doing so would cause the women unrelieved pain (North Dakota) or harm and unrelieved pain (Kentucky, Pennsylvania, and South Dakota). Pennsylvania's law regarding pregnancy is especially interesting for the legislature backed up its restriction with a promissory note, agreeing—as part of the living-will law—to cover all medical costs for maintaining an incompetent and severely ill pregnant woman who is not covered for medical expenses by a third-party payer.[15]

In addition to these restrictive positions, there is also silence. No mention of pregnancy is made at all in eleven jurisdictions (including the District of Columbia, where the Angela Carder case was heard). It is beyond the scope of this inquiry to delve into legislative hearings and debate records from these jurisdictions to determine whether such omissions were intentional or the product of simple oversight. In liberal California, the Catholic Conference is said to have extracted a promise that pregnancy would not be addressed (Glick, 1992, p. 96). Oversight might explain the behavior of the Louisiana legislature: Given this state's conservative record on the abortion question, it is hard to imagine that Louisiana legislators purposely dodged the pregnancy issue. In the remaining states, it is more difficult to speculate on whether omission was a product of simple oversight or political accommodation.

The one notable exception in all of this is New Jersey. There, the legislature has turned in an entirely different and much more liberal direction by granting that "a female declarant may include in an advanced directive executed by her, information as to what effect the advanced directive shall have if she is pregnant" (New Jersey Act [1972]). This language (pregnancy is not mentioned in any other context elsewhere in the legislation) suggests that the New Jersey legislature intended to grant the declarant primary control over the fetus—a clear and marked departure from the approach taken in the other states. This course is much more in tune with the two major court decisions to date. Both the New York court (*In re Klein*) and the D.C. court of appeals (*In re A. C.*) found that the women did, in fact, have the right to die, pregnant or not.[16]

At this point, it might be reasonable to ask why, except in the case of New Jersey, the states have decided to strike out in this area of right-to-die legislation when they have been sluggish in almost every other respect. After making a preliminary investigation, we have concluded that interest-group dynamics are at the heart of the matter.

As we have noted, there is a distinctive lack of pressure from parties who might be interested in advancing policy in this area: parents of severely handicapped infants, those interested in increasing the pool of harvestable organs, and women's rights activists (who are probably too worried about *Roe* v. *Wade* to spend much time or political capital on this issue). Instead, the only actively engaged interest groups seem to be those arrayed on the prolife side of the ledger—the various state Catholic conferences and the antiabortion lobby. Representatives of these groups generally demand and get a seat at the table when it comes time to hammer out compromises in right-to-die legislation.

For some of these groups, pregnancy considerations have become something of a cause célèbre. In most states, these right-to-life groups have lobbied actively, even tenaciously, for an "incubator" amendment to living-will laws currently being considered.[17] As the data on legislative provisions suggest, in most cases, these right-to-life groups have had their way with both the legislatures and the legislation. Ultimately, then, maybe the better question is this: How did New Jersey get away with its radical departure on the pregnancy question?[18]

Trends in Statutory Law

In spite of all the diversity among the states on the key issues reviewed here, there are some clear and marked trends in state legislative activity that represent something of a convergence for statutory law across the states. In almost all cases, the legislatures are finding that convergence means moving toward the general consensus of the state courts. States recently adopting living-will legislation tend to incorporate more leniency in their laws than those that did so earlier. Moreover, states that have amended their existing laws tend almost exclusively to do so in a generally liberal (what Glick [1992, p. 184] calls "facilitative") direction.

First, it appears that the state legislatures are becoming more liberal in their definition and conceptualization of a "terminal" condition. Second, most legislatures are becoming increasingly liberal in their treatment of artificial nutrition and hydration. Third, provisions for the designation of proxy decisionmakers are becoming more comprehensive. Fourth, pregnancy as a disqualifying condition may be getting a more liberal treatment, though the evidence on this score is far from definitive. And fifth, there are a number of generally liberal perfecting amendments now wending their way through the state legislative labyrinth.

Qualifying Conditions Revisited. First and probably most significant is the general tendency of the states to liberalize conditions that apply under living-will statutes. On the definitional front, the first seven years of legislative activity were dominated by the use of conservative definitions of the "terminal" prognosis. In contrast, all nine state laws using the liberal construction—in which death is imminent "regardless" of whether life support is continued or not—have been enacted or amended to reflect the liberal approach sometime in the past seven years.

With regard to the PVS question, we note that a number of states recently passed laws or amendments to existing laws that have added permanent unconsciousness as a qualifying right-to-die classification. Three of the thirteen states that allow life support to be withdrawn from PVS patients (Ohio, Pennsylvania, and South Dakota) have passed living-will laws to that effect in the past two years. Five more of these thirteen states (Arizona, New Hampshire, Connecticut, South Carolina, and Virginia) have amended their existing statutes to include PVS in the same time frame.

In addition, two states currently debating living-will legislation (New York and Michigan) include PVS in the bills now being considered. And finally, a number of other states (Oregon, Tennessee, Georgia, Washington, Florida, North Carolina, and Hawaii) are actively considering or have recently considered amendments that would accomplish the same end if adopted. In both the definitional and PVS reforms, the state legislatures seem to be playing catch-up with the state courts. The courts have never been troubled by the fine distinctions that have proved so vexing for the legislatures to this point, but clearly, the legislatures are on their way to coming around.

ANH Revisited. Second in order of importance is the generally liberal course the states have been taking in the matter of withdrawing artificial nutrition and hydration. To this point, twenty states have passed provisions, several just recently, that allow for withholding or withdrawing ANH under certain conditions. Five of the six states to pass living-will laws since 1990 are among this group (Kentucky, New Jersey, Ohio, Pennsylvania, and South Dakota), and two other states (Connecticut and Virginia) have passed amendments to this effect in the same time frame. Other states (Georgia, Indiana, North Carolina, and Washington among them) are actively considering moving in this direction. Efforts to amend the living-will statutes in Oregon, Hawaii, and South Carolina to allow for the withdrawal of ANH also were considered in the early 1990s.[19]

Pennsylvania, in the most liberal move to date along these lines, passed a living-will law in 1992 that provides a checklist of procedures a declarant could use to indicate exactly what he or she would wish to receive or refuse in the way of medical interventions (Pennsylvania Advance Directive for Health Care Act [1991]). In addition to ANH, the list includes cardiac resuscitation (mixing the DNR philosophy with the living will), receipt of blood products, artificial respiration, kidney dialysis, surgery, and antibiotics. Though it is not clear how much weight a patient's declaration would carry (for example, in cases where antibiotics were checked off as something the declarant wished to refuse), the fact that such a checklist exists at all is indicative of a more general trend toward individual autonomy in medical decisionmaking.

Indeed, only one state has seemed to be swimming against this legislative (and judicial) tide in recent years: Montana. There, the legislature recently amended a statute to expressly prohibit the withdrawal or withholding of nutrition and hydration (Montana Code, 1991). Otherwise, however, the states once again seem to be taking their lead from the courts, which, at least since New Jersey's *Conroy* decision in 1985, have firmly supported the right to withdraw artificially provided nutrition and hydration.

Proxies Revisited. Provisions that regularize the assignment of proxies—both prospectively by the declarant and automatically according to a priority list— have also undergone something of a convergence. Unlike PVS and ANH provisions, however, proxy provisions have not yet become the subject of a ground swell of legislative interest. Still, given current trends, we should expect that states without proxy provisions (Alaska, Nebraska, and Oklahoma) and states with incomplete proxy provisions (see Figure 8.2) will amend their statutes over the course of time to accommodate the declaration and assignment of surrogate decisionmakers, as recommended by the Uniform Law Commissioners' (ULC) amendments of 1989 and subsequently adopted, in one form or another, by a number of other states.

This is where the courts and the legislatures are more closely matched. The issue of surrogacy really opens up a whole new arena of problems and policies, and neither the courts nor the legislatures have been very successful in (1) determining *who* should make decisions when there is no clear evidence of patient intent or (2) establishing criteria for guiding *how* those decisions should be made. For their part, the courts have dabbled with the "who" question and spent a good deal of time trying to establish rules that would guide behavior, in response to the "how" question (e.g., the substituted-judgment and best-interests standards). Meanwhile, the state legislatures have taken a swipe at the "who" question (by providing for ad hoc proxies if none are designated in advance directives, for example), but as a group, they seem to have left the "how" question for another day. We suspect that surrogate decisionmaking for incompetents will remain a primary source of contention for both the courts and the legislatures in the years to come. But the courts can be expected to lead the way where, apparently, the legislatures fear to tread.

Pregnancy Revisited. Currently, New Jersey (the last state to pass a living-will law) and Arizona (which recently amended its law) are the only two states that explicitly empower women with the right to make medical decisions for themselves should they be pregnant at the time they become enmeshed in a right-to-die scenario. But these two states may be part of an emerging trend. All four states that hedge their positions by suggesting that the disposition of the fetus may be determined, in part, by the effect the continued pregnancy would have on the mother (North Dakota in 1989, Kentucky in 1990, South Dakota in 1991, and Pennsylvania in 1992) are among the group of eight states to have passed living will laws since 1989.

One might see, in the actions of these six states taken together, the beginning of a predisposition to liberalize right-to-die laws along the lines of individual autonomy or at least individual deference. At the same time, the two states actively con-

sidering passage of a living-will law muddy the picture a bit. The New York statute currently being weighed does not mention pregnancy, and the Michigan draft
explicitly excludes pregnant women from protection. There can be little doubt
that most states will want to wait on the pregnancy question until they have time
to assess the long-term impact of the Supreme Court's ruling on the Pennsylvania
Abortion Control Act (*Planned Parenthood of Southeastern Pennsylvania* v. *Casey*
[1992])—a decision that, on its face, seemed to swing open the door to further
"reasonable" state restrictions on the right to privacy. One cannot help but think
the states will also be watching closely to see what further direction(s) the Supreme Court takes on *Roe* v. *Wade* before they expend much political capital in
this religiously charged and highly controversial area of public policy.

Perfecting Amendments. There are some other minor and more technical areas in the living-will arena where relatively noncontroversial, perfecting alter-
ations in legislation may presage future, generally liberalizing trends. For example, the recently passed New Jersey law attempts to bring living-will declarations
into compliance with hospital-based DNR policies. The Joint Commission on Accreditation for Hospital Organizations has, for several years, required their member hospitals to formulate DNR policies. Since there is so much overlap between
state living-will laws and these institutionally promulgated DNR policies, the
logic and, ultimately, the necessity of reconciling procedures associated with these
two kinds of medical directives may prove compelling.

North Dakota's contribution to the ongoing living-will debate involves the ex-
emption of emergency medical personnel (EMS) from liability for failing to comply with an advance directive (North Dakota, 1991). The rationale here is self-evident. Operating almost entirely outside the institutional setting and in crisis
situations, EMS personnel cannot be expected to know what an individual patient's advance directive states. Nor should they be expected, while on an emergency call, to find out if an advance directive exists and what (if one does exist) it
says, at the expense of caring for the patient. Pennsylvania's recently passed law
provides EMS personnel with this kind of protective umbrella.

In one of the most dramatic and progressive right-to-die developments to date,
twenty-one states have managed to combine the philosophy of the DNR order
with concerns about the ability of EMTs to act in accordance with advance directives. The product of this interest and concern is an entirely new right-to-die instrument: the nonhospital DNR, made legitimate either by statute (in Arizona,
Colorado, Florida, Georgia, Illinois, Maryland, Montana, New Mexico, New York,
Pennsylvania, Rhode Island, Tennessee, Utah, Virginia, Washington, West Virginia, and Wyoming) or by legislative protocol (in California, New Hampshire,
and Vermont). The nonhospital DNR makes it possible for individuals to indicate
their desire not to be resuscitated in an emergency situation by using brightly col-
ored forms (Arizona's form is printed on orange paper), wallet cards, or—as in
California—Medic Alert–style bracelets or necklaces bearing the inscription "Do

Not Resuscitate—EMS" ("Hospitals Establish Policies," 1993). As with living-will legislation, the substance of these laws (regarding those who qualify to execute a nonhospital DNR, for example), varies tremendously from state to state. But clearly these new instruments, taken as a group, provide more options for individuals to express their end-of-life intentions and additional safeguards to ensure that those end-of-life intentions are honored.

As for perfecting the living will a number of other states have picked up on the California provision requiring that one of the two witnesses to an advance directive made by a resident of a long-term care facility be an ombudsman from outside the institution. This seems to be a logical and self-evident protection against abuses of the living-will laws. We only wonder why other states did not follow California's lead in this more quickly.

The issue of dispute resolution also raises some interesting questions. When an individual has executed both a living will and a durable power of attorney, which document controls? Most states are silent on this question. But a few have made their preferences explicit. In Illinois, the durable power of attorney trumps all declarations, but according to the recently passed law in South Dakota, the latest signed document controls. In Kansas, the living will controls, and in Nevada, the proxy's decisions are required by law to conform with the intentions of the principal as expressed in the living will. As conflicts arise between living wills and durable powers of attorney for health care, more states, no doubt, will follow the lead of those in which the order of priority is made clear.

Lastly, there seems to be a movement afoot to increase the availability of living-will information. For example, Maine now requires that living-will forms be provided to applicants for driver's licenses and hunting licenses. And Oregon requires health-care facilities to give patients advance directive materials. The Patient Self-Determination Act only requires that institutions inform patients of their rights under state law and offer to help obtain further information on advance directives if requested. Oregon has taken the next step and required that living-will forms be provided whether requested or not. In an innovative twist, Illinois driver's licenses now note whether the driver has a current advance directive or not. Clearly, the dissemination of information—with regard to both formulating and implementing advance directives—is the key here, given the arcane state of legislative language and the sensitive nature of the issues involved. Therefore, these developments promise to add their own measure of policy activism to the right-to-die milieu.

Explaining Legislative Behavior

When all is said and done, there are really three kinds of legislative behaviors that bear explaining. First, why do the states pass living-will laws in clusters with so much in common (at least with regard to the rudiments)? Second, why has the substance of those laws diverged so fundamentally from the general consensus positions taken in the state courts regarding the really important issues, like ANH, PVS, and pregnancy? And finally, what is behind the more recent, generally liberal trend toward convergence between the legislatures and the courts?

Answering these questions is no mean feat due to the rich diversity of political cultures and idiosyncratic dynamics that are the hallmarks of legislature behaviors across the fifty states. Still a number of overlapping generalizations that cut across state borders can be used to explain, in a general way, the behavior of the state legislatures as bodies of mediation in the right-to-die debate.

Explaining Common Ground

The concept of "policy diffusion" has been the topic of a stream of literature in policy studies since Jack Walker's seminal work on the subject, "The Diffusion of Innovations Among the American States," was published in 1969. Policy diffusion in the legislative context speaks to the issue of convergence among state legislatures on new and emerging issues of public policy (just as judicial policy diffusion speaks to the forces that edge courts toward consensus in innovative policy arenas). According to observers of representative assemblies in the states, a small group of legislatures have the reputation for being "policy innovators"—"beacons of legislative activity" that cut a policy-making path that other states follow (borrowing from Chapter 7, where innovative state courts were called "beacons of jurisprudence").

The ranks of these legislative beacons are thought to be dominated (again, as with the court innovators) by populous, urban, industrialized and affluent states with independent political cultures (like California, New York, New Jersey, Michigan, Massachusetts, and Pennsylvania). Usually, with their complex and diverse societies, such states are among the first to adopt progressive legislative policy innovations (Glick, 1992, pp. 43–44; Walker, 1969), and other less populous, less urban, and more homogeneous states within a "beacon" state's region or sphere of influence tend to fall in line only after the trail has been blazed.

The fact that California's legislature was the first to adopt a living-will law fits nicely into this framework. So, too, does the fact that in the year following adoption of California's Natural Death Act (NDA), five of the seven states to pass living-will laws were in the West (Idaho, Nevada, New Mexico, Oregon, and Texas). Moreover, three of those Western states within California's sphere of influence passed laws that were substantially similar to the California act. Indeed, the living-will bill sponsor in Nevada put the matter quite explicitly, stating that the purpose of his proposed measure was "to bring our law into conformity with California" (cited in Glick, 1992, p. 169).

Sometimes, according to experts on diffusion, states do not follow each other so much as they follow the lead of respected third parties. This dynamic, too, seems to help explain the commonalities among the states' living-will codes. Just as the courts were found to derive ideas and support from third parties (on the President's Commission report and the AMA policy statement, see Chapter 7), so have the legislatures looked beyond their own realm for guidance.

They found it in the form of a model living-will bill—the Uniform Rights of the Terminally Ill Act (URTIA)—developed through 1984 and officially released in 1985 by the National Conference Commission on Uniform State Laws (NCCUSL).[20] Bill sponsors in fully half of the states enacting living-will laws in this period claimed to have been "stimulated" by the NCCUSL, ultimately basing their own bills on its uniform law (Glick, 1992, p. 173). Indeed, large portions of the URTIA are evident in the bills passed in Alaska, Arkansas (amendments to the 1977 law), Iowa, Maine, Missouri, Montana, and Oklahoma.[21] Publication of the URTIA, with the 1983 release of the President's Commission report supporting comprehensive living-will legislation, and the AMA endorsement of patient self-determination, also in 1983, all helped to chart a course for legislative advocates in the twenty states that successfully passed legislation in 1984 and 1985.

In addition to the NCCUSL, a number of other third parties—primarily interest groups and national associations—played a role in leading state lawmakers to the legislative well. For example, the Society for the Right to Die published its own version of a model living-will bill, the Medical Treatment Decision Act (MTDA), for state consideration in the early 1980s. Although no state adopted the MTDA in toto, a number of living-will laws were influenced by MTDA provisions, including statutes in Alabama, the District of Columbia, Florida, Illinois, Indiana, Kansas, Louisiana, New Hampshire, Oregon, South Carolina, Virginia, Washington, West Virginia, and Wyoming (Meisel, 1989, pp. 336–337). Professional organizations that serve the interests of state legislatures, such as the National Conference of State Legislatures (NCSL) and the American Legislative Exchange Council (ALEC), also play a role in the diffusion process.[22]

Sometimes, innovative ideas travel across state boundaries via regional and national news programs, nationally read newspapers (such as the *New York Times* and *Wall Street Journal*), or weekly news magazines. State legislators use these media to look at other legislatures in search of analogies between the situations they find themselves in and those of another state where the policy issue has already been successfully resolved. When searching for a solution, legislators engage in the "politics of the possible" by pirating ideas from other states, then rationalizing this behavior to their colleagues, their constituents, and themselves by asking, rhetorically, "If it works great in state X, why not here?"

Once an innovation finds its way into a number of states, the new policy tends to gain a momentum of its own, becoming something "every state should have" (Walker, 1969, p. 890). Recalcitrant legislatures are eventually forced (some might say "shamed") into adopting trendy solutions by media coverage of legislative in-action in the home state. Thus, an element of interstate competition enters into the picture for those states who are slow to mediate solutions to perceived prob-lems.

The state legislatures, like the state courts, are under no obligation to borrow precedents from their neighbors. But like the courts, the legislatures seem predis-posed to use each other's laws, while also looking to respected third parties like the Uniform Commissioners as guides for their own policy mediation purposes. Clearly, then, policy diffusion is in play here, helping to explain the existence of a common ground among state laws.

At the same time, the state legislatures exhibit some unexpected behaviors in this regard. For example, it took New Jersey and Pennsylvania fourteen and fif-teen years, respectively, to follow in California's footsteps in passing living-will legislation, while forty-three other states stepped in line ahead of these two "in-novative" states. In addition, three of the four states that have yet to pass a living-will law—New York, Massachusetts, and Michigan—are supposedly innovative states. Even more surprising, when Henry Glick ran correlations between a state's tendency to be innovative (liberal) and the speed with which it passed a right-to-die law, he found a mild relationship—in the unexpected direction! That is, the more liberal the policies in a given state, the less likely the state's legislature was to have passed a living-will law.

Digging deeper into this seeming paradox, Glick (1992, p. 177) found a state's policy liberalism to be closely related to the percentage of the population claiming to be Catholic, and it seems that the Catholic variable as a force of restraint over-whelms any predisposition to exhibit liberalism on the right-to-die question. Glick summarizes his findings by noting that "the larger a state's Catholic popula-tion, the less likely states are to adopt living will laws." According to him, religion is more important than ideology in this instance since the right to die is an issue that is viewed primarily in moral, as opposed to economic, terms (even though economic issues lie just beneath the surface).[23] Glick sums up the matter bluntly: "No other interest group has been as concerned with these laws as the Catholic church, nor have they had the impact. It appears that the Catholic church was able to prevent the enactment of living will laws in most states for many years" (1992, p. 202).[24]

Explaining Divergence

Just as the lack of legislative activity on the right to die can be attributed to the Catholic church, the ultimate passage of conservative laws that diverge from the generally liberal positions taken by the courts can be traced to Catholic influences on the legislative process. As trends in popular opinion, popular and professional publications, and court agitation increased pressure on state legislators to act through the early 1980s, Catholic elites shifted ground. In these years, the passage of living-will laws became increasingly inevitable and, from the Catholic point of view, maybe even desirable. In the face of the judicial activism represented by the parade of liberal court decisions that were being issued,[25] Catholics found that they could no longer afford the luxury of outright resistance. Some Catholic activists even began to see legislative innovation as a vehicle for rolling back some of the advances made by the courts on the right-to-die front.

Ultimately, fearing that continued resistance would shut them out of the process completely, Catholic elites made the strategic decision to soften their stand and either endorse or agree not to oppose passage of limited living-will laws that incorporated important restrictions that were key to the Catholic position (e.g., pregnancy exclusions, ANH restrictions, and applicable conditions that were narrowly defined). The authoritative pronouncement was made in 1984, when the National Conference of Catholic Bishops officially abandoned its blanket opposition to living-will legislation. Not coincidentally, seven states passed laws that same year to end something of a drought in legislative activity, and thirteen more states joined the fold the following year, creating the biggest watershed in legislative activity regarding the right to die in the issue's entire history.

Not all the credit (or blame) for the passage of conservative right-to-die laws in the states can be laid at the feet of Catholic elites, however, for at least some of the legislative resistance on the right-to-die issue can be attributed to the general forces of restraint laid out in Chapters 1 and 2. Legislatures are simply collections of individuals who presumably share a common cultural framework with their constituents. Understandably, then, if Americans tend to fear death and deny their own mortality, their legislative representatives will, as well. For most—legislators included—the notion that death can be "managed" through consideration of living-will laws is even more difficult to cope with.

We have made a case in Chapters 3 through 6 that the forces of activism are on the rise, to the point where they are beginning to overwhelm the forces of restraint. But policy mediators are not all affected the same way by such policy dynamics. To date, the courts have been especially sensitive to the forces of right-to-die activism. Advances in medicine have created right-to-die scenarios for a small but growing number of individuals who, because of changes in the social structure, have become increasingly distrustful of their caretakers and increasingly bullish about bringing their own rights-based claims to court. The courts have had no choice, really; they were obliged to respond.

Legislatures are another story, however. Legislators have been slow to deal with critical right-to-die issues because they, like most of their constituents, are still reluctant to get involved with an issue whose status remains nothing short of taboo in many quarters. Even if legislators were predisposed to act boldly on this front, constituents have not yet offered much in the way of electoral payoffs for toiling in this thorny vineyard. Thus, there was very little incentive for legislators to make bold political strokes through the 1980s. The courts took the heat—and relieved the pressure—created by individuals who advanced rights-based claims, while generally conservative instincts, buttressed by the considerable influence of the Catholic church, were allowed to hold sway in the legislatures. Forty states and the District of Columbia passed living-will laws prior to 1990, but whether that body of statutory law was of much help to those who found themselves in right-to-die situations is another matter entirely. Indeed, when conflicts arose in any but the most routine right-to-die situations,[26] the individuals involved found themselves forced to repair to the courts in order to enjoy what the courts have considered a constitutionally protected right for the better part of a decade.

Explaining Convergence

Although the early and middle 1980s were marked by the passage of generally conservative state laws, a general trend toward a convergence with the more liberal consensus positions established by the state courts has been in evidence more recently. This can be explained, at least in part, as the result of a wearing down of restraint by the broad-based forces of activism. Entreaties by the courts are finally taking their toll, as individuals become more rights-conscious and more comfortable with considering what it would mean to manage a "happy death." Meanwhile, medical technology marches onward, creating more right-to-die scenarios daily—scenarios that demand increasingly precious resources that governments and private insurers are less and less willing and able to underwrite.

All the while, the Catholic influence that was so much a part of the explanation for conservative legislation through the 1980s has been on the wane more recently, freeing up legislators (and constituents) to pursue a more liberal path as they see fit. With impetus in full swing and obstacles melting away, liberalizing trends should have fairly smooth sailing in the years to come, though the forces of restraint cannot be discounted: Imbedded cultural attitudes such as those associated with death and dying do not fade away overnight.

Case Studies

A good deal of generalization has been laid on the table to this point, but not much context or detail has been rendered. Are generalizations evident in individual cases? Do the experiences of individual states support the general rules that have been offered as explanations for legislative behavior? A review of the experience of Pennsylvania (the last state to pass a law) and briefer looks at California (the first state to pass a law), Florida (with a law passed in 1984), and Massachusetts (still with no living-will law on the books) will help to answer these questions in the affirmative.

Pennsylvania. Pennsylvania's Advance Directive for Health Care Act includes the same curious mix of conservative and liberal positions evident in so many of the state laws now in force.[27] These conflicting messages may, in part, have something to do with the forces of activism (policy diffusion) and restraint (the Catholic influence) that tugged and hauled at the bill over the course of its entire seven-year history.

Living-will legislation was not even introduced in Pennsylvania until 1985, eight years after the first wave of such legislation passed in the wake of the New Jersey *Quinlan* decision. By that time, bills had been introduced in nearly every other state, and by the end of that year, thirty-six states would have legislation on the books. So the story in Pennsylvania starts with restraint—a not very surprising beginning, really, given its large, ethnic-Catholic population.

State Representative Frank Pistella (D-Pittsburgh) first proposed the legislation in response to a right-to-die scenario he experienced some years prior to his election. During the Christmas season of 1973, Pistella's father suffered a period of memory loss: The elder Pistella could not even remember the Christmas festivities the entire family had enjoyed just a few days before. He had a relapse of memory loss in the fall of 1974, and soon afterward, he slipped into a coma and died.

This personal exposure to a right-to-die scenario ultimately served as a force of activism in the Pennsylvania legislature for upon entering the house of representatives after his father's death, the younger Pistella tried to legislate guidance for families placed in scenarios like the one he had found himself in with his father. Working with Professor Alan Meisel of the University of Pittsburgh School of Law and drawing from legislation already on the books in other states, Pistella devised and introduced a bill. He sent his handiwork to the House Public Health and Welfare Committee, where the forces of restraint were sufficient to guarantee that his bill would never see the light of legislative day.

The Pistella bill never got out of the house committee due to pressures exerted by two extremely influential groups: the Pennsylvania Catholic Conference and the Pro-Life Federation. Many areas of the state of Pennsylvania are religiously conservative, and the legislature counts among its ranks some staunchly conservative Catholics who gravitate to positions held by the Catholic Conference and other prolife groups.[28] Passage of Pennsylvania's abortion-control law in 1990— one of the most conservative pieces of legislation of its kind in the country—is testament to that. Legislative staffers mince no words in explaining that it is nearly impossible to pass legislation if (as in the case of the Pistella bill) the Catholics and their sympathizers in the legislature are opposed to it.[29]

Pistella eventually gave less and less attention to the living-will matter because he eyed a leadership position in his party. The issues surrounding the legislation, especially the link with abortion (something the Catholic Conference continued to harp on), were enough to divide the ranks of his party, and Pistella avoided pressing an issue that could have knocked him out of the running for the Democratic house leadership (a kind of political concern that judges, as a rule, do not have to worry about).

Undaunted by these forces of restraint, State Senator John Stauffer picked up on Pistella's idea in 1986 and went ahead with a bill of his own in the senate.[30] The Stauffer bill, virtually identical to Pistella's measure, was introduced after senior citizens in his district urged him to follow up on the groundwork already laid by Pistella (back to the forces activism, again). The Stauffer bill passed the senate by a 45 to 5 vote in 1987 but died in the same house committee in which the Pistella bill had been bottled up.

The next legislator to raise the issue was State Senator Roy Wilt, the newly appointed chair of the Senate Public Health and Welfare Committee. Wilt sponsored his own piece of legislation in 1989 and pushed it hard, at least in part, out of embarrassment. Wilt spoke to his colleagues of a "Good Morning America" program featuring Arthur Miller, a respected Boston attorney who criticized Pennsylvania for suppressing living-will legislation by weighing it down with extraneous issues (policy diffusion).

Ultimately, however, Wilt's staunch advocacy was no match for the forces of restraint in the house. His bill easily passed the senate by a 46 to 1 vote but was quickly slowed down upon reaching the house floor, where interest ebbed with the coming of general elections in November 1990. The pregnancy issue in particular was seen as a political hot potato that most legislators preferred to steer clear of, and so they did. The Wilt bill was amended by conservative representatives three times on the floor of the house before being passed. But by then, it was late November 1990, too late for the measure to be fully reconsidered by the senate, which adjourned a few hours after receiving the amended bill. This ended the 1989–1990 legislative session and effectively killed Wilt's bill in the process.[30]

The new legislative session brought Senator John Peterson to the chairmanship of the Senate Public Health and Welfare Committee. Peterson, motivated by the U.S. Supreme Court's 1990 *Cruzan* decision (back to the forces of policy activism), was determined to get something passed. He called together a coalition of the staffs from the Democrat and Republican caucuses of both the house and senate to establish some common ground and chart a legislative course for passage of a living-will bill. Next, he turned to the interest groups who were perceived to have a stake in this matter.

Peterson called on representatives of the health-care community, including individuals from the Pennsylvania Department of Health, the Pennsylvania Nurses Association, the Pennsylvania Medical Society, the Pennsylvania Association of Non-Profit Nursing Homes, and the Hospital Association of Pennsylvania. He also touched base with the legal community by inviting representatives from the Philadelphia and Pennsylvania bar associations to the table. Several religious denominations were also called in—representatives from Tressler Lutheran Services, the Pennsylvania Jewish Coalition, the Pennsylvania Council of Churches, and, last but certainly not least, the Pennsylvania Catholic Conference. To round out the pluralist chorus, representatives from organizations representing the interests of the elderly—the American Association of Retired People, the Pennsylvania Department of Aging, the Pennsylvania Council on Aging, and the Coalition for the Rights of the Infirm Elderly—were invited to take part in the deliberations.

This unprecedented coalition met eighteen times over the course of a year and a half to hammer out the final language of the latest proposed legislation. On the activist side of the negotiations, legislators, advocates for the elderly, and medical interest groups pushed for the bill's adoption. The primary force of restraint was, not surprisingly, the Pennsylvania Catholic Conference, which continued to lobby hard on issues of pregnancy (demanding an "incubator" amendment) and ANH (preferring that legislation prohibit its withdrawal). In the end, the Catholic Conference caved in to a degree by offering not to block the legislation with further restrictive amendments in exchange for a watered-down pregnancy exclusion and a conservative reading of the concept "terminal." Senator Peterson and others on the coalition gave in to the Catholics' demands, knowing their opposition was the only thing standing in the way of concluding the long battle.

With the concessions made, the bill passed without much more wrangling. When it did, Pennsylvania became the forty-sixth state in the union to imbue the right to die with the force of statutory law. It did so seven years after living-will legislation was first introduced, sixteen years after California set the pace by passing the first law, and twenty-three years after an otherwise anonymous Florida legislator, Dr. Walter Sackett, sponsored the first living-will bill ever introduced in the United States. To be sure, the forces of restraint proved to be formidable in Pennsylvania. Slowly but surely, however, they yielded to the forces of activism as Pennsylvania finally joined the ranks of the legislative policy mediators by passing a relatively liberal piece of legislation.

California, Florida, and Massachusetts. In *The Right to Die: Policy Innovation and Its Consequences,* Henry Glick (1992) conducted studies in three other states—California, Florida, and Massachusetts—and the similarities between the experiences of those states and the Pennsylvania case are striking. In all four cases, living-will legislation was spurred on by one or two advocates who had either personal or professional experience with lingering death. And in each of the four cases, the state's respective Catholic Conference played a large role in policy restraint by stalling passage and extracting concessions from legislative entrepreneurs.

Barry Keene was a California lawyer who had helped a neighbor cope with withdrawing medical treatment from the neighbor's wife, who was suffering with terminal cancer. He became involved with the issue again in 1972 when he found his mother-in-law in the same predicament. Consequently, when Keene was elected to the California State Senate in 1974, he took on living-will legislation as something of a personal crusade. The California Medical Association (CMA) was opposed to the bill at first. But CMA resistance evaporated after its executive director was sensitized to the need for such a bill by having to personally intervene in his father's medical treatment to prevent a protracted death (Glick, 1992, p. 97).

The California Catholic Conference was strong, however, and it was able to extract a number of important concessions before agreeing not to oppose the bill. These concessions included (1) backing away from the pregnancy issue, (2) limiting coverage to terminal illness, conservatively defined, (3) requiring a fourteen-day waiting period following a terminal diagnosis before a living will could be made, and (4) limiting validity of the document to five years from date of signature. The California law has stood unamended since being passed in 1976 as the most restrictive living-will law in the United States. The powerful influences of the Catholic Conference and other fundamentalist religious organizations, combined with the ideologically conservative predispositions of George Deukmejian (the Republican governor who, in 1988, vetoed a liberal rewrite of the 1976 law) have ensured that California's restrictive code would stand the test of time.

In Florida, Representatives Walker Sackett and Richard Hodes—both medical doctors with close personal experiences with death—played crucial roles in putting and keeping living-will legislation on the legislative agenda during the 1970s. Neither was directly responsible for final passage, but both helped to raise the issue's profile and soften up resistance, thereby setting the stage for passage. A living-will law finally passed in Florida in 1984, but only after the Florida Catholic Conference extracted three key concessions: (1) that ANH must always be provided,[31] (2) that coverage be limited to terminal patients (with no coverage for PVS), and (3) that the living will be nullified in the case of pregnancy.

An early sponsor of legislation in Massachusetts also was moved to act by personal experience: his knowledge of a brain-dead teenager in his district, the victim of an automobile accident, who was being kept alive on life-support systems (Glick, 1992, p. 120). Later, another legislator, Richard Voke, became a key player largely because his mother was a registered nurse and very interested in the right to die due to her long hospital experience (Glick, 1992, p. 123). As in other states, however, the Catholic Conference has been a formidable opponent in Massachusetts. In fact, according to Glick (1992, p. 120), the right to die in Massachusetts is largely the story of the Catholic church and its key spokesman in the state's upper chamber—Senate President William M. Bulger.

In Massachusetts, the Catholic hierarchy is much more conservative and the population is more religiously homogeneous than elsewhere. Catholics constitute over 50 percent of the population in the Bay State, ranking it second only to Rhode Island in that category. More importantly, Senator Bulger, a Catholic representing a working-class, socially conservative district in south Boston, flatly opposes living-will legislation. A powerful legislator and adept tactician, Bulger has almost single-handedly prevented living-will legislation from proceeding. As one staffer close to the Senator put it in 1991, there simply will be no living-will law in Massachusetts as long as Bulger is senate president (personal communication). Since then, however, some observers suggest that Bulger has become more receptive to legislation after a personal experience of his own—the death of his mother (Glick, 1992, p. 126).

Cases in Perspective

The review of case materials from Pennsylvania, California, Florida, and Massachusetts helps to bring into sharper focus an explanation for the legislative behavior regarding right-to-die legislation. In the end, one can see all three policy dynamics—policy diffusion, religious restraint, and liberal trends—at work.

As stated, Pennsylvania used the laws of other states as a starting point in building its own legislation. Pressures brought to bear by (1) activism in other state legislatures, as broadcast on a morning news program (horizontal diffusion within the same branch of government), and (2) activism at the Supreme Court level, as rendered in the *Cruzan* decision (vertical policy diffusion across branches of government), were also evident in the Pennsylvania case. In addition, as already noted, a particular kind of activism was at work in each state studied: In all four cases, it was the impetus provided by firsthand experience that motivated legislators to act (activism akin to that discussed in Chapters 5 and 6). As Quill (1993, p. 22) notes, it is just this kind of "firsthand experience with such tragedy [that] makes one more fearful of a difficult death, and also wary of a profession that does not openly acknowledge or respond to its possibility."

At the same time, there was plenty of religiously motivated restraint to go around, causing divergence between what the legislatures were able to muster and what the courts were willing to grant in the way of rights protections. The influence wielded by the Catholic lobby was sufficient in each case reviewed to either slow passage of a law (Florida and Pennsylvania), prevent passage of a law (Massachusetts), or prevent an amended law from passing (California). In each of the three cases where a living will did pass, the Catholic Conference helped to shape a more conservative bill than would have emerged otherwise. Ultimately, even though Catholic elites seemed to acquiesce in "allowing" passage of living-will laws during the 1980s (usually by agreeing not to oppose legislation), they were careful to do so only after extracting key concessions—concessions that, in some cases, eviscerated the substance of what was being passed, state-court decisions to the contrary notwithstanding.

Religion is still important as a force of restraint, but the influence of the Catholic lobby and other religious organizations is on the wane now as the forces of policy activism lead the legislatures in a more liberal direction. Florida dropped its conservative, religiously inspired ANH restriction after the courts found the ANH rule unconstitutional (in *Corbett* v. *D'Alessandro* and, later, in *Satz* v.

Perlmutter). And Pennsylvania, a state where the Catholic lobby was strong enough to stall legislation for years, recently passed a relatively liberal law that allows withdrawal of ANH, covers PVS, and even makes concessions toward women on the pregnancy issue. The Catholic lobby never would have had to stand for that five years ago. But today, the forces of activism are painting an entirely different picture and opening up a set of entirely new possibilities on the living-will front.

Summary: Policy Forces and Policy Mediation

If anything is clear from this review of right-to-die case law and statutory provisions, it is this: The right to die is an area that does not lend itself to straightforward resolutions. Cultural taboos, religious rites, legal liabilities, and society's deference (albeit waning) to physician autonomy combine to make end-of-life decisions an extraordinarily complicated policy area to negotiate. Increasingly sophisticated medical technologies will not deliver Americans from right-to-die dilemmas, either. Indeed, the advances in medical management of seriously ill patients is a primary cause of the current situation. Consequently, we should not expect that future advances in medical technology will do anything but add to the complexities of the conundrums the state legislatures now face.

Something else is clear as well: Political consensus among and within state legislatures has been difficult to muster. The forty-seven living-will laws that have passed are generally rife with contradiction, especially with regard to qualifying conditions. On many of the most controversial issues (e.g., pregnancy and ANH), more than a few states have chosen simply to remain silent. In the end and aside from the basics, muddle and confusion—with just a hint of emerging trends— seem to be the only patterns of behavior that spring from this hodgepodge of legislative activity and languor across the fifty states.

The courts have labored as well. But they have been more successful in forging an enduring interstate consensus for they are more insulated from the religious and political interest-group pressures that have slowed progress in the legislative arena. In fact, when the state legislatures have acted, they have taken their lead from the courts. One should expect this modus operandi to continue.

In the end, state-court judges can continue to exhort their policy mediation counterparts in the legislatures to take the initiative, but one might wonder why they would bother. The courts have, in effect, established a fait accompli with their right-to-die pronouncements, then sat back to see if the legislatures would act on them. When the legislatures fail to act or act outside the boundaries set by the courts (that is, when the legislators do anything but ratify prevailing court decisions), justices have tended, in a fashion that has become typical for them in recent decades, to trump the statutory law, replacing legislative provisions with their own reading of rights and liberties.

In a way, the state courts are in a "buck-stops-here" situation: They cannot go out of their way to make policy, but when something like the right to die falls in their lap, they are obliged to deal with it. The legislatures have a good deal more latitude in this regard. Of course, they can and often do take the lead in making policy when problems emerge, when policy alternatives surface, and when political conditions are amenable to action all at the same time. But legislatures also enjoy the luxury of benign neglect when these conditions fail to emerge coincidentally. That is, when clear policy solutions to problems do not present themselves together with political impetus for policymaking, then the legislatures can defer to the courts. In terms of right-to-die policy, most legislatures have often done just that.

But by failing to act or acting in ways inimicable to constitutional and common-law prescriptions, the state lawmakers have, in effect, ceded their role as primary legislators to the judiciary.[32] Referring in particular to the controversy over withdrawing artificial food and nutrition, the Florida court stated that such issues are "more suitably addressed in the legislative forum. ... Nevertheless, preferences for legislative treatment cannot shackle the courts when legally protected interests are at stake. ... Legislative action cannot serve to close the doors of the courtrooms ... to ... citizens who assert cognizable Constitutional rights" (cited in Glick, 1992, p. 110).

Indeed, of the 100-plus court decisions rendered in right-to-die cases, only two—one in Missouri (*Cruzan*) and one in Ohio (*Couture* v. *Couture*)—have taken their lead from the legislatures. The rest have followed each other, often in direct contradiction to their respective state legislatures. This state of affairs is not without its costs or risks, however, as Justice Felix Frankfurter so aptly pointed out in 1951 when he stated: "History teaches that the independence of the judiciary is jeopardized when the courts become embroiled in the passions of the day and assume primary responsibility in choosing between competing political, economic, and social pressures" (cited in Krantz, 1977, p. 28).

At the same time, even though the legislatures, generally speaking, have been slow to respond and incremental in their responses, progress is being made. A significant convergence with the courts on some of the central right-to-die issues—the right to designate proxies for end-of-life decisionmaking, the right to withdraw food and fluids, the right to die for patients in a persistent vegetative state, and, down the road, maybe even the right to an assisted suicide—seems to be evolving.[33]

All this may be fine for those who will not have to face the right-to-die scenario until progressive trends prevail in their state or for those who, in the meantime, have the resources and predisposition to take their right-to-die cases to the courts. But for everyone else, legislative lassitude leaves the right to die in limbo, exactly where those who are in a position to make end-of-life decisions would rather not be. So it is, and so it will continue to be, it seems, until the legislatures take the initiative back from the courts in setting a legally and constitutionally sound course in what is, at least chronologically, the ultimate arena of civil rights: the right to die.

9

Policy Activism, Restraint, Mediation, and the Right to Die

IN THIS POLICY PRIMER on the right to die, we have attempted to deal with two fundamental questions. First, what forces of restraint and activism have shaped the right to die into an important policy issue in the United States today? And second, how have the institutions of policy mediation responded? We have fashioned answers to these core questions by resorting to an inspection of American culture, medical professionalism, social activism, state-court case law, and legislative activity across the fifty states.

Activism and Restraint

In looking for answers to the first question, we begin by noting that issues of public policy appear on the agenda not by accident but because a confluence of forces make an issue's rise something of an inevitability. Problems are always cropping up, but if they are ever to see the light of day, they must survive the competition between clashing forces of policy activism (forces that push problems onto the agenda) and policy restraint (forces that keep problems off the agenda).

If a problem survives the battle of activism versus restraint, then policy alternatives are fashioned and applied by policy mediators. Occasionally, these alternatives represent something innovative, but more often, they come from ideas that have been floating around in some form or another (e.g., in the Constitution, in the common law, or in the laws of some other state) in what John Kingdon (1984) calls the "policy primeval soup." Ultimately, policy is formed by the convergence of a problem, a policy, and politics; that is when a policy issue's time has come. Clearly, the right to die is such an issue.

At the same time, it is clear that the right to die is an area in which the conflict between individual self-determination and state interests in preserving life does not lend itself to straightforward resolutions. Cultural forces of restraint—the denial of mortality, exacerbated by individualism, an abiding faith in technology, the entitlement syndrome, and religious taboos—continue to have an effect, turning policymaking into an extraordinarily muddled and incremental process. The forces of activism—technology, the rights culture, the happy-death movement, and the changing nature of the relationship between medical professionals and those they care for—have forced mediators to deal with the right to die. But the forces of restraint keep them from going too far and too fast in codifying the rules that would guide the exercise of those rights.

Forces of Policy Restraint

The forces of activism may have unwittingly conspired to create a policy issue, but the nature of American culture has helped keep the right-to-die debate submerged as an item of extensive public discussion until recently. More than citizens of other countries, Americans tend to be obsessed with death, to the point of denying their own mortality. As Walter Smith (1985, p. 283) notes, "Often the things that concern us the most deeply are the very things we talk about the least. Death certainly figures prominently among these topics."

Americans do not plan for death. They do not talk about death, except in hushed and euphemistic tones. They do not accept death as part of the life cycle. And as a result, they have not—as a group—pressured the popularly elected representatives in government to take bold steps in this policy area. In short, the right to die will be a sticky issue to resolve in this country, despite the forces of activism, because Americans typically avoid what they perceive as a very personal, private, and emotionally disconcerting subject.

It seems, then, that forces of activism have precipitated an issue that the public seems loath to put on the public-policy agenda. When it has come up in the past, the only organized political forces with an interest were those arrayed on the prolife side, suppressing the issue at every turn. Indeed, antiabortion groups have begun to adopt the right to die as a cause célèbre, as have disability-rights groups such as the National Legal Center for the Medically Dependent and Disabled and, to a decreasing degree, the Catholic church.[1]

The unbounded faith that Americans put in technology is another force of policy restraint that the forces of activism have had trouble overwhelming. Instead of facing up to tough choices, Americans tend to demand that the latest technology be available and employed in every case, to every extent, almost as if access to such advanced medical procedures were a right of citizenship. And giving up on life may be viewed by some as almost unpatriotic. As Arnold Toynbee has noted (cited in Charmaz, 1980, p. 96), "Death is 'un-American'; for if the fact of death were once admitted to be a reality even in the U.S., then it would also have to be admitted that the U.S. is not the earthly paradise that it is deemed to be."

In the end, these cultural, societal, and professional pressures conspire to stifle public discussion of right-to-die questions. Privately and individually, decisions to end the lives of terminally ill patients have been made for years at hospital bedsides and in doctors' offices. But in public, general discussion about when someone should be allowed to die borders on the taboo. Rather, the question usually is framed: What more can be done to save the life of a terminally ill individual? That, it seems, is the American way.

Forces of Policy Activism

Probably the most important force of policy activism in the right-to-die area is medical technology. Advances here have made it possible for health-care providers to sustain life and postpone death for days, months, and even years beyond the point at which someone would have died, naturally, just a few decades ago. Procedures ranging from the mundane (use of antibiotics, tube feeding, and artificial respiration) to the exotic (organ transplant and kidney dialysis) are now common means of artificially prolonging life when death would otherwise be imminent. Today, with the world's most advanced equipment, drugs, therapies, and operative procedures in play, life—even if severely degraded—can be preserved, sometimes indefinitely. And that is when right-to-die questions inevitably surface.

The changing nature of the American family also has had a marked effect in precipitating right-to-die scenarios. For many senior citizens, the combined impact of Social Security and Medicare makes it more likely that they will live independently and apart from their children. And when these elderly individuals contract long-term illnesses, they are more likely than ever to receive institutional care (in a hospital or nursing home) in which life-saving and life-prolonging therapies are apt to be rendered on a routine basis. Two generations ago, most elderly parents would die quickly and quietly at home (where they probably lived with or were taken care of by their children) from simple causes: pneumonia (sometimes called "the old man's friend"), infections, and serious falls. Those were the days when 80 percent of all deaths occurred in the home and sickness took its toll with some dispatch (DeSpelder and Strickland, 1992, p. 19). Today, the tables are turned: Some 80 percent of all deaths now take place in an institutional setting, where the dying may linger with chronic illnesses for weeks, months, years, and, in some cases, even decades.

As professional caregivers have supplanted family members, the close network of support within the family has broken down, leaving the old to die slow, lonely, institutional deaths. It is no wonder that the suicide rate for the elderly is the fastest growing rate for any age group (Douglas, 1992). The old have seen firsthand and within their peer group the aggregate picture painted by the National Center for Health Statistics (NCHS), in which the last year of life is often characterized by loneliness, poverty, and physical helplessness ("Last Year," 1992). About half of all individuals in this category need help to bathe, walk, dress, and use the toilet. And more than one-third are likely to need assistance in eating. When life ends like that, it is no wonder that the elderly are increasingly taking right-to-die matters into their own hands, sometimes literally.

Meanwhile, doctors are medically trained, culturally predisposed, and legally required (or at least they believe so) to keep individuals alive at all costs, literally. So, rather than allowing patients near death to slip over the edge, they are more likely to keep the terminally ill alive, literally at all costs and sometimes with insufficient pain medication (for fear that overprescribing drugs may precipitate death). This, too, causes right-to-die scenarios to emerge.

The "deep-pockets" nature of health-care finance in the United States has also helped turn the right to die into a policy problem. Most other developed nations have public systems of health-care finance, making it possible (and necessary) to cap overall expenditures. Setting explicit expenditure limits makes it necessary to ration care in some general fashion by distributing resources according to some rule—a rule usually grounded firmly in the principle of medical efficacy. In the United States, where private, third-party insurers play such an important role in the finance of health care, money is spent at rates that are controlled not by government or medicine but by markets. But when private insurance markets cannot bear the costs of keeping terminally ill individuals alive for extended periods of time—and some suggest that this time is rapidly approaching—then questions about the right to die (or the "duty to die," as former Colorado Governor Richard Lamm might prefer to put it—see Chapter 3) are likely to be raised with increased frequency.

As the time has grown ripe for right-to-die scenarios to emerge, patients seem to have become more estranged from their health-care system than at any time in the past. The bureaucratization of the hospital, combined with an increasingly specialized medical corps, has led to a breakdown in the doctor-patient relationship. Nearly all care is now provided outside the home, usually by overworked, often superspecialized professionals who may or may not know the patient's first name. And in today's world, where physicians tend to be strangers and hospitals tend to be strange places, the natural bond of trust between doctor and patient has weakened substantially.

This all fuels existing trends of consumerism in health care. Patients are more likely than ever to shop around for physicians and second opinions. Emboldened by media exposés of physician incompetency and wrongdoing, patients are encouraged to ask questions and demand answers of their caretakers. And with the passage of the Patient Self-Determination Act, they may become even more informed about just what their rights are. The impact of the PSDA has been minimal to date, but it would be surprising if, over time, the act did not encourage more patients to take greater advantage of their rights as provided for by state law. As DeSpelder and Strickland (1992, p. 392) note, "Matters that were once the province of fate have now become a matter of human choice." The end of life has become something to manage, and patients will be participating in the process to a far greater degree. Death, we suspect, will never again be quite the same.

The emergence of the happy-death movement is having an effect, as well. No one expects the home funeral parlor to reemerge any time soon, but people are talking about death, writing about death, agitating for the right to die, and voting on assisted-suicide initiatives in record numbers.[2] Some individuals—most noticeably, members of the Quinlan and Cruzan families—have become so perturbed about the right to die that they have taken their cases to court, and the impact those cases have, thanks to extensive media coverage, reaches far beyond the courtroom to feed back into the activism loop.

In the end, the right to die is not an issue because anybody in particular wants it to be. It is an issue by default, the inevitable result of a confluence of activism forces. Moreover, the subject is here to stay. As Margaret Battin, a philosopher at the University of Utah, has noted, "We've crossed over the river now. ... But if you think the abortion issue was emotional, just wait until we get fully into euthanasia and death. Unlike abortion, [these issues] confront everyone and through their parents, probably several times" (cited in Malcolm, 1990a). Indeed, because death is something everyone must confront, any developments in this area will have a natural, broad-based constituency. And as Americans age and more and more of us are touched by right-to-die scenarios through the experiences of grandparents, parents, siblings, and spouses, the intensity of interest in the right to die is only likely to increase.

Policy Mediation

Bold strokes of policy emerge only when the forces of activism are sufficient to overwhelm the forces of restraint. Where restraint prevails, there is no cause for policy mediation. And where the forces of activism are roughly equal to the forces of restraint, halfway policy measures emerge from the legislatures and attention turns to the courts. That, it seems, is where we are with the right to die.

Courts and Legislatures

Where the forces of activism have generated a policy problem, American culture has stifled public debate. As a result, much of the mediation in the right-to-die arena has occurred in the venue of last resort—the courts—where private parties have chosen to sue in order to ensure that their perceived civil rights to self-determination are respected. The courts have been relatively successful and accommodating in forging an enduring interstate consensus for they are relatively insulated from the political and cultural forces that have slowed progress in the legislative arena. But that does not mean justices in the state courts like playing the role of policymaker.

Indeed, state judges have beseeched their legislatures time and again to take up the right-to-die cause and lay down some ground rules. But the state legislatures have struggled with the right to die because of their increased sensitivity to the forces of restraint. When legislatures have acted, they have lagged behind the courts either by responding to court cases slowly and erratically, then simply ratifying what the state courts have decided, or by trying to put the brakes on court decisions in some areas that seem to be especially sensitive (such as legitimizing the right to withdraw artificially provided food and water).

In the first instance, the state legislatures might be viewed as redundant, legitimizing for the body politic the rights the courts have already granted to individuals. In the second instance, the state legislatures have become almost irrelevant since when they attempt to put the brakes on the courts, the judiciary trumps the legislature to reinstate whatever rights were originally granted in the case law. Thus, it seems that, until recently, the forces of activism have forced the courts to deal with right-to-die scenarios, but the cultural pressures of policy restraint and the apparent lack of political leadership have left the state legislatures in position to play only a sideline role in mediating the right-to-die debate.

Bedside Policy Mediation

State-court decisions and the body of statutory law notwithstanding, a vast amount of policy discretion remains in the hands of bedside physicians. Physicians decide what to tell the families, what not to tell them, and how to advise them about what they ought to do. The old saw "knowledge is power" could not be more appropriate in the right-to-die arena, where, in spite of consumerist tendencies in the general population, there is still a tremendous disparity in knowledge between the clinician and client.

Saying that physicians have power does not tell us much about what the fate of right-to-die policy will be, however, because physicians tend to make determinations in private, on a case-by-case basis. Moreover, they face a maze of conflicting sentiments: They are guided by healing instincts that are tempered by sympathy for their patients, they are guided by a fear of legal liability that is tempered by pride in the autonomous nature of their craft, and they are sometimes guided by financial considerations that are tempered by an emerging ethos of responsibility to do only those things that are medically necessary. It is difficult to predict where those clashing impulses will take right-to-die policy in the years to come.

At the same time, we should note that there does seem to be a sea change under way in the prevailing medical ethos about caring for seriously ill patients. Today, even though patients may not control their destiny to the degree that the court cases and legislation suggest they might, physicians have begun to look at cases more in terms of what a patient might logically want, as opposed to what is technologically possible. Warm-water pediatric drownings are a good example.[3] Ten years ago, a child suffering this fate would almost surely be treated with heroic measures in an attempt to resuscitate the body. But today, there is more sensitivity to the idea that if the brain is gone, it might not make any sense to keep the child alive. Physicians may have pulled the plug clandestinely in the past, but today, such decisions are more likely to be made, talked about, and accepted openly as physicians weigh all the possibilities.

Living-will legislation has had some effect in this regard. Physicians may claim that living-will laws have not changed the nature of their practices. They may claim that end-of-life decisions have been made for years, in conjunction with the patient's wishes. But the ethic of bringing the patient and family into the decision-making process—even if their role is largely controlled and pro forma at this stage of the game—represents a substantial shift from years past. Together, living-will legislation and the Patient Self-Determination Act have changed the context in which decisions are made. Ultimately, this has all tended to legitimize the notion that taking aggressive measures might not be—by definition—the right way to go.[4]

At the same time, some argue that there is much work still to be done. As Fenella Rouse, executive director of the National Council on Death and Dying, says, "The practical reality is very spotty. ... In many hospitals you still can't get a respirator removed from a terminally ill patient" (cited in Malcolm, 1990a). When physicians, family, and patients have a long-standing, intimate relationship or when hospitals are committed to accommodating a wide range of patient preferences, legal directives are usually unnecessary. Otherwise, until physician hegemony breaks down more completely and until legislative waffling gives way to laws with some teeth in them, most Americans will not know much about what degree of autonomy they will eventually enjoy at the end of life. This will be true, it seems, until the medical profession openly embraces patient autonomy, and the legislatures find it expedient to overcome the inertia brought on by the forces of restraint.

Summary: The Last Word

Those interested in advancing the right to die may feel that they have been swimming against the current for years. In many ways, they have been because the current—American culture—has been flowing in the opposite direction. It is not that the culture rejects the right to die in particular so much as it rejects discussion of death at any level.

Yet, death is now on the public agenda, and private individuals, medical professionals, hospital administrators, and state legislators will have to find a way to cope. Technological advances, consumer-rights activism, happy-death advocates, and disgruntled individuals willing to sue for the right to die are combining to slowly overcome countervailing pressures of restraint that have helped to keep the right to die off the agenda until recently. Currently, the forces of restraint are strong enough only to limit the scope of right-to-die policy and slow its development.

Issues associated with the right to die will be difficult to resolve, however. This is because policy mediation is all about establishing general rules and drawing lines to distinguish right from wrong, appropriate from inappropriate, and legal from illegal. That is hard to do in right-to-die matters for the line between meaningful life and death is so blurry. Indeed, the very nature of the distinction inhibits the formulation of generalizations, and the search for enduring policy is continuously confounded. Rules will be tough to establish—and maybe even tougher to follow—in a policy environment like this.

Nonetheless, it is important to remember that dramatic social transformations such as those involved in establishing the right to die usually come incrementally, in a two-steps-forward-one-step-back fashion, with the passing of generations. We are only now—seventeen years after *Quinlan*—near the end of the first "right-to-die generation," and the number of people affected by right-to-die scenarios is still relatively small. We suspect, however, that as the second right-to-die generation matures and as the number of right-to-die scenarios increase, death will no longer be considered a taboo subject. Perhaps then we will find enduring answers about what exactly is entailed when people proclaim that, given their grave medical condition, they would like to exercise what for all Americans will eventually become a recognized and protected deathright.

Notes

Chapter 1

1. The most common symbol of condolence in the greeting-card studies was flowers: They appeared on 80 percent of the specimens McGee analyzed. Live flowers also serve as a common vehicle for conveying sympathies when words seem inadequate. Funeral parlors typically overflow with flowers, and the American Society of Florists estimates that between 20 percent to 25 percent of business nationwide can be attributed to what is euphemistically called "sympathy sales" (personal communication).

2. Unfortunately, explains one cryonics advocate, individuals who were suspended when the technology was new left the responsibility for covering the annual maintenance fee (required for cooling and storage) in the hands of surviving family members, many of whom tired of keeping up with the payments after a few years. As a result, storage facilities have been forced to foreclose on the estates of about half of those who have been suspended to date. The bodies of these individuals have since been thawed out and disposed of in a more traditional fashion.

Chapter 2

1. Some believe that Halloween was conceived, at least in part, as a way to familiarize children in this country with the idea of death.

2. Americans deny taxes in the sense that they continue to subscribe to the myth of the free lunch. It seems that liberals and conservatives alike have a nearly insatiable appetite for public programs that benefit them directly. Yet no one seems very willing to pay the tab, which is why America sets the low-end standard for tax burden among the industrial nations of the world. Our enormous public debt—currently well over $4 trillion and growing at a rate of about $7,000 per second, every second, minute, hour, and day of the year—is clear evidence of that phenomenon.

3. "Low-ingredient" offerings (low fat, sodium, sugar, cholesterol, etc.), "light-food" products (e.g., light beer, wine, popcorn, ice cream, and even cat and dog food), and "ingredient-free" product lines (sugar-free, caffeine-free, alcohol-free, cholesterol-free, sulfide-free, etc.) are ubiquitous in the modern American grocery store. New eating trends—the search for that food that will enhance our immortality—are also part of the food fad craze. Fiber, oat bran, fish, chicken, pasta, wine (much to the delight of many), and vegetarian regimens have all been touted as culinary routes to a long and healthy life in recent

years. Interest in organic growing methods (no use of pesticides or herbicides), herbal teas (purported to have significant medicinal benefits), home-canned produce, and "all-natu-ral" foods (whatever that means) of every description have also been marketed as means to similar ends.

4. The water diet, the liquid diet, the Atkins diet, the Scarsdale diet, the Stillman diet, the high-protein diet, the high-carbohydrate diet, and the grapefruit diet are just a few ex-amples. Various food manufacturers offer ready-to-microwave entrées for people who do not have time to prepare their own dietetically correct meals. Diet powders and pills are another option for those who are a bit more desperate for results.

5. Having the meals prepared for pickup or delivery—provided in conjunction with in-house counseling—is a popular option that has helped the diet business blossom in the last two decades from a minor enterprise into a major industry with $33 billion in annual sales. Americans have spent about $2 billion of that total patronizing a variety of dieting pro-grams that offer weight-reduction services, even though these businesses have been subject to federal investigation for advertising programs that have no proven, long-term effect. Ac-cording to some university-based researchers, the diet plans pushed by these retailers may even be dangerous. At best, researchers agree that the long-term success rates for the 7.9 million people who have enrolled in such programs is astoundingly low (E. Rosenthal, 1992).

The ever-popular self-help groups also stand ready to pitch in. Some adults even pa-tronize weight-loss hypnotists, and others repair to residential fat farms. Even husky kids have an option along these lines: the summer camp for overweight children.

6. Some, obsessed with their figures and unable to achieve the results they desire through dieting and exercise, end up with anorexia nervosa, the deliberate self-starvation that arises from an obsession with food that leads to unhealthy and potentially life-threat-ening weight loss. Bulimia, involving recurrent episodes of binge eating followed by purg-ing through use of diuretics, laxatives, and/or self-induced vomiting, is another such disor-der. Figures vary, but it is generally thought that anorexia afflicts approximately 1 percent of Americans and that as many as 8 percent of American women are bulimic. According to psychologist Christine Ganis, approximately 85 percent of those who suffer from these sorts of eating disorders are either in the normal weight range or underweight already (cited in Jacobsen, 1992).

7. Meanwhile, tanning parlors have proliferated in the last decade or so. Many Ameri-cans patronize these salons in an attempt to add a golden glow to their pale bodies, despite increasing evidence about the link between skin cancer and ultraviolet radiation.

8. Also, by 1969, when Neil Armstrong took that first big step for mankind, Americans had conveniently forgotten the catastrophic rocket failures that marked the first few years of the race into space, incidents that flew in the face of American ingenuity. That all helps explain why when technological tragedy struck again with the *Challenger* disaster in 1986, Americans reacted with shock and confusion: "How could this have happened? Our rock-ets are not supposed to blow up."

9. There is also the issue of the tens of thousands of Iraqi children who have died since the war for lack of pure water. That story did not get very much play either: Why should it when "surgical" air strikes on water purification plants by Stealth bombers are good by def-inition, according to scientistic American thinking.

Chapter 3

1. Janus, the Roman god of comings and goings, is a figure with two faces, one looking left and one looking right. It was common for the Janus figure to be located near doorways, the mark of both an entrance and an exit. We invoke Janus here to describe the two-faced nature of medical technology. On the one hand, it feeds into scientism and thereby fuels the forces of restraint. On the other hand, technology is responsible for creating medical scenarios where right-to-die activism comes into play.

2. Tomography (from the Greek *tomos*, "a cut," and the Greek *graphein*, "to write") creates three-dimensional pictures oriented along the body's axis, running from head to toe. Patients are injected with a dye that is sensed by the scanner, which produces relatively detailed images of the body in slices, like rings of a cut-up pineapple.

3. Using the same principle that is applied in submarine sonar, ultrasound is now used for imaging various body parts. Probably the most popular use today is for monitoring fetal development. Somewhere between 30 percent and 50 percent of all pregnant women in the United States have at least one ultrasound during gestation, and ultrasounds are required of women in Great Britain and Germany.

4. MRIs detect the chemical composition of structures within the body by introducing that body to an electromagnetic field, then scanning for any resulting electromagnetic resonation emanating from body tissues. The principle is parallel to that in play when a tuning fork is struck, then brought within close proximity of a second tuning fork. If the two forks are of the same size, the first fork's vibrations will induce the second to begin humming in resonance. So it is with the MRI: If one is attempting to detect the presence of hydrogen in the body's tissues, the MRI can be set to generate a magnetic field that will excite or resonate with hydrogen nuclei. Then, a radio frequency sensor detects resonances in the body and traces them out as a visual image of where the hydrogen is located in the body.

5. Scopes and instruments are inserted through small openings in the leg. Then, with the patient under local anesthesia, the equipment is threaded up through a blood vessel to the heart, two to three feet away, where the major arteries can be assayed and unclogged using inflatable balloons.

6. Cupping involved placing partially evacuated cups on the skin near areas of affliction in order to draw blood toward or through the skin and out of the body. The average adult body holds about five quarts of blood.

7. Kidneys are transplanted five times more often than all other organs combined.

8. Indeed, to the dismay of most ethicists, a lucrative black market for kidneys has emerged in the Third World on the heels of organ-transplant advances. Prices vary, depending on the condition of the donor and the desperation of the potential recipient, but $5,000 is not out of line as a price for a kidney today.

9. Defibrillators are designed to restore a steady, rhythmic heartbeat in a person suffering a heart attack by discharging a large DC current through metal paddles placed on the individual's chest.

10. Elaine Esposito, the longest-surviving PVS patient to date, never recovered consciousness after receiving anesthesia on August 6, 1941. She finally died on the Sunday after Thanksgiving in 1978, 37 years and 111 days later (President's Commission, 1983, p. 177).

11. The few patients that have recovered consciousness after prolonged periods of unconsciousness were severely disabled. The degree of permanent damage varies, but most are unable to speak or see, and many suffer from permanent distortion of the limbs and paralysis.

12. It is interesting to note that when doctors began treating infants with spina bifida aggressively, the number of recorded "stillbirths" dropped drastically (Rothman, 1991, p. 191).

13. After the fact, the Florida Supreme Court decided to hear the case after all and in November 1992 issued its ruling. That decision affirmed the lower court's ruling that prevented physicians from declaring baby Campo legally dead for purposes of transplanting its organs. That ruling was upheld, according to the court, on the grounds that there was not enough proof that such donations saved lives to rationalize making a radical departure from the standard brain-death criteria ("Florida Court Rejects," 1992).

14. The viability of organs for donation deteriorates rapidly after a body expires, making it important to harvest them as close to the time of death as possible.

15. Americans spend about $2,651 per person annually in public funding of medical services for the over-sixty-five age group. Spending on those under sixty-five amounts to only about one-tenth of that amount—about $265 per person annually (Hahn and Lefkowitz, 1992).

16. This is a relatively small number, considering that Americans spend over $800 billion annually on health care, but $5 billion is still more than twice the amount spent on all public maternity and child-health programs in the United States combined (N. Clark, 1992).

17. Some critics find it especially hard to rationalize spending so much to avoid death in the seriously ill and elderly when so little attention—relative to that in other developed countries—is paid to preventing death (and treating the less serious illnesses) of those who are still very much alive, especially the young. The United States ranks tenth out of ten Western countries in the percentage of preschool children with full polio, diphtheria-tetanus-pertussis (DPT), and measles immunizations (Shapiro, 1992, p. 21). The U.S. infant mortality rates top those in any other developed country (Shapiro, 1992, p. 18). The United States also leads the way in the percentage of infants born at low birth weight (Shapiro, 1992, p. 19). The fact is that this country devotes less than 5 percent of health-care spending to prevention efforts in any given year, while spending billions on those who, from a medical standpoint, are lost causes.

18. Only about 580,000 individuals were eighty-five or older in 1950, but that number swelled to 3.1 million in 1990 and is expected to expand another 70 percent to 5.3 million by the year 2005.

19. This pattern of resource allocation in Great Britain is common to most other European countries, as well (Jennet, cited in Bronzino, Smith, and Wade, 1990, p. 252).

20. That works out to about $800 billion annually, or about $2,500 for every second of every minute of every hour of every day of the year. On an annual, per-capita basis, that is about $2,700 for every man, woman, and child in the country.

Chapter 4

1. The first Nobel Prize laureate, Wilhelm Conrad Roentgen, discovered the X ray in November 1895 when he "viewed with stunned amazement the bones in his hand with the crude device he had fashioned" (Bronzino, Smith, and Wade, 1990, p. 417).

2. This was done partly out of necessity. Catholic and Jewish doctors were regularly discriminated against in Protestant and secular institutions, and so the only route of advancement open to them was through their own denominational hospital system.

3. Two hundred seventy community hospitals were closed in just the ten-year period from 1977 to 1987, a rate of about twenty-five closings per year (Rolde, 1992, p. 55).

4. In one study of 8,758 families in 18 states, 56 percent of visits between 1928 and 1931 involved house calls (cited in Rothman, 1991, p. 112).

5. The transportation revolution had an impact, as well. The improvement of roads and the proliferation of automobiles made it easier to go to an office or hospital for care.

6. Although Westerners accept the orthodoxy of specialization and compartmentalization as the ideal, it is by no means clear that the attitude is well founded. Eastern medical orthodoxy continues to embrace a more holistic approach, and, at least in some cases, this alternative seems better able to produce the desired effects that one has come to expect of modern medical practice.

7. The future of the general practice in the United States looks even gloomier: Only 18 percent of current medical school students surveyed say they are planing to go on to generalist graduate training ("Overspecialized Doctors," 1992). The remaining 82 percent will choose from among twenty-five specialties and fifty-six subspecialties, thirty-five of which have been recognized in only the past five years ("Overspecialized Doctors," 1992). In contrast, over half of all Canadian doctors continue in the general practice of medicine.

8. Not surprisingly, the overwhelming percentage of malpractice lawsuits filed in the United States are filed against specialists. Of course, there are more specialists than generalists, and specialists are more apt to apply riskier technologies and deal with more problematic cases. But part of the reason for the disproportionate number of suits filed against specialists surely has to do with the social distance—and commensurate lack of trust—between specialist and patient.

9. According to Starr (1982), specialists and subspecialists tend to treat their patients as organisms suffering from a collection of special and subspecial problems rather than as people suffering from general maladies, and that tends to distance the clinicians from the clients in human terms. Moreover, as specialists and subspecialists learn more about microscopic body parts and processes, their knowledge and language becomes more foreign to the average patient. Physicians and patients grow more distant as the information gap widens and as the language of interaction become more objective and technical. Patients, especially in the research setting, may tend to lose their humanity in the eyes of highly trained specialists by being objectifiable as "clinical material."

10. Some have even suggested that those who choose to go into the health-care fields are a self-selected group of individuals who have a heightened sense of denial as a common denominator (W. Smith, 1985, pp. 284–285). These individuals choose to become experts on health care, so the argument goes, out of a deep-seated need to gain some measure of immortality by acquiring the kind of knowledge that would help pave that path (Schulz and Aderman, 1980, p. 134).

11. One survey of medical publications in the years 1960–1971 failed to turn up even one article documenting instruction concerning death and dying for medical students, and Bugen (1979) suggests that the situation has not improved much in the intervening years.

12. Nursing schools have done a bit better along these lines. According to William Smith, "Most professional literature related to the psychosocial care of the dying is written by

nurses. The dichotomy between nursing and medicine is striking in this regard" (W. Smith, 1985, p. 284; also see Charmaz, 1980, p. 236).

13. According to Schulz and Aderman (1980, p. 142), the dying patient is a deviant in the medical subculture, and as a result, dying patients elicit aversive attitudes from caretakers. Less charitably, Schoenfeld (1978, p. 53) suggests that physicians avoid the dying because dying patients "simply will not feed the doctor's narcissism by responding and getting well. Their care is demanding, frustrating, and far from helpful to the medical magician's self-esteem."

14. As Walter Smith (1985, p. 286) notes, "The contemporary practice of medicine is seriously compromised by the herculean demands made on physicians, nurses, and other allied health professionals. The volume of work required of these persons, coupled with the urgency, gravity, and intensity of the demands of medical intervention, seriously affect their ability to manage equally well all the important dimensions of effective patient care. Providing medical care is an emotionally complex task. The profession places great strain on its members in terms of personal investment, effort, and energy as well as commitment of time."

15. Some claimed that the unvarnished truth would be too much for their patients. That truth is described as "a death sentence," "torture," or "hitting the patients with a baseball bat." Expressions of concern about the psychological damage that could ensue from such revelations were common, even though there was no empirical evidence to support the claim (indeed, there may be evidence to the contrary). Others cited "therapeutic privilege" as a reason for exempting themselves from the requirements of informed consent when caring for terminally ill patients (President's Commission, 1983, pp. 52–53).

16. One study conducted in 1953 revealed that over two-thirds of the 442 Philadelphia physicians sampled never disclosed diagnoses of terminal cancer (DeSpelder and Strickland, 1992; see also Oken, 1961). A 1960 national study of physicians revealed that 84 percent withheld information from patients about their incurable cancers at least some of the time, with 22 percent admitting that they withheld such information all of the time. In three other studies, conducted between 1953 and 1961, it was reported that 69 percent to 90 percent of physicians routinely failed to inform cancer patients of their diagnoses.

17. According to Raymond Carey and Emil Posavac's (1980, p. 145) study of physician attitudes in the late 1970s, 29 percent of physicians and fully 45 percent of nurses agreed that the physician should give complete and honest information regarding the terminal condition without waiting for the patient to ask. In addition, 42 percent of physicians and 43 percent of nurses agreed that doctors should go ahead and reveal terminal condition information if a patient asks (see also Carey and Posavac, 1978–1979, and Rea, Greenspoon, and Spinka, 1975, both cited in Charmaz, 1980, p. 137). These are only self-reported attitudes, however, that may or may not have much to do with actual behavior.

18. Such fears are not necessarily unfounded. A third of all physicians, half of all surgeons, and three quarters of all obstetrician/gynecologists will be sued at least once in their professional careers (Shapiro, 1992, pp. 28–29). Physicians in the United States are five times more likely to be sued than physicians in either the United Kingdom or Canada.

19. Malpractice suits represent not so much a lack of faith in doctors as, in the first instance, an abiding faith in both doctors and technology—a faith shared with doctors, fueled by a physician's aggressive treatment impulses. Malpractice suits are not so much a manifestation of faithlessness as they are a manifestation of a faith—scientism, magnified by the technological imperative—that has been broken.

20. One motivation we have not examined very deeply is avarice. Some suggest that certain physicians may overtreat their patients out of simple greed. To be sure, there is not much money to be made in death: Sustaining lives is much more lucrative for all parties in a position to bill and receive payment for their services. But greed alone is not enough to account for doctors overtreating patients in medically futile situations. It is only one reason for some to choose to sustain life, rather than help to manage death, in accordance with the technological imperative (see Pelligrino, 1991).

21. One only need look at the relatively dramatic changes that have taken place in childbirth in recent years to find evidence of this trend toward demedicalization. Fifty years ago, during the early days of medicalization, doctors participating in home deliveries were threatened with the loss of hospital privileges, and midwives in some states (California, for one) were prosecuted for practicing medicine without a license (Starr, 1982, p. 392). Home deliveries have not returned, but most hospitals now offer the next best thing: birthing rooms with homey decor, rocking chairs, and comfortable beds that can be adjusted for the delivery. There is also a resurgent interest in midwifery. And prospective parents are no longer kept in the dark about what to expect. Instead, the father- and mother-to-be take classes on natural childbirth, as a team. Preadmittance tours of the hospital are offered in many communities, and when the delivery time comes, the father is welcomed in the delivery theater, no longer relegated to nervous pacing in the waiting room.

22. Not as much progress has been made at the end of life, but advances are evident, with the hospice movement providing the most conspicuous changes. Not only have residential hospices been set up, many areas now offer hospice care in the home. And many large hospitals provide a special hospice area, where dying patients can get the medical attention they need while enjoying relaxed bureaucratic rules involving visitation, diet, and decor.

23. At the same time, patients or their surrogate decisionmakers who try to break with the physician-autonomy mold typically have a rough go of it. The story of Norman Paradis (1992) is illustrative. Paradis, director of emergency medicine research at New York University-Bellevue Hospital, and his brother, an attorney, found themselves with no control whatsoever over treatment decisions for their incompetent, terminally ill father (himself a physician for nearly fifty years). Despite clear instructions to the contrary, the physicians attending the elder Paradis continued for weeks to perform invasive diagnostic procedures and therapies. As Norman Paradis lamented, in closing his story, "If a doctor and a lawyer could not get decent care for a doctor, what chance does the public have?"

24. The Joint Commission on Accreditation for Hospital Organizations is a nonprofit credentialing organization contracted by the federal government to certify hospitals as worthy of reimbursement under Medicare and Medicaid.

25. For example, in New York, the state legislature essentially passed the technological imperative into law with passage of an act that requires that all patients be resuscitated in the absence of a DNR order to the contrary (Joint Commission, 1987, p. 90).

26. Anesthesiologists present one important exception to DNR policies that tend to empower patients with the right to decide their own medical fate. This group of specialists see resuscitation as part of their "standard of care" in dealing with the necessary and anticipated cardiorespiratory effects of anesthesia. For that reason, they typically will decline to honor the DNR in the operating room. With the backing of their national professional association, anesthesiologists prefer not to honor the DNR because the drugs they administer may be directly responsible for precipitating the arrest. In addition, since they have the

knowledge and skill to execute the resuscitation in the heavily monitored, controlled, and well-equipped environs of the operating room, the chances of successful resuscitation are relatively high (American Hospital Association, 1992, pp. 1–5).

27. In one study done at Duke University, researchers followed 146 CPR patients from 1988 through 1991 and found that only about half (84 patients, or 58 percent) were successfully resuscitated, and only 5 percent (7 patients) got well enough to leave the hospital. Subsequently, these patients were responsible for over $1 million in health-care expenditures, which amounts to about $150,000 per discharged patient ("Common Use of CPR," 1993).

28. Still, the fact that 41 percent of the ethics committees that existed in 1983 were located in New Jersey suggests that the *Quinlan* decision had at least something to do with the proliferation of such bodies.

29. Advance directives were conceived of as state laws that would allow for both the execution of a living will (stating a patient's treatment preferences if terminally ill) and health-care proxy laws (giving others the right to make decisions for the patient when the patient becomes incompetent).

30. Several other recommendations were made, as well. The commission exhorted the medical profession to do everything possible to renew respect for the concept of informed consent. According to the commission's report, the patient (or legal proxy) should have both the right to the latest, most comprehensive information regarding the medical situation of the patient and the right to refuse treatment. Finally, the commission boldly raised the resource-scarcity issue and recommended that it would be inappropriate to expend resources on "lost causes" if such expenditures would preclude the use of those resources in another case with a better prognosis.

31. Data from various studies also suggest that female physicians are apt to spend more time with patients than their male counterparts (Angier, 1992). In one study, male physicians were found to spend ten minutes or more with a patient less than half the time, whereas female physicians were found to spend more than ten minutes with two-thirds of their patients. Candace West, a sociologist specializing in this area, found that male physicians interrupted their patients twice as often as patients interrupted them. If the patient was a woman, male physicians were much more likely to interrupt than if the patient was a man.

32. Dubler (1993, p. 25) argues that hospital counsels regularly exaggerate this fear out of all proportion to case-law realities.

33. There are other reasons why advance directives may not be honored. Sometimes, patients dying at home go into arrest, and despite the patient's expressed wishes, the family panics and calls 911. Emergency medical personnel, not wanting to waste time in a crisis situation, are likely to go ahead and initiate resuscitation, waiting to sort out advance directives after the fact. And sometimes, advance directives simply are not available even under more controlled conditions in a hospital if, during a medical crisis, a treatment/no treatment decision has to be made without delay.

Chapter 5

1. The homeopathic philosophy flourished in Europe in the late eighteenth century and early nineteenth century. And the popularity of homeopathy has remained high there, especially in France, according to the National Center for Homeopathy, with 32 percent of

family physicians adhering to this approach and with homeopathic prescriptions covered by the national health-care system.

2. Relaxation techniques, chiropractic massage, imagery, and spiritual healing were among the common therapies tried. Herbal medicine and folk remedies, biofeedback, hypnosis, and self-help groups were also mentioned (Haney, 1993).

3. The National Welfare Rights Organization is dedicated to promoting and advocating the rights of the poor in the areas of health, education, and welfare.

4. Increasingly sophisticated attempts to measure and report on quality of care have continued through the 1980s. The Health Care Financing Administration began issuing Medicare mortality analyses for selected hospitals across the country in 1986, and other state agencies have followed suit by publishing reports on the status and quality of institutionally based medical care within their respective jurisdictions. New York State's Department of Health and Pennsylvania's Health Care Cost Containment Council have both begun collecting and reporting data on health-care charges and mortality rates for individual physicians and hospitals in selected treatment categories, and other states are expected to do so in the future. Although it is difficult to measure the impact of such reports, banner headlines about higher-than-expected mortality rates—with individual physicians and hospitals identified by name (at least in Pennsylvania)—cannot help but cause further erosion of public confidence in the medical profession.

5. Women, according to Hippocratic writings, were governed by their womb and were therefore incapable of logic and reason. In addition, spiritual deficiencies were supposed to have laid them open to temptation by the devil. During the Middle Ages, intellectual deficiencies were added to the list of flaws presumed to plague the female character. And twentieth-century critics argued that women were simply too physically frail, insufficiently dedicated, and temperamentally ill suited to the study and practice of medicine. When women did survive the gauntlet of medical education to become certified to practice, they were discredited for overemphasizing sympathy over science (The Boston Women's Health Book Collective, 1984, p. 592).

6. The Dalkon Shield was an interuterine device (IUD) marketed by A. H. Robbins and prescribed by American physicians from 1971 to 1974. This contraceptive device was implicated in many cases of pelvic inflammatory disorder (PID) and miscarriages that led to at least seventeen documented deaths. The Dalkon Shield was taken off the market in 1974, but devices already sold were not recalled, so that, in the early 1980s, it was estimated that 50,000 American women still had them in place (with another 500,000 women using the device in other countries).

7. Even though the number of women using the pill peaked at ten million in 1973, it is still the most widely used reversible contraceptive both in the United States and worldwide (The Boston Women's Health Book Collective, 1984, p. 237).

8. Not only did the pill help spawn a sexual revolution, it also facilitated a revolution in the labor force, as more women found it possible to enter the work force when they were more in control of their own reproductive mechanisms. This was an empowering experience in itself for the experience women have gained in the workplace has helped them become more confident of their abilities and more comfortable in dealing with—and challenging—authority figures.

9. Estimates of sex abuse in the general physician population run as high as 5 to 10 percent. In one survey of health-care professionals in California, published in a 1973 edition of the *American Journal of Psychiatry*, 36 percent of psychiatrists and 46 percent of psycholo-

gists reported having sex with at least one of their patients (cited in The Boston Women's Health Book Collective, 1984, pp. 562–563). Such breaches of confidence, often magnified out of proportion by the media, served to put women on guard.

10. This was a position that made delivery more difficult and painful for the mother, but it was (and in many places still is) used because the more natural position—with upper body more vertical and the vagina tipped downward—forces medical personnel to crouch.

11. Approximately 90 percent of first-time mothers delivering in major U.S. hospitals undergo episiotomies (Davis-Floyd, 1992, p. 168). Physicians continue to argue that this procedure prevents damage to the baby's head, vaginal tearing, and other internal damage, even though there is little clinical evidence to support those claims (The Boston Women's Health Book Collective, 1984, p. 383; also Michaelson, 1988, p. 13).

12. The cesarean rate is significantly higher in profit-making hospitals and with women covered by private health insurance ("U.S. Says 349,000 Caesareans," 1993).

13. The average cesarean costs $7,826, compared with $4,720 for a vaginal delivery ("U.S. Says 349,000 Caesareans," 1993).

14. Studies by the federal Center for Disease Control suggest that the chances of death during childbirth are two to four times greater for women delivering by cesarean than for women delivering vaginally, and the National Institute of Health suggests that somewhere between 33 percent and 75 percent of cesareans are not necessary (cited in The Boston Women's Health Book Collective, 1984, p. 385). Approximately 30 percent of these cesareans are performed on women who have already had them, even though there is little hard evidence to indicate such a course of action.

15. Not surprisingly, perhaps, hysterectomies occur far less frequently under prepaid plans, such as HMOs, than under more traditional fee-for-service insurance plans like Blue Shield (The Boston Women's Health Book Collective, 1984, p. 511). Some go so far as to suggest that the number of hysterectomies has gone up as the birth rate has declined because obstetrician/gynecologists have scrambled to maintain the cash flow of their practices. (Fees run $3,000 to $6,000 per operation, adding up to about $5 billion worth of operations annually in the United States).

16. There was a medical committee to review experiments with human subjects (essentially everything that was done within the hospital), but it was rarely consulted. Instead, professionals were left to regulate themselves. As one institute director put it, "The usual patient [wants] to avoid the necessity of grappling with painful facts related to his own welfare. He prefers (and in a real sense he has no other choice) to depend on the overriding faith that the physician and institution will safeguard his interests above any other consideration" (cited in Rothman, 1991, p. 58).

17. The very fact that researchers would defend the practices Beecher questioned and explicitly reject the notion that ethical protocols could even be developed, much less be of any use, speaks volumes about the potential for dissonance between the medical research community and the general public during this period.

18. We should note that the very coverage by the popular press of articles (like Beecher's) that had appeared in professional medical journals was somewhat unique at the time, which is one reason why, to that point, medical researchers had been able to report their questionable research protocols in the medical journals without prompting much second-guessing. But the ethic of consumerism, the blossoming rights culture, and the general distrust of authority figures made both the reporting of and the response to articles about the abuse of the public trust by medical researchers almost inevitable.

19. Given this mood, the public understandably moved beyond criticism of research protocols and began to question the very motives of medical researchers. In the past, the disciples of Hippocrates were accorded almost saintly status. They were assumed a priori to be acting in the best interests of their patients. But now, a more complex and realistic set of motivations seemed to emerge. The profit motive (from the marketing of new drugs and technologies), glory, academic prizes, lucrative research grants, career advancement (all the spoils of successful research projects), and power (regarding the lives and deaths of patients in their care) were added to the purely humanitarian motives that were assumed to drive the medical researcher's behavior.

Chapter 6

1. According to Lofland (1978, p. 87), the happy-death movement deserves to be called a movement because, as with the women's rights movement and the ecology movement, it creates new patterns of thinking about the world on a mass scale. The movement phenomenon does not necessarily require an organized, entirely conscious effort on the part of some dedicated core of participants. Rather, such movements represent a "sprawling, diverse, multi-structured, diffuse assemblage of persons" who act "independently and as part of organizations, engaging in a multiplicity of largely uncoordinated activities and in possession of varying degrees of 'consciousness' relative to their participation in the movement" (Lofland, 1978, pp. 75–76).

2. Indeed, Fletcher's work is widely acknowledged as the first modern work on medical ethics to be issued outside the stream of writings by Catholic theologians (Glick, 1992, p. 59).

3. College classrooms provided an important venue for increasing Americans' exposure to death. That exposure is also crucial to right-to-die activism because many who take a course in death and dying will become inoculated, to varying degrees, with social stigmas and cultural taboos relating to death. These students will have read about, talked about, and written about death in ways their parents would not have dreamed of. Many of these students may well go on to inoculate their own progeny, creating yet another level of geometric growth in sensitivity to death and dying as a natural part of living. In the end, what goes on in U.S. institutions of higher education has the potential for far-reaching effects, well outside the purely academic realm.

4. It is probably safe to say that the seminal works on death published between the mid-1950s and the mid-1970s were more important for what they led to than what they accomplished in and of themselves. This is because, in addition to securing their own positions in academe, their authors encouraged others to work in the area of death. Fletcher, Gorer, Feifel, Kübler-Ross, Becker, Templer, Weisman, and their colleagues set a course for others to follow and provided the intellectual foundation—new theoretical frameworks, new concepts, and old methodologies applied in new ways—on which others could build. From there, the increase in publications, the proliferation of college courses, and the expansion of the general interest in death issues became something of an inevitability.

5. In fact, litigation in the United States accounts for fully 2.5 percent of the gross domestic product (GDP), a rate that puts this country in a category of its own. Belgium, France, and Austria tie for second place with only 0.6 percent of GDP devoted to litigation (Shapiro, 1992, p. 136).

6. Surely, the emergence of the rights culture, fueled by the enduring nature of American individualism, can help explain this litigiousness. In addition, the explosion in the lawyer population (today, there are 310 lawyers for every 100,000 Americans) has been partly responsible for increases in legal activity. In Great Britain, the percentage of attorneys in the population is less than half what it is in the States (Shapiro, 1992, p. 136). The related shift toward activism on the part of the courts also plays a major role in the increased legal activity.

7. Clearly, decisions about this sort of care were being made routinely without formal court review. Indeed, the Supreme Court of New Jersey recited at some length the testimony of a physician witness indicating that problems such as these had "long existed and ordinarily had been handled without the involvement of people or social institutions other than the patient's family, physicians, and possibly hospital administrators. The witness endorsed the practice, which he termed 'judicious neglect'" (President's Commission, 1983, p. 155).

8. Since that time, the number of articles published in the medical literature in a given year has never dropped below 30 and has climbed steadily since 1984 to nearly 175 in 1990 alone. Material on publications presented here is derived from the analysis by Glick (1992, pp. 53–91).

9. Part of the devotion to the right to die in the scholarly and popular literature, beginning in 1976, can be attributed to passage of the nation's first living-will law that same year: California's Natural Death Act. Aside from being the first such law, however, there is nothing particularly radical or controversial about the California NDA. Indeed, it was and continues to be a very conservative and restrictive measure that, unlike *Quinlan*, does little to advance the right to die in a substantive way (see Chapter 8 for more details on the NDA). In contrast, the *Quinlan* decision involved an identifiable set of actors and represented a marked departure from past thinking on the right to die (see Chapter 7 for more details on *Quinlan*). Passage of the NDA was important and noteworthy, but the *Quinlan* decision represented the real turning point for the happy-death movement.

10. To be sure, the courts had been involved in medical cases before *Quinlan*, but inevitably, doctors were found without fault as long as they could demonstrate that they had acted in good faith and in accordance with "accepted medical practice." Accepted medical practice was the carte blanche that always had been invoked to defend physician autonomy, and generally speaking, this defense had carried the day to that point. But when lawyers for Quinlan's physicians attempted the same tack, they were rebuffed. The physicians' lawyers also advanced another common pre-*Quinlan* argument about the Hippocratic commitment to do no harm. This rationale, too, was found wanting by the New Jersey court in the face of overriding family interests.

11. The Patient Self-Determination Act, sometimes referred to as providing the medical equivalent of Miranda rights, took effect on December 1, 1991. It requires that all hospitals receiving reimbursement from Medicare or Medicaid inform incoming patients about their rights to make advance directives (e.g., living wills and durable powers of attorney) about health-care decisions, including the decision to accept or refuse life-sustaining treatments. Hospitals can design their own method of informing patients about advance directives, and they need only inform patients of their rights under state law. But they must broach the subject in a timely manner and provide guidance along the way to those who wish to execute instructions about what therapies, if any, they would prefer to refuse and under what conditions.

12. For some patients, questions about advance directives will be dismissed as just more bureaucratic probing in an already belabored admissions process. For others, however, information about the right to refuse medical treatment, provided pursuant to the PSDA, may be an empowering dose of reality. We suspect that, as time passes and as more Americans cycle through the hospital, more individuals will become informed about and comfortable with their rights to make advance directives, thanks to the impact of the PSDA.

13. Busalacchi was talking with physicians at the Hennepin County Medical Center, the Minnesota institution that went to court to stop medical treatments for Helga Wanglie; see Chapter 3.

14. Both were young women from Missouri, both were victims of automobile accidents, and both were diagnosed to be in a persistent vegetative state. At one point, they were both treated in the same Missouri institution.

15. *Euthanasia*, literally translated, means "good death," from the Greek *eu*, "good," and *thanos*, "death."

16. Members of the new group thought it important to drop the "E" word—*euthanasia*—due to its negative connotations.

17. Humphry divorced Wickett several years later in a messy and well-publicized split after she was found to have terminal breast cancer. Wickett took her own life—using techniques espoused by the Hemlock Society—in the solitude of the Oregon backcountry. Given Humphry's high profile, that story, too, made headlines.

18. Humphry's book also advises that patients devise a backup plan, such as tying a plastic bag around the head—should the ingested drugs be vomited up before they have the intended effect.

19. His comments were made in response to questions submitted to him by Dr. Bruon Haid, a Catholic himself and chief of anesthesia at the University of Innsbruck surgical clinic (Reiser, 1977, p. 47).

20. Significantly, the positions of these two organizations are the only full-text statements by such groups that the authors of the Presidential Commission report chose to provide in their 500-page treatise on forgoing life-sustaining treatments.

21. The Catholic position seems to have softened on the issue of pain management, as well. In the past, Catholic elites discouraged the extensive use of sedating drugs for at least two reasons. First, pain and suffering were thought to be useful vehicles of redemption. And second, sedating patients too extensively might bring on unconsciousness, robbing the patient of the opportunity to mentally and religiously prepare for death. Pope Paul's 1980 statement on the subject represented a more accepting view regarding the use of sedatives to manage pain, even if such use brought on unconsciousness, and possibly even depressed vital bodily functions to the point where death was hastened (Glick, 1992, p. 61).

22. The Catholic Health Association, the national service organization comprising Catholic hospitals and long-term care facilities, was very supportive of the PSDA concept, lobbying for and testifying in favor of its passage during hearings before the Senate Finance Committee's Subcommittee on Medicare and Long Term Care (Catholic Health Association, 1991).

23. There is really only one important distinction to be made between assisted suicide and mercy killing. With assisted suicide, the dying principal takes an active part in the death and is only assisted by a second party. With mercy killing, the second party takes on primary responsibility for causing the death of the principal. Both assisted suicide and

mercy killing are considered "active euthanasia" because individuals take an active role in precipitating death. By way of contrast, "passive euthanasia" involves allowing an individual to die: Medical treatments may be withheld or withdrawn, after which "nature" is allowed to take its course.

24. In May 1992, after Proposition 119 went down to defeat, the United Methodist church, representing nine million Methodists nationwide, went partway down the trail cut by its Northwest Conference. It approved a resolution that, though not endorsing any specific assisted-suicide legislation, expressed a general sense of understanding regarding the plight of persons in a medically hopeless situation. "When the natural process of dying is extended by application of medical technology, the emotional, economic, and relational consequences for self and others may lead a responsible person seriously to question whether continued living is faithful stewardship of the gift of life. Churches need to provide preparation in dealing with these complex issues" (United Methodist church, 1992, p. 144).

25. Kevorkian had been writing for decades about what he calls "medicide," a word he invented to describe orchestrating the deaths both of condemned criminals (in earlier writings) and of those wishing to end their lives because of some overwhelming physical ailment (a more recent interest). The aim of medicide, according to Kevorkian, is to advance a wholly new specialty: *obitiatry* (pronounced "oh-bit-eye-a-tree," another Kevorkian term). This new category of medicine would involve the conducting of live human experimentation (under deep and irreversible anesthesia) and the harvesting of organs and tissues.

26. This line of thinking holds that the Pythagoreans, who were vehemently opposed to abortion, falsely attributed their oath to Hippocrates in hopes that recruiting the father of medicine as the author post mortem would lend credibility to their views on this and other controversial subjects. (The Hippocratic Oath does forbid doctors from conducting abortions.) The fact that Hippocrates was a common name at the time, coupled with the lack of copyright law, meant that few eyebrows were raised when the Pythagoreans first began promulgating an oath under that name, several score years after Hippocrates' death.

27. Some draw a parallel between human and animal life here. There are ethical norms in society, argue proponents of assisted suicide, with regard to putting animals "to sleep" when they are in great pain or near the end of life. Few would argue about the propriety or even the expediency of putting animals out of their misery in such situations. But if it is inhumane, and maybe even illegal, to make animals suffer needlessly, how can a failure to provide humans with moral and legal protections against end-of-life suffering be considered ethical or humane? What happens to humanity, argue those who advance the assisted-suicide alternative, when humans are doing the suffering?

28. As Kevorkian notes, just as with "back-alley abortions," if the suicide is done improperly, in haste, or sloppily, a person can end up in a substantially worse condition than before the attempt was made.

29. Although the activities of the two doctors have many similarities, there is at least one primary and important difference between them: Quill readily admits to being ethically challenged by the prospect of assisted suicide, whereas Kevorkian seems cocksure. For many, Kevorkian seems to lack an appropriate sense of discomfort with the entire idea of assisted suicide; he seems not to appreciate the departure from standard practice that publicly acknowledged assisted-suicide represents. In short, Kevorkian seems ideologically wed to a purpose whose ends many might agree with but whose means become problematic for the potential for abuse is nightmarish.

Chapter 7

1. Material for Chapters 7 and 8 is drawn, in part, from an article entitled "The Right to Die: State Courts Lead the Way Where State Legislatures Fear to Tread" (Hoefler and Kamoie, 1992).

2. The privacy cases commonly referred to by the courts included: *Einstadt* v. *Baird* (affirming the right of access to contraceptives by unmarried persons, including minors, 405 U.S. 438 [1972]), *Loving* v. *Virginia* (affirming the right to interracial marriage; 388 U.S. 1 [1967]), *Pierce* v. *Society of Sisters* (affirming the right to attend private school; 286 U.S. 510 [1925]), and *Meyer* v. *Nebraska* (affirming the right to learn a foreign language, 262 U.S. 390 [1923]). It is beyond the scope of this inquiry to discuss the specific privacy questions raised in each case. It is sufficient for present purposes simply to note that these cases were significant for dealing with the privacy interest in an increasingly broad area of life activity (Borst, 1985, p. 905).

3. Commenting on the extension of the privacy right to right-to-die cases, Vincent Borst suggests that "abortion decisions can be viewed, therefore, as a reaffirmation of the principle that the constitutional right to privacy protects an individual's autonomy in making decisions which involve intimate matters. No decision is more intimate than to terminate one's own life" (Borst, 1985, pp. 905–906).

4. *Cruzan* was the first right-to-die case of its sort to be heard by the Supreme Court. Thus, the justices could not possibly have held that the right of privacy encompassed the right to refuse treatment.

5. Extending his line of reasoning, Rehnquist argued that, on the one hand, erroneous decisions to maintain life are correctable or can be negated in a number of ways: discovery of new evidence regarding the patient's intent, medical advances that would alleviate the patient's condition, or the unexpected death of the individual, despite the continuance of life-sustaining treatments, for example. On the other hand, an erroneous decision to withdraw treatment is not susceptible to correction. Therefore, it is not unreasonable for the state to require petitioners to satisfy elevated evidentiary standards before allowing the withdrawal of life support.

6. The significance of *Saikewicz* in this regard should not be overemphasized. The Massachusetts court later modified (although it never explicitly rejected) this policy. And significantly, it has been rejected by all states that have raised the issue, save for an Ohio appellate court (Glick, 1992, p. 147).

7. We should note that items (1) and (3) seem to borrow from the best-interest standard, and item (2) derives from the substituted-judgment standard. It is not uncommon for courts to mix and match the two as they see fit, in finding their way to the decision they have in mind.

8. Generally speaking, according to the National Center for State Courts (1992, p. 177), a "coma is a sleep-like (eyes closed) unarousable condition resulting from impairment of brain stem functions." The most profound coma is described as "brain death," in which the coma is both irreversible and severe to the point that there are no brain-stem functions whatsoever. Unlike those in a coma, individuals in a PVS have their eyes open, even though their neocortical functions have ceased. It is not uncommon for someone in a coma (eyes closed) to "evolve" into an eyes-open PVS. In both cases, patients can be considered to be "neocortally dead" because their brain stems—the center of all thinking and sensory activity—is permanently and irreversibly damaged. However, under the currently accepted def-

inition of legal death, these individuals are still alive because their brain stems, controlling involuntary motor functions and internal organ functions, continue to operate. Patients in either of these conditions have ceased to have any sensory, thinking existence, but they continue to live on—at least in the legal sense of the word—in either an eyes-open (PVS), or eyes-closed (coma) state. As a matter of fact, these patients cannot even be described as terminally ill, even though there is absolutely no medical reason to hope for recovery in most cases. This is the case because they may be maintained, with proper medical care, for years and even decades (the longest recorded survival being thirty-seven years [Meisel, 1989, p. 139]; for more on PVS and brain death, see our Chapter 3).

9. To this point, the only possible exception is the decision in *Couture* v. *Couture* (48 Ohio App. 3d 208, 549 N.E.2d 571 [1989]; see National Center for State Courts, 1992, p. 168).

10. The National Center for State Courts (NCSC, 1992) lists 105 state and federal cases addressing the initiation, maintenance, and removal of life-sustaining treatment, beginning with *Quinlan* in 1976 and carrying through *Busalacchi* in 1992. Our analysis, based on data contained within that report, suggests that the prototypical right-to-die case involves family members who are asking permission to withdraw ANH from an incompetent principal somewhere in his or her seventies.

11. Many of these incompetent individuals were characterized as being in a persistent vegetative state (41 cases out of 108), even though that specific term was not always used (other terms included *chronic vegetative state* and *semicomatose*). Patients were considered to be fully comatose in another 12 instances and brain dead in another 6. This brings the total of those who were essentially in a persistent vegetative state to well over half the total of 108.

Only 16 out of 108 cases heard to date involved patients who were considered to be completely competent to make decisions for themselves. In all but 2 of these cases, the petitioners won. In 1 of the 2 cases in which the petitioner was unsuccessful, the court refused to make a prospective decision regarding a hypothetical case, arguing that it had to wait until an actual case arose (*A.B.* v. *C.*, 1984).

Donaldson v. *Van de Kamp* (1992) was the other failed right-to-die case involving a competent patient. Here, the petitioner was asking the court for relief far outside the mainstream of jurisprudence to that point. Donaldson was the individual referred to in Chapter 1 who asked that he be allowed to undergo decapitation while still alive for purposes of cryogenically suspending his head before his inoperable brain tumor could do any more damage. The court dismissed the request, arguing that the petitioner had "no constitutional right to either pre-mortem cryogenic suspension or assistance in committing suicide" (NCSC, 1992, p. 158).

12. Artificial respiration came in a close second as the procedure most likely to be involved in court cases, at 35 percent (38 out of 108 cases). Refusing surgery (mostly amputations) was cited as the central issue in 14 cases, and refusing therapy (e.g., hemodialysis and chemotherapy) was an issue in 6 other instances. In 5 other situations, the removal of "life-support procedures" was referred to in general terms. (The total does not add up to 108 because some cases involved more than a single procedure.)

13. As noted, Massachusetts wanted final decisionmaking in right-to-die cases to rest with the courts, whereas New Jersey advocated the use of ethics committees, thinking the court would become the final arbiter only in cases with extenuating circumstances or unresolvable disagreements. For its part, the New York court raised the evidentiary standard for right-to-die cases set by *Quinlan* by requiring that guardians produce "clear and convinc-

ing evidence" that terminating life support was consistent with a principal's desires. New Jersey had adopted the more lenient standard, in which guardians had only to demonstrate that the termination of life could reasonably be expected to be the wish of the principal.

14. New Jersey has its *Quinlan, Colyer,* and *Conroy* decisions; Massachusetts is cited for authoring the *Spring, Saikewicz,* and *Hier* decisions; New York has its *Eichner, Storar,* and *Klein* decisions; and California rounds out the group with decisions in the *Barber, Bouvia,* and *Donaldson* cases.

15. In addition to its two right-to-die precedents, the New Jersey court has been noted for a variety of rights-based rulings, including (1) its ruling that the local system of school finance unconstitutionally discriminated against children in poor districts, (2) its attack on zoning ordinances designed to exclude low-income housing, and (3) its strengthening of protections against illegal searches and seizures by rejecting the "good faith" exception.

Chapter 8

1. The statutory information we assembled for analysis here constitutes a "snapshot" of right-to-die law in the fifty states as it existed during the time the of our research (beginning in the summer of 1991 and ending in the spring of 1992). Admittedly, many states have amended their laws since that time, making some of the details of our analysis a bit outdated. At the same time, we feel the general theme of the analysis holds up quite well: The state courts have led and continue to lead the way on right-to-die policymaking, and the state legislatures struggle to resist but ultimately converge with the consensus position carved out by the state courts.

2. Durable powers of attorney for health-care provisions give the principal a way to empower a second party with the right to make health-care decisions for the principal when he or she becomes incompetent. These new kinds of provisions have been required because regular powers of attorney are not typically applicable in right-to-die situations for two reasons. First, powers of attorney traditionally become void when the principal becomes incompetent; making powers of attorney "durable" resolves this defect. Second, traditional powers of attorney have been thought to cover only estate and fiduciary matters, making it necessary to pass perfecting legislation in which the coverage of the power of attorney is specifically extended to health-care decisionmaking.

3. Glick (1992) notes that the *Quinlan* decision did not directly motivate the California legislature to act for the issue had been on the decision agenda in that state for several years. What *Quinlan* did was provide right-to-die advocates with a window of opportunity, which helped them finally push the bill over the top.

4. The state law in Washington provides a good, typical example (see Washington Natural Death Act [1979]).

5. In an effort to distinguish acts associated with allowing terminal patients to die from the acts suggested by the controversial terms *mercy killing* and *euthanasia,* the Alaska statute goes so far as to coin a new term—*mercy dying*—to describe what the statute condones.

6. In a departure from this norm, California requires living wills to be reauthorized every five years and reexecuted within four months after an individual is declared terminally ill. In another minor departure from the norm, Georgia requires reauthorization every seven years.

7. The Patient Self-Determination Act of 1991 represents a significant development along these lines at the federal level. The PSDA—somewhat like the Nevada law that pre-

dated it—requires hospitals, hospices, nursing homes, HMOs, and other health-care facilities receiving reimbursement under either Medicare or Medicaid to provide written information to patients upon admission regarding the extent of their legal rights (in accordance with their respective state laws) to refuse medical treatment should they become incapacitated. Hospitals must also note the patient's preferences on his or her medical records. The act also requires the Department of Health and Human Services to conduct a nationwide campaign to educate the public about right-to-die legal options.

8. In apparently the only "wrongful life" case heard to date, an Ohio court dismissed all charges against St. Francis-St. George Hospital, where Edgar Winter, an eighty-four-year-old heart patient, was resuscitated after a heart attack, against his wishes ("Wrongful Life Suit," 1991).

9. Residents of Mississippi should take note of their state's one exception to the liability shield: Physicians involved in removing a patient's organs for purposes of transplantation are prohibited from participating in the withdrawal of life support from that patient.

10. Some public officials, including U.S. Representative Pat Schroeder (D-Colorado), suggest that it would make good economic sense to give premium discounts to those who were willing to sign advance directives. Though the ethical arguments against such a move may seem prohibitive at this time, this is an option that no doubt will receive more attention in the future, unless spiraling health-care costs can be brought under control some other way.

11. To be sure, some degree of variation among the state laws is no evidence of their weakness as a whole. Indeed, those arguing from a "states' rights" or "new federalism" perspective would celebrate what diversity exists, while demurring at the prospect that state laws should be measured against some national standard for living-will legislation. At the same time, there may be some fundamental aspects of the right to die, grounded both in common law, and in the U.S. Constitution, that would supersede legislative prerogatives. It is the degree to which the state laws impinge on rights with those kinds of foundations that may, indeed, be taken as a measure of the state legislatures' deficiency as a whole in dealing with the right-to-die issue.

12. Use of the terms *conservative* and *liberal* is not meant to necessarily suggest that these categories of linguistic construction represent positions endorsed by individuals of those respective ideological persuasions.

13. The named individual(s) must be willing and competent to make decisions for the incompetent patient. Otherwise, decision-making authority devolves to the next class listed.

14. The Uniform Law Commissioners provide guidance on only two important issues, stating that (1) a failure to reach consensus does not authorize the next class in line to decide and (2) the proxy decision cannot conflict with the previously expressed intentions of the individual (National Conference of Commissioners on Uniform State Laws, 1989, pp. 12–13). Even when the states have modeled their laws after the URTIA, however, it is not always clear that these two understandings have been adopted.

15. This is significant because of a recent New York case, even though pregnancy was not an issue. In that case, Murray Elbaum had requested that the feeding tube in his comatose wife's stomach be removed, arguing that his wife had asked him repeatedly not to keep her alive if she should become comatose. The New York court, operating under the strict "clear and convincing" test charted in *Eichner* and *Storar,* refused Elbaum's request on the grounds that his wife's private pleas to her husband did not satisfy the required evidentiary

standard. After losing his case, Elbaum refused to continue paying for his wife's care, but an appellate division of the state supreme court eventually ordered him to do so: a sum amounting to $100,000 by the time the decision was rendered (Belkin, 1992).

16. In the Washington, D.C., opinion, the more significant of the two given the advanced stage of Carder's pregnancy (twenty-six weeks), the judges stated that "respect for patient autonomy compels us to accede to the decisions of a pregnant patient whenever possible" (cited in Greenhouse, 1990).

17. *Incubator* is a generally pejorative, shorthand term used by women's rights advocates to describe the nature of pregnancy exclusion provisions—provisions they see as reducing women to the status of an incubator if they are prohibited from exercising the right to die when pregnant.

18. The law was co-sponsored by several female legislators. And, if the New Jersey court is any indication, there is a tradition of liberal policy mediation in the state. At the same time, New Jersey has a relatively high percentage of Catholics. And with a 90 percent male membership, New Jersey has one of the most male-dominated legislatures in the country. Why, then, did the New Jersey legislature do what it did? One lobbyist for the state's Catholic Conference gave the impression that the conference in particular, and the pro-life movement in general, simply ran out of steam in a state that has traditionally taken relatively liberal stands on such issues (personal interview).

19. Using regression-analysis techniques, Glick (1992, pp. 182–184) finds just the opposite relationship: The more recent the passage of the bill or amendment, the more likely it is that ANH will be excluded as a procedure that can be withheld or withdrawn. We suspect, however, that the low number of states on which the analysis was based made the regression overly sensitive to a few exceptional cases. Regression is problematic as a method of comparative state analysis even when all fifty states are involved. When the number of states drops below fifty, results become even more questionable. In this case, nine states had no living-will laws in force when Glick did his analysis, and nineteen others did not mention ANH one way or another. Two more states equivocated on the issue, leaving a total sample of twenty states on which to run an analysis. Five of the six states to pass laws in the last three years have included ANH as a procedure that can be withheld or withdrawn, and two other states have amended their laws to allow for ANH withdrawal since Glick's analysis was conducted. The sensitivity of Glick's original analysis to a few atypical cases, combined with developments that have taken place since that analysis, help explain the divergence of conclusions on the ANH issue between Glick's analysis and ours.

20. The National Conference of Commissioners on Uniform State Laws (NCCUSL) is an interstate legislative body consisting of two representatives appointed by the governor from each state. Its stated mission involves drafting model pieces of legislation for all states to adopt. The NCCUSL is a well placed, well connected, and widely respected body, and as such, it is a source of legislative policy diffusion in a league of its own.

21. The commissioners updated the URTIA in 1989, and that, too, had a substantial impact on legislation across the country: The revised code was adopted, essentially in toto, in Alaska, Iowa, Maine, Missouri, Montana, and Oklahoma.

22. These groups issue interstate analyses of legislative initiatives and act as information clearinghouses for other issues. Such organizations also publish newsletters and magazines that facilitate the exchange of ideas and increase awareness of legislative developments. In addition, they hold conferences where legislators can exchange ideas face to face.

23. David Fairbanks (1980, p. 104) described the same phenomenon in 1980. He conducted policy innovation research on a range of issues that, like the right to die, have a distinctively moral (as opposed to economic) dimension to them and found that "most efforts to regulate morality are based on religious beliefs, and measures of religious culture provide the single best predictor of the type of morality policies a state will pursue."

24. Indeed, in states in which the Catholic population is large and the church is especially powerful (e.g., New York, Massachusetts, New Jersey), living-will laws have been slow in coming, if they have come at all. These states may traditionally be very innovative with regard to economic policy trends, "but in this particular policy, it strongly appears that the Catholic church has successfully blocked legislation" (Glick, 1992, p. 159).

25. For example, the following cases all gave Catholic elites cause for concern: *Saikewicz* in 1980, *Eichner* in 1981, *Bouvia* in 1982, *Colyer* in 1983, *Hier* in 1984, and in one of the most serious blows to the Catholic position, *Conroy* in 1985 (New Jersey's liberal decision allowing the withdrawal of ANH).

26. In this context, routine means that the principal is competent but not pregnant, that ANH is not involved, and that a valid, unambiguous living will has been executed.

27. On the one hand, the new law allows for the withdrawal of artificial nutrition and hydration, the designation of proxy decisionmakers, and the right to die for individuals in a persistent vegetative state; Pennsylvania's law also bends ever so slightly in the liberal direction regarding the rights of pregnant women. On the other hand, Pennsylvania adopted the old, conservative definition of the concept "terminal condition" that was more popular with legislatures in the later 1970s and early 1980s.

28. The current governor, Robert Casey, can be included here. Although a committed Democrat, Casey is extremely sensitive to conservative Catholic positions.

29. The Catholic Conference and the Pro-Life Federation worked to keep the issue off of the legislative agenda first by linking the right to die to abortion and then by spreading fear that legislation would open the door to euthanasia and the legalization of death by lethal injection. The divisiveness of the issues surrounding the right to die and the link to abortion ensured it would never receive serious consideration.

30. It is often said of legislatures that "the power to delay is the power to kill" (Oleszek, 1989). Clearly, the power of the house to delay consideration of right-to-die legislation, combined with the power to take the time to load a bill down with conservative amendments, turned out to be sufficient to kill living-will legislation in Pennsylvania for five years running.

31. The Florida law has since been amended to allow for the withdrawal of artificial nutrition and hydration, under certain conditions.

32. For example, in at least five cases, state courts have specifically rejected state statutory provisions that precluded the withdrawal of artificial nutrition and hydration: *Barber* v. *Superior Court* (California), *Corbett* v. *D'Alessandro* and *Satz* v. *Perlmutter* (Florida), *In re Gardner* (Maine), and *McConnell* v. *Beverly Enterprises, Inc.* (Connecticut). In each case, the courts made it clear that statutes could not limit an individual's constitutional right to refuse medical treatment (Glick, 1992, p. 161).

In California, the court has also explicitly criticized the legislature's Natural Death Act for requiring a fourteen-day waiting period after a patient has been declared terminally ill before a living will can be executed. By that time, the court argued, many individuals—as many as half—would be unable to complete such a document (Glick, 1992, pp. 179–180).

33. The right to die for pregnant women may prove more problematic, however, even though the beginnings of a progressive trend are detectable. This will be the case, it seems fair to say, as long as abortion rights themselves remain in question.

Chapter 9

1. Catholics argue that the right to die is inimical to the sanctity-of-life principle. Prolife groups see the fight against the right to die as a natural extension of their interests in prohibiting abortions. Disabled rights groups are worried that the right to die will someday degenerate into the right to take the lives of disabled individuals whose lives do not seem, in the eyes of some third parties, to be worth living (or supporting with public funds). The loud and persistent protests carried out by these kinds of groups—both outside hospitals and long-term care facilities where right-to-die scenarios are being played out, and inside courtrooms and legislative hearing rooms where rights to die are being considered—generally have retarded the mediation process.

2. Even *Mad* magazine has circulated its version of a model living will, including the stipulation: "While I am not morally or ethically opposed to so-called 'life-sustaining treatment,' I am vehemently opposed to the concept of hooking up such machinery to 'The Clapper.'"

3. Warm-water drownings are more problematic than cold-water drownings. In warm water, the lack of oxygen seriously and irreparably damages the brain and other organs after just a short time (a couple of minutes). In the case of a cold-water drowning, however, the body core temperature drops substantially, and metabolic rates slow to the point where the brain (and other organs) can be sustained without a supply of oxygen for extended periods of time (twenty minutes or longer, in some cases). If warming and resuscitation of a young cold-water drowning victim is completed under controlled conditions with medical supervision, the child—if he or she was healthy prior to the incident—can recuperate with little or no long-term damage.

4. Increasingly, patients, families, and physicians are conspiring to make bold decisions about forgoing life-sustaining treatments. According to American Hospital Association, many of the "6,000 deaths that occur in this country every day are somehow timed or negotiated by patients, families, and doctors who ... armed with an amazing array of death-delaying technology ... reach a very painful and a very private consensus not to do all that they can do and let a dying patient die" (Malcolm, 1990a).

References

Altman, Lawrence K. 1991a. "More Physicians Broach Forbidden Subject of Euthanasia," *New York Times*. March 12.

———. 1991b. "Jury Declines to Indict a Doctor Who Said He Aided in a Suicide," *New York Times*. July 27.

———. 1993a. "Doctors Report Signs of Progress in Patient Who Got Baboon Liver," *New York Times*. January 27.

———. 1993b. "A Focus on Curing as Well as Caring: Doctors Should Be Trained to Give Patients Active Role, a Health Official Says," *New York Times*. August 15.

American Association of Retired Persons. 1988. *Tomorrow's Choices*. Washington, D.C.: American Association of Retired Persons.

American Hospital Association. 1992. "New Views Define Appropriate Resuscitation Circumstances." *Hospital Ethics*. Vol. 8, No.1. January/February, pp. 1–5.

American Medical Association. 1989. *Current Opinions of the Council on Ethical and Judicial Affairs*. §2.20, at 13.

American Medical Association, Council on Ethical and Judicial Affairs. 1992. *Current Opinions of the Council on Ethical and Judicial Affairs, American Medical Association*. Chicago, Ill.: American Medical Association.

Anderson, Kelly L. 1992. "All Charges Dismissed in Dr. Kevorkian Case," *Harrisburg* (Pa.) *Patriot-News*. July 22.

Angier, Natalie. 1992. "Bedside Manners Improve as More Women Enter Medicine," *New York Times*. June 21.

———. 1993a. "U.S. Opens the Door Just a Crack to Alternative Forms of Medicine," *New York Times*. January 10.

———. 1993b. "Unusual Therapy Gains Popularity," *New York Times*. January 28.

Annas, G. J., 1975. In *Changing Attitudes Toward Euthanasia: Excerpts from Papers Presented at the Eighth Annual Euthanasia Conference, New York, N.Y., December 6, 1975*. New York: The Euthanasia Educational Council, pp. 9, 10.

"Another Right-to-Die Case Poses New Questions." 1991. *New York Times*. January 2.

Anton, Thomas J. 1989. *American Federalism & Public Policy: How the System Works*. Philadelphia: Temple University Press.

———. 1991. "Jury Declines to Indict a Doctor Who Said He Aided in Suicide," *New York Times*. July 27.

Aseer, M. Adil Al. 1990. "An Islamic Perspective on Terminating Life-Sustaining Measures." In Arthur S. Berger and Joyce Berger, eds., *To Die or Not to Die?* New York: Praeger Press.

"Baby Born Without Brain Dies, but Legal Struggle Will Continue." 1992. *New York Times.* March 31.

Barasch, Douglas S. 1992. "The Mainstreaming of Alternative Medicine," *New York Times: The Good Health Magazine.* October 4.

Barrington, Mary R. 1990. "Euthanasia: An English Perspective." In Arthur S. Berger and Joyce Berger, eds., *To Die or Not to Die?* New York: Praeger Press, pp. 85–102.

Beck, M., Beachy, L., Wilson, L., Hager, M., and Dickey, C. 1990. "Peddling Youth over the Counter," *Newsweek.* March 5.

Becker, Ernest. 1973. *The Denial of Death.* New York: Free Press.

Beecher, Henry K. 1966. "Ethics and Clinical Research." *New England Journal of Medicine.* Vol. 74, pp. 1354–1360.

Behnke, J. A., and Bok, S., eds. 1975. *The Dilemmas of Euthanasia.* New York: Doubleday.

Belkin, Lisa. 1992. "In Right-to-Die Fight, Court Finds Family Liable for Care," *New York Times.* September 24.

_____. 1993. "There's No Simple Suicide," *New York Times Magazine.* November 14.

Benson, Herbert, and Klipper, Miriam Z. 1975. *The Relaxation Response.* New York: Avon.

Berger, Arthur S. 1990. "Last Rights: The View from a U.S. Courthouse." In Arthur S. Berger and Joyce Berger, eds. *To Die or Not to Die?* New York: Praeger Press, pp. 129–151.

Berger, Arthur S., and Berger, Joyce, eds. 1990. *To Die or Not to Die?* New York: Praeger Press.

Blank, Robert H. 1988. *Life, Death, and Public Policy.* De Kalb: Northern Illinois University Press.

Blauner, Robert. 1966. "Death and Social Structure." *Psychiatry.* Vol. 24, pp. 378–394.

Blumstein, James F., and Sloan, Frank A., eds. 1989. *Organ Transplantation Policy: Issues and Prospects.* Durham, N.C.: Duke University Press.

Bok, Sissela. 1987. "Euthanasia and Care for the Dying." In J. A. Behnke and S. Bok, eds., *The Dilemmas of Euthanasia.* New York: Doubleday.

Bopp, James Jr., ed. 1987. *The Medical Treatment Rights of Children with Disabilities: A Litigation Manual.* Indianapolis, Ind.: National Legal Center for the Medically Dependent and Disabled.

Borst, Vincent T. 1985. "The Right to Die: An Extension of the Right to Privacy." *John Marshall Law Review.* Vol. 18, pp. 895–914.

The Boston Women's Health Book Collective. 1984. *The New Our Bodies, Ourselves.* New York: Simon and Schuster.

Brody, Jane E. 1993a. "Standing Up for a Dying Patient's Rights," *New York Times.* January 27.

_____. 1993b. "Is Doctor-Assisted Suicide Ever Acceptable?" *New York Times.* March 17.

Bronzino, Joseph D., Smith, Vincent H., and Wade, Maurice L. 1990. *Medical Technology and Society: An Interdisciplinary Perspective.* Cambridge, Mass.: MIT Press.

Bugen, Larry A. 1979. *Death and Dying.* Dubuque, Iowa: Wm. C. Brown.

Bulger, Roger J. 1988. *Technology, Bureaucracy, and Healing in America.* Iowa City: University of Iowa Press.

Caldiera, Gregory. 1985. "The Transmission of Legal Precedent: A Study of State Supreme Courts." *American Political Science Review.* Vol. 79, pp. 178–193.

Callahan, Daniel. 1983. "On Feeding the Dying." *Hastings Center Report.* October, p. 22.

_____. 1990. *What Kind of Life? The Limits of Medical Progress.* New York: Simon and Schuster.

Canon, Bradley, and Baum, Lawrence. 1981. "Patterns of Tort Law Innovations: An Application of Diffusion Theory to Judicial Doctrines." *American Political Science Review.* Vol. 75, pp. 975–987.

Cantor, Norman L. 1987. *Legal Frontiers of Death and Dying.* Bloomington: Indiana University Press.

Carey, Raymond G., and Posavac, Emil J. 1980. "Attitudes of Physicians on Disclosing Information to and Maintaining Life for Terminal Patients." In Richard A. Kalish, ed., *Perspectives on Death and Dying: Vol. 2. Caring Relationships: The Dying and the Bereaved.* New York: Baywood, pp. 145–154.

Carse, James P., and Dallery, Arlene B., eds. 1977. *Death and Society: A Book of Reading and Sources.* New York: Harcourt Brace Jovanovich.

Carson, Rachel. 1962. *Silent Spring.* Boston: Houghton Mifflin.

Catholic Bishops of Pennsylvania. 1991. "Nutrition and Hydration: Moral Considerations." Harrisburg: Pennsylvania Catholic Conference.

Catholic Health Association (CHA). 1991. "The Patient Self-Determination Act: Healthcare Decisions in Advance." St. Louis, Mo.: Catholic Health Association.

Chang, H.H.B., and Chang, C. K. 1980. "The Denying of Death: A Social Psychological Study." *Journal of Sociology and Social Welfare.* Vol. 7, No. 5, pp. 742–754.

Charmaz, Kathy. 1980. *The Social Reality of Death.* Reading, Mass.: Addison-Wesley.

Chartrand, Sabra. 1992. "Baby Missing Part of Brain Challenges Legal Definition of Death," *New York Times.* March 29.

Cieply, Michael. 1991. "Marine Fighting in Gulf Takes Out Afterlife Policy," *Los Angeles Times.* February 27.

Clark, Jill. 1985. "Policy Diffusion and Program Scope: Research Directions." *Publius.* Vol. 15, No. 4, pp. 61–70.

Clark, Nicola. 1992. "The High Costs of Dying," *Wall Street Journal.* February 26.

Cohn, Victor. 1989. "When Death Is Near," *Washington Post Magazine.* August 29.

Collins, Peggy L. 1987. "The Foundations of the Right to Die." *West Virginia Law Review.* Vol. 90.

"Common Use of CPR in Hospitals Questioned." 1993. *Carlisle* (Pa.) *Sentinel.* March 17.

Conroy, Pat. 1987. *The Prince of Tides.* New York: Bantam Books.

"Cost of Heart Revival Put at $150,000 per Survivor." 1993. *New York Times.* March 21.

Counts, David R. 1980. "The Good Death in Kaliai: Preparation for Death in Western New Britain." In Richard A. Kalish, ed., *Perspectives on Death and Dying: Vol. 1. Death and Dying: Views from Many Cultures.* New York: Baywood.

Crane, Diana. 1975. *The Sanctity of Life: Physicians' Treatment of Critically Ill Patients.* New York: Russell Sage Foundation.

Cranford, Ronald. 1991. "Helga Wanglie's Ventilator." *Hastings Center Report.* July–August, pp. 23–25.

Cranston, Sylvia, and Williams, Carey. 1984. *Reincarnation: A New Horizon in Science, Religion, and Society.* New York: Julian Press.

Danforth, John. 1992. Personal communication to Catholic Health Association, December 1.

Danis, M., Southland, L. I., Garrett, J. M., Smith, J. L., Hielema, F., Pickard, C. G., Egner, D. M., and Patrick, D. I. 1991. "A Prospective Study of Advance Directives for Life-Sustaining Care." *New England Journal of Medicine.* Vol. 324, pp. 882–888.

"Dartmouth Redesigns Medical Training To Give Future Doctors A Human Touch." 1992. *New York Times.* September 2.

Davis-Floyd, Robbie E. 1992. *Birth as an American Rite of Passage.* Berkeley: University of California Press.

"The Death of Nancy Cruzan." 1992. "Frontline" (PBS Television). March 24.

DeSpelder, Lynne Ann, and Strickland, Albert Lee. 1992. *The Last Dance: Encountering Death and Dying.* Mountain View, Calif.: Mayfield Press.

"Doctor Assists 2 More Suicides in Michigan." 1992. *New York Times.* December 16.

"Doctors Want to Pull Plug; Husband Says No." 1990. *Carlisle* (Pa.) *Sentinel.* January 10.

Domenici, Pete, and Koop, C. Everett. 1991. "Sue the Doctor? There's a Better Way," *New York Times.* June 6.

Douglas, William. 1992. "Elderly's Suicide Rate Fastest-Growing of Any Age Group," *Harrisburg* (Pa.) *Patriot-News.* December 11.

"Dr. Ponce de Leon." 1990. *U.S. News & World Report.* July 16.

Dubler, Nancy N. 1993. "Commentary: Balancing Life and Death—Proceed with Caution." *American Journal of Public Health.* Vol. 83, No.1. January, pp. 23–25.

Dychtwald, Ken. 1989. *Age Wave.* Los Angeles: Jeremy P. Tarcher.

Dye, Thomas R., and Gray, Virginia, eds. 1980. *The Determinants of Public Policy.* Lexington, Mass.: D. C. Heath.

Ebert, Robert H. 1977. "Medical Education in the United States." In John H. Knowles, ed., *Doing Better and Feeling Worse.* New York: W. W. Norton, pp. 171–184.

Eckholm, Erik. 1990. "Haunting Issue for U.S.: Caring for the Elderly Ill," *New York Times.* March 27.

Edelstein, Ludwig. 1943. *The Hippocratic Oath: Text, Translation, and Interpretation.* Baltimore: Johns Hopkins Press.

Elazar, Daniel J. 1984. *American Federalism: A View from the States.* New York: Harper & Row.

Emanuel, Linda L., Barry, J. M., Stoeckle, J. D., Ettelson, L. M., and Emanuel, E. J. 1991. "Advance Directives for Medical Care: A Case for Greater Use." *New England Journal of Medicine.* Vol. 324, pp. 889–895.

Ettinger, Mae A. 1992. "What Is an Immortalist?" *The Immortalist* (newsletter of the Immortalist Society and the American Cryonics Society). Vol. 23, No. 6, p. 1.

Ettinger, Robert C.W. 1964. *The Prospect of Immortality.* Garden City, N.Y.: Doubleday.

Eyestone, Robert. 1977. "Confusion, Diffusion, and Innovation." *American Political Science Review.* Vol. 71, pp. 441–477.

Fairbanks, David J. 1980. "Politics, Economics, and the Public Morality: Why Some States are More Moral than Others." In Thomas R. Dye and Virginia Gray, eds., *The Determinants of Public Policy.* Lexington, Mass.: D. C. Heath, pp. 95–105.

Faludi, Susan. 1991. *Backlash: The Undeclared War Against American Women.* New York: Crown.

Feifel, Herman, ed. 1959. *The Meaning of Death.* New York: McGraw-Hill.

"Film Gets Upbeat Ending for American Audiences." 1992. *Harrisburg* (Pa.) *Patriot-News*. February 12.

Fletcher, Joseph Francis. 1954. *Morals and Medicine; The Moral Problems of: The Patient's Right to Know the Truth, Contraception, Artificial Insemination, Sterilization, Euthanasia*. Princeton, N.J.: Princeton University Press.

"Florida Court Rejects New Death Definition." 1992. *New York Times*. November 14.

Foderaro, Lisa. 1991. "New York Will Not Discipline Doctor for His Role in Suicide," *New York Times*. August 17.

"The Forgotten Talent Pool." 1992. *New York Times*. April 27.

Frederickson, Donald S. 1977. "The Responsibility of the Individual." In John H. Knowles, ed., *Doing Better and Feeling Worse*. New York: W. W. Norton, pp. 159–170.

Freud, Anna. 1976. "The Doctor-Patient Relationship." In Samuel Gorovitz, *Moral Problems in Medicine*. Englewood Cliffs, N.J.: Prentice-Hall, pp. 200–203.

Freudenheim, Milt. 1992a. "Managed Care: Is it Effective?" *New York Times*. September 1.

_____. 1992b. "A Squeeze Hurts a Health Niche," *New York Times*. September 2.

Friedman, Meyer, and Rosenman, Ray H. 1974. *The Type A Behavior and Your Heart*. New York: Knopf.

Fumento, M. 1991. "The Dying Dutchman: Coming Soon to a Nursing Home Near You." *The American Spectator*. Vol. 24, October, pp. 18–22.

Garrett, Thomas, Baillie, Harold W., and Garrett, Rosellen M. 1989. *Health Care Ethics: Principles and Problems*. Englewood Cliffs, N.J.: Prentice-Hall.

Gates, John B., and Johnson, Charles A., eds. 1991. *The American Courts: A Critical Assessment*. Washington, D.C.: Congressional Quarterly Press.

General Accounting Office (GAO). 1991. *Canadian Health Insurance: Lessons for the United States*. Washington, D.C.: U.S. GAO.

Gelman, David, and Hager, Mary. 1989. "The Brain Killer," *Newsweek*. December 18.

Gerbner, George. 1993. Comments made during the Dickinson College Public Affairs Symposium, "Violence: Society Under Siege." Carlisle, Penn., February 15.

Gibbs, Nancy. 1990. "Love and Let Die," *Time*. March 19.

Glaberson, William. 1991. "Jurors to Decide: Should a Doctor Who Aided Suicide Face Trial?" *New York Times*. July 22.

Glick, Henry J. 1990. "Policy Making and State Supreme Courts." In John B. Gates and Charles A. Johnson, eds. *The American Courts: A Critical Assessment*. Washington, D.C.: Congressional Quarterly Press.

_____. 1992. *The Right to Die: Policy Innovation and Its Consequences*. New York: Columbia University Press.

Glick, Henry J., and Hays, Scott. 1991. "Innovation and Reinvention in State Policymaking: Theory and the Evolution of Living Will Laws." *Journal of Politics*. Vol. 53, No. 3, pp. 835–850.

Gorer, Geoffrey. 1956. "The Pornography of Death." In W. Phillips and P. Rahv, eds., *Modern Writing*. New York: Berkeley.

_____. 1965. *Death, Grief, and Mourning in Contemporary Britain*. London: Cresset Press.

Gorman, James. 1992. "Take a Little Deadly Nightshade and You'll Feel Better," *New York Times*. August 30.

Gorovitz, Samuel. 1976. *Moral Problems in Medicine*. Englewood Cliffs, N.J.: Prentice-Hall.

"Governor Signs Ban After 2 More Assisted Suicides." 1992. *Carlisle* (Pa.) *Sentinel.* December 16.

Gray, Virginia. 1973. "Innovation in the States: A Diffusion Study." *American Political Science Review.* Vol. 71, pp. 1174–1186.

Green, Judith Strupp. 1980. "The Days of the Dead in Oaxaca, Mexico: An Historical Inquiry." In Richard A. Kalish, ed., *Perspectives on Death and Dying: Vol. 1. Death and Dying: Views from Many Cultures.* New York: Baywood, pp. 56–71.

Greenhouse, Linda. 1990. "Hospital Sets Policy on Pregnant Patients' Rights," *New York Times.* November 29.

Gross, Jane. 1991. "Voters Turn Down Legal Euthanasia," *New York Times.* November 7.

Gutman, David. 1977. "Dying to Power: Death and the Search for Self-Esteem." In Herman Feifel, ed., *New Meanings of Death.* New York: McGraw-Hill, pp. 335–347.

_____. 1991. "Reclaimed Powers: A Cross-Cultural Look at Aging," *Los Angeles Times Magazine.* November 17.

Hahn, B., and Lefkowitz, B. 1992. "Annual Expenses and Sources of Payment for Health Care Services" (APHCR Pub. No. 93-0007). *National Medical Expenditure Finding 14,* Agency for Health Care Policy Research. Rockville, Md.: Public Health Service.

Haney, Daniel Q. 1993. "Unorthodox Care Common in Study," *Harrisburg* (Pa.) *Patriot-News.* January 28.

Harmer, Ruth Mulvey. 1963. *The High Cost of Dying.* New York: Crowell-Collier Press.

Haug, Marie, and Levin, Bebe. 1983. *Consumerism in Medicine: Challenging Physician Authority.* Beverly Hills, Calif.: Sage Publications.

Health Smart. 1992. Newsletter of Holy Spirit Hospital, Camp Hill, Penn. February.

"He Fills Need with Pet Burial Business." 1992. *Carlisle* (Pa.) *Sentinel.* November 16.

Hilts, Philip. 1992. "Quality and Low Cost of Medical Care Lure Americans on Border to Mexico," *New York Times.* November 23.

Hinton, John. 1976. *Dying.* England: Penguin Books.

Hoefler, J., and Kamoie, B. 1992. "The Right to Die: State Courts Lead Where Legislatures Fear to Tread." *Law & Policy.* Vol. 14, No. 4. October, pp. 337–380.

"Hospitals Establish Policies to Limit Futile Care." 1993. *Hospital Ethics.* September-October, pp. 10–15.

Humphry, Derek, and Wickett, Ann. 1986. *The Right to Die: Understanding Euthanasia.* New York: Harper & Row.

"Indiana Court Backs Family in Allowing Daughter to Die." 1991. *New York Times.* September 17.

Jackson, Charles O. 1980. "Death Shall Have No Dominion: The Passing of the World of the Dead in America." In Richard A. Kalish, ed., *Perspectives on Death and Dying: Vol. 1. Death and Dying: Views from Many Cultures.* New York: Baywood, pp. 47–55.

Jacobsen, Cynthia. 1992. "Mother, Daughter Share Story Of Struggle," *Carlisle* (Pa.) *Sentinel.* December 12.

Janini, Jose. 1958. "La Operation Quirurgica, Remedio Ordinario." *Revista Espanola de Teologia.* Vol. 335.

Johnson, Gretchen L., ed. 1987. *Voluntary Euthanasia: A Comprehensive Bibliography.* Los Angeles: National Hemlock Society.

Joint Commission on Accreditation for Hospital Organizations (JCAHO). 1987 and 1992. *Manual of Hospitals.* Chicago: JCAHO.

"Judge Rejects Request by Doctors to Remove a Patient's Respirator." 1991. *New York Times.* July 2.

"Judge Strikes Down Michigan's Assisted-Suicide Ban." 1993. *Carlisle* (Pa.) *Sentinel.* May 21.

Kalish, Richard A., ed. 1980a. *Death and Dying: Views from Many Cultures.* New York: Baywood.

_____. 1980b. *Death, Dying, Transcending.* New York: Baywood.

_____. 1980c. *Caring Relationships: The Dying and the Bereaved.* New York: Baywood.

Kalish, Richard A., and Reynolds, David K. 1976. *Death and Ethnicity: A Psychocultural Study.* Los Angeles: University of Southern California Press.

Kastenbaum, Robert, and Kastenbaum, Beatrice. 1989. *The Encyclopedia of Death.* Phoenix, Ariz.: Oryx Press.

Kato, Shigeru. 1990. "Japanese Perspectives on Euthanasia." In Arthur S. Berger and Joyce Berger, eds. *To Die or Not to Die?* New York: Praeger Press.

Katzman, Abner. 1992. "Report Proposes Infant Mercy-Killing," *Harrisburg* (Pa.) *Patriot-News.* July 30.

Kay, W. J., Nieburg, H. A., Kutscher, A. H., Grey, R. M., and Fudin, C. E., eds. 1984. *Pet Loss and Human Bereavement.* Ames: Iowa State University Press.

Kelly, Alfred Hinsey, and Harbison, Winfred A. 1976. *The American Constitution: Its Origins and Development.* 5th ed. New York: W. W. Norton.

Kelly, Gerald. 1958. *Medico-Moral Problems.* St. Louis: Catholic Hospital Association.

Kenney, Stephen C. 1990. "Death and Life Decisions: Who Is in Control?" *Loyola of Los Angeles Law Review,* Vol. 23, pp. 791–828.

"Kevorkian at Suicide Scene." 1993. *Carlisle* (Pa.) *Sentinel.* September 10.

"Kevorkian Criticizes Proposed Assisted Suicide Ban." 1992. *Carlisle* (Pa.) *Sentinel.* December 5.

Kevorkian, Jack. 1991. *Prescription: Medicine.* Buffalo, N.Y.: Prometheus Books.

_____. 1992. Comments made before the National Press Club, Washington, D.C., October 27.

Kingdon, John W. 1984. *Agendas, Alternatives, and Public Policies.* Boston: Little, Brown.

Klawans, Harold L. 1992. *Life, Death, and In Between: Tales of Clinical Neurology.* New York: Paragon House.

Knowles, John H., ed. 1977a. *Doing Better and Feeling Worse.* New York: W. W. Norton.

_____. 1977b. "The Responsibility of the Individual." In John H. Knowles, ed., *Doing Better and Feeling Worse.* New York: W. W. Norton.

Kolata, Gina. 1992a. "A Malformed Infant's Brief Life Forces an Issue of Medical Ethics," *New York Times.* April 5.

_____. 1992b. "Ethicists Debate New Definition of Death," *New York Times.* April 29.

Krantz, S. 1977. *Supplement to the Law of Corrections and Prisoners' Rights.* Sec. 2, chap. 6, p. 28. St. Paul, Minn.: West Publishing.

Krauthammer, Charles. 1992. "The Case of Baby Theresa," *Washington Post.* April 3.

Kronmiller, Wendy Ann. 1988. "A Necessary Compromise: The Right to Forego Artificial Nutrition and Hydration Under Maryland's Life-Sustaining Procedures Act." *Maryland Law Review.* Vol. 47, pp. 1188–1218.

Krucoff, Nancy. 1992. "Fit over 40: Can Exercise Fight the Effects of Aging?" *Washington Post: Health.* January 7.

Kübler-Ross, Elisabeth. 1969. *On Death and Dying.* New York: Macmillan.

Kushner, Harold. 1981. *When Bad Things Happen to Good People.* New York: Avon.

LaFleur, W. R. 1974. "Japan." In F. H. Holck, ed., *Death and Eastern Thought: Understanding Death in Eastern Religions and Philosophies.* Nashville, Tenn.: Abingdon Press, pp. 226–256.

"Last Year Often Poor, Lonely." 1992. *Carlisle* (Pa.) *Sentinel.* December 30.

Lear, Martha W. 1993. "Should Doctors Tell the Truth? The Case Against Terminal Candor," *New York Times Magazine.* January 24.

Leone, Bruno, ed. 1987. *Opposing Viewpoints Sources: Death/Dying.* St. Paul, Minn.: Greenhaven Press.

Lerner, Monroe. 1977. "When, Why, and Where People Die." In James P. Carse and Arlene B. Dallery, eds., *Death and Society: A Book of Reading and Sources.* New York: Harcourt Brace Jovanovich, pp. 441–464.

"Let the Patient Decide." 1990. *Washington Post.* December 3.

Levin, Betty W. 1988. "The Cultural Context of Decision Making for Catastrophically Ill Newborns: The Case of Baby Jane Doe." In Karen L. Michaelson, *Childbirth in America: Anthropological Perspectives.* South Hadley, Mass.: Bergin and Garvey, pp. 178–193.

Lewin, Tamar. 1990. "Doctor Cleared of Murdering Woman with Suicide Machine," *New York Times.* December 14.

———. 1991. "Despite Daughter's Death, Parents Pursue Right to Die," *New York Times.* July 28.

———. 1993. "Man Is Allowed to Let Daughter Die," *New York Times.* January 27.

Lofland, Lyn H. 1978. *The Craft of Dying.* Beverly Hills, Calif.: Sage Publications.

Lueck, Thomas. 1992. "2 Convicted of Mail Fraud in Pet Burials." *New York Times,* January 17.

Lutz, Helene A. 1990. "Ethical Perspectives on the Right to Die: A Case Study." In Arthur S. Berger and Joyce Berger, eds., *To Die or Not to Die?* New York: Praeger Press.

Lyall, Sarah. 1991. "Pet Burials Rivaling Some for People," *New York Times.* July 1.

Maguire, Daniel C. 1974. *Death by Choice.* Garden City, N.Y.: Doubleday.

Malcolm, Andrew. 1990a. "Giving Death a Hand: Rending Issue," *New York Times.* June 9.

———. 1990b. "Judge Allows Feeding-Tube Removal," *New York Times.* December 15.

Margolick, David. 1993. "New Level of Debate Arising over Doctor-Assisted Suicide," *New York Times.* February 22.

Mayo, Thomas Wm. 1990. "Constitutionalizing the Right to Die." *Maryland Law Review.* Vol. 49, pp. 103–155.

McLean, Barbara G., and Townsend, Pegeen. 1990. *The Right to Die.* Legislative Report Series. Vol. 8, No. 2. Annapolis, Md.: Research Division of Legislative Reference, State of Maryland.

Meisel, Alan. 1989. *The Right to Die.* New York: John Wiley & Sons.

Melville, Keith. 1992. *The Health Care Crisis.* New York: McGraw-Hill.

Michaelson, Karen L. 1988. *Childbirth in America: Anthropological Perspectives.* South Hadley, Mass.: Bergin & Garvey.

"Michigan Doctor at Side of 4th Suicide." 1992. *New York Times.* May 16.

Miles, Steven H. 1991. "Informed Demand for Non-Beneficial Medical Treatment." *New England Journal of Medicine*. Vol. 325, No. 7. August 15, pp. 512–515.

"Missouri Court Rejects Moving Comatose Woman." 1991. *New York Times*. March 6.

"Missouri Justices Get Father's Case." 1991. *New York Times*. April 22.

Mitford, Jessica. 1963. *The American Way of Death*. New York: Simon and Schuster.

———. 1973. *Kind and Usual Punishment: The Prison Business*. New York: Knopf.

Mollaret, P., and Goulon, M. 1959. "Le Coma Dépassé." *Review of Neurology*, Vol. 101, pp. 3–18.

Moody, Raymond. 1975. *Life After Death*. Covington, Ga.: Mockingbird Books.

Morgan, John D. 1989. "Death Themes Through History." In Robert Kastenbaum and Beatrice Kastenbaum, *Encyclopedia of Death*. Phoenix, Ariz.: Oryx Press.

Morganthau, Tom, Barrett, Todd, and Washington, Frank. 1993. "Dr. Kevorkian's Death Wish," *Newsweek*. March 8.

Nader, Ralph. 1965. *Unsafe at Any Speed*. New York: Grossman.

National Center for State Courts (NCSC). 1992. *Guidelines for State Court Decision Making in Life-Sustaining Medical Treatment Cases*. 2d ed. Williamsburg, Va.: NCSC.

National Conference of Commissioners on Uniform State Laws. 1989. "Uniform Rights of the Terminally Ill Act." Presented at the Uniform Law Commissioners Annual Conference, Kauai, Hawaii, July 28–August 4.

The National Hemlock Society. 1993. Membership application and promotional brochure. Eugene, Ore.: The National Hemlock Society.

Newman, Marvin E. 1990. "Active Euthanasia in the Netherlands." In Arthur S. Berger and Joyce Berger, eds. *To Die or Not to Die?* New York: Praeger Press.

"New Review in Missouri Right-to-Die Case." 1991. *New York Times*. December 2.

Nordheimer, Jon. 1990. "High-Tech Medicine at High-Rise Costs Is Keeping Pets Fit," *New York Times*. September 17.

Oken, Donald. 1961. "What to Tell Cancer Patients: A Study of Medical Attitudes." *Journal of the American Medical Association*. Vol. 175, pp. 86–94.

Olen, Helaine. 1991. "Studies Challenge AMA View on Evils of Malpractice Suits," *Los Angeles Times*. October 29.

Oleszek, Walter J. 1989. *Congressional Procedures and the Policy Process*. Washington, D.C.: Congressional Quarterly Press.

Opperman, Kathleen M. 1988. "Termination of Life-Sustaining Treatment: Who and How to Decide?" *New York Law School Review*. Vol. 33, pp. 469–507.

"Organ Donations Barred by Judge." 1992. *New York Times*. March 28.

"Overspecialized Doctors Raise Costs, Group Says." 1992. *Carlisle* (Pa.) *Sentinel*. September 2.

"Pair Get $1.2 Million over Pet Grave." 1992. *Carlisle* (Pa.) *Sentinel*. September 1.

Paradis, Norman. 1992. "Making a Living off the Dying," *New York Times*. April 25.

"Patient Rights." 1992. In *Accreditation Manual for Hospitals*. Chicago: Joint Commission on Accreditation for Hospital Organizations, pp. 103–105.

Pearson, Durk, and Shaw, Sandy. 1982. *Life Extension: A Practical Scientific Approach*. New York: Warner Books.

———. 1984. *Life Extension Companion*. New York: Warner Books.

Pelligrino, E. D. 1991. Public comments made during symposium, "Health Care: A Right or a Privilege?" Thomas Jefferson University Hospital, Philadelphia, Pa., April 6, 1991.

"Peri Picks." 1992. *Newsweek.* August 17.

Physicians' Desk Reference for Nonprescription Drugs. 1992. Oradell, N.J.: Medical Economics.

Physician's Desk Reference to Pharmaceutical Specialties and Biologicals. Oradell, N.J.: Medical Economics.

Pine, Vanderlyn R. 1980. "Social Organization and Death." In Richard A. Kalish, ed., *Perspectives on Death and Dying: Vol. 3. Death, Dying, Transcending.* New York: Baywood, pp. 88–92.

Plough, Alonzo L. 1986. *Borrowed Time.* Philadelphia: Temple University Press.

Pollock, Stewart G. 1985. "Adequate and Independent State Grounds as a Means of Balancing the Relationship Between State and Federal Courts." *Texas Law Review.* Vol. 63, pp. 977–993.

President's Commission for the Study of Ethical Problems in Medicine and Biomedical and Behavioral Research. 1981. *Defining Death.* Washington, D.C.: U.S. Government Printing Office.

———. 1983. *Deciding to Forego Life-Sustaining Treatment.* Washington, D.C.: U.S. Government Printing Office.

Prodis, Julia. 1993. "Kevorkian Hospitalized After Release from Jail," *Harrisburg* (Pa.) *Patriot-News.* December 18.

Quill, Timothy E. 1991. "Death and Dignity: A Case of Individualized Decision Making." *New England Journal of Medicine.* Vol. 324, No. 10, pp. 691–694.

———. 1993. *Death and Dignity: Making Choices and Taking Charge.* New York: W. W. Norton.

Ray, Robert B. 1985. *A Certain Tendency of the Hollywood Cinema, 1930–1980.* Princeton, N.J.: Princeton University Press.

Reinhold, Robert. 1992. "California to Decide if Doctors Can Aid in Suicide," *New York Times.* October 9.

Reiser, Stanley Joel. 1977. "Therapeutic Choice and Moral Doubt in a Technological Age." In John H. Knowles, ed., *Doing Better and Feeling Worse.* New York: W. W. Norton, pp. 47–56.

Roan, Shari. 1991. "Doctor Describes Aiding Cancer Patient's Suicide," *Los Angeles Times.* March 8.

Robertson, Douglas K. 1985. "Washington's Judicial Development of the Right to Die." *Willamette Law Review.* Vol. 21, pp. 847–884.

Rogers, Carla. 1992. Minutes of the Thomas Jefferson University Hospital Ethics Committee. April 7, pp. 1–2.

Rogo, D. Scott. 1985. *The Search for Yesterday.* Englewood Cliffs, N.J.: Prentice-Hall.

Rolde, Neil. 1992. *Your Money or Your Health: America's Cruel Bureaucratic, and Horrendously Expensive Health Care System—How It Got That Way and What to Do About It.* New York: Paragon House.

Rosenbaum, Jerry. 1992. Personal communication.

Rosenblatt, Stanley M. 1992. *Murder of Mercy: Euthanasia on Trial.* Buffalo, N.Y.: Prometheus Books.

Rosenthal, Alan. 1981. *Legislative Life.* New York: Harper & Row.

Rosenthal, Elisabeth. 1991. "In Matters of Life and Death, The Dying Take Control," *New York Times.* August 18.

———. 1992. "Commercial Diets Lack Proof of Their Long Term Success," *New York Times.* November 24.

Rothman, David. 1991. *Strangers at the Bedside.* New York: Basic Books.

———. 1992. "Rationing Life." *New York Review of Books.* March 5.

Sabatino, Charles P. 1990. "Health Care Powers of Attorney: An Introduction and Sample Form." American Bar Association Commission on Legal Problems of the Elderly. Washington, D.C.: American Bar Association.

Savage, Robert L. 1984. "When a Policy's Time Has Come: Cases of Rapid Policy Diffusion." *Publius.* Vol. 15, No. 3, pp. 111–125.

———. 1985. "Diffusion Research Traditions and the Spread of Policy Innovations in a Federal System." *Publius.* Vol. 15, No. 4, pp. 1–27.

Schapira, David V. 1990. "The Right to Die: Perspectives of the Patient, the Family, and the Health Care Provider." In Arthur S. Berger and Joyce Berger, eds., *To Die or Not to Die?* New York: Praeger Press, pp. 3–12.

Scheuerle, James. 1989. "The Present Status of the Right-to-Die in Michigan: Decision-Making for Incompetent Individuals." *Detroit College of Law Review.* Vol. 1989, pp. 715–736.

Schneiderman, Lawrence J., and Spragg, Roger G. 1988. "Ethical Decisions in Discontinuing Mechanical Ventilation." *New England Journal of Medicine.* Vol. 318, pp. 984–988.

Schoenfeld, C. G. 1978. "Mercy Killing and the Law: A Psychoanalytically Oriented Analysis." *Journals of Psychiatry and Law.* Vol. 6(2), pp. 48–57.

Schulz, Richard, and Anderman, David. 1980. "How the Medical Staff Copes with Dying Patients: A Critical Review." In Richard A. Kalish, ed., *Perspectives on Death and Dying: Vol. 2. Caring Relationships: The Dying and the Bereaved.* New York: Baywood, pp. 134–144.

"Second Missouri Father Blocked from Letting Comatose Daughter Die." 1990. *New York Times.* December 31.

Shapiro, Andrew L. 1992. *We're Number One: Where America Stands—and Falls—in the New World Order.* New York: Vintage.

Shurkin, Joel. 1992. "Eat Less, Live Longer," *Los Angeles Times: Health Horizons.* March 29.

Simons, Marlise. 1993. "Dutch Parliament Approves Law Permitting Euthanasia," *New York Times.* February 10.

Sinclair, Upton. 1988. *The Jungle.* New York: New American Library.

Smith, John M. 1992. *Women and Doctors.* New York: Atlantic Monthly Press.

Smith, Walter J. 1985. *Dying in the Human Life Cycle.* New York: Holt, Rinehart and Winston.

Society for the Right to Die. 1991. *State Law Governing Durable Power of Attorney, Health Care Agents, Proxy Appointments.* New York: Society for the Right to Die.

Solomon, M. Z., O'Donnell, L., Jennings, B., Guilfoy, V., Wolf, S., Nolan, K., Jackson, R., Koch-Weser, D., and Donnelley, S. 1993. "Decisions Near the End of Life: Professional Views on Life-Sustaining Treatments." *American Journal of Public Health.* Vol. 83, No. 1. January, pp. 14–23.

Sprung, Charles L. 1990. "Changing Attitudes and Practices in Forgoing Life-Sustaining Treatments." *Journal of the American Medical Association.* Vol. 263, No. 16, pp. 2211–2215.

Starr, Paul. 1982. *The Social Transformation of American Medicine.* New York: Basic Books.

"State Makes Public Videotape in Right-to-Die Case." 1991. *New York Times.* February 5.

Stein, Howard F. 1990. *American Medicine as Culture.* Boulder, Colo.: Westview Press.

Stinson, Robert, and Stinson, Peggy. 1983 (originally published in 1976). *The Long Dying of Baby Andrew.* Boston, Mass.: Little, Brown.

Stout, Hilary. 1993. "Clinton's Health Plan Must Face Huge Costs of a Person's Last Days," *Wall Street Journal.* March 22.

Strauss, B. V. 1977 (1951). "The Role of the Physician's Personality in Medical Practice (Psychotherapeutic Medicine)." *New York State Journal of Medicine,* Vol. 51. Reprinted in *Elmcrest Classic of the Month* (Elmhurst Psychiatric Institute. Portland, Conn.) 1977. Vol. 2, No. 6. June, p. 2.

"Suicide Assistance Gains New Backing." 1992. *New York Times.* November 5.

"Suicide Law Struck Down, But Kevorkian Stays Jailed." 1993. *New York Times.* December 14.

"Suicide Tried to Back Out?" 1993. *Carlisle* (Pa.) *Sentinel.* February 26.

Sullivan, Joseph. 1990. "New Jersey Court Seen as Leader on Rights," *New York Times.* July 18.

Templer, Donald Irvin. 1970. "The Construction and Validation of a Death Anxiety Scale." *Journal of General Psychology,* Vol. 82.

United Methodist Church. 1992. "Understanding Living and Dying as Faithful Christians." In *The Book of Resolutions of the United Methodist Church: 1992.* Nashville, Tenn.: United Methodist Publishing House, Abingdon Press, pp. 140–150.

"U.S. Says 349,000 Caesareans Last Year Were Unnecessary." 1993. *New York Times.* April 23.

Vorenberg, James. 1991. "Going Gently, with Dignity," *New York Times.* November 5.

"Waiting List Soars While Donor Rate Stagnates." 1993. *The Bank Account.* Vol. 14, No. 2. Summer, p. 1.

Walker, Jack. 1969. "The Diffusion of Innovations Among the American States." *American Political Science Review.* Vol. 63, pp. 880–899.

Walsh, Edward. 1991. "Recasting Right to Die," *Washington Post.* May 29.

Wanzer, Sidney H. et al. 1989. "The Physician's Responsibility Toward Hopelessly Ill Patients: A Second Look." *New England Journal of Medicine.* March 30, pp. 844–849.

"Washington State Voters to Address Euthanasia." 1991. *Carlisle* (Pa.) *Sentinel.* October 23.

Weisman, Avery D. 1972. *On Dying and Denying: A Psychiatric Study of Terminality.* New York: Behavioral Publications.

Wentworth, Patricia A. 1988. "Termination of Life-Prolonging Medical Treatment: An Analysis of Pennsylvania's Proposed Medical Treatment Decision Act." *Dickinson Law Review.* Vol. 92, pp. 839–862.

White, Mary Modenbach. 1984. "Right to Die—A Current Look." *Loyola Law Review.* Vol. 30, pp. 139–178.

Wildavsky, Aaron. 1977. "Doing Better and Feeling Worse: The Political Pathology of Health Policy." In John H. Knowles, ed., *Doing Better and Feeling Worse.* New York: W. W. Norton, pp. 105–124.

Wilson, J. B. 1975. *Death by Decision: The Medical, Moral, and Legal Dilemmas of Euthanasia.* Philadelphia: Westminster Press.

Wiredu, Kwasi. 1990. "On the Question of the Right to Die: An African View." In Arthur S. Berger, and Joyce Berger, eds. *To Die or Not to Die?* New York: Praeger Press.

Worsnop, Richard. 1992. "Assisted Suicide." *Congressional Quarterly Reporter.* February 21, pp. 147–167.

"Wrongful Life Suit Dismissed in Cincinnati." 1991. *Harrisburg* (Pa.) *Patriot-News.* July 31.

Case-Law Citations*

Alabama
Camp v. *White,* 510 So.2d 166 (Ala. 1987)

Arizona
Rasmussen v. *Fleming,* 154 Ariz. 207, 741 P.2d 674 (1987)

California
Barber v. *Super. Ct. of Los Angeles County,* 147 Cal. App. 3d 1006, 195 Cal. Rptr. 484 (Ct. App. 1983)

Dority v. *Super. Ct. of San Bernardino County,* 145 Cal. App. 3d 273, 193 Cal. Rptr. 288 (Ct. App. 1983)

Bartling v. *Super. Ct. of Los Angeles County* (Bartling I), 163 Cal. App. 3d 186, 209 Cal. Rptr. 220 (Ct. App. 1984)

Bartling v. *Glendale Adventist Medical Center* (Bartling II), 184 Cal. App. 3d 97, 228 Cal. Rptr. 847 (Ct. App. 1986)

Bartling v. *Glendale Adventist Medical Center* (Bartling III), 184 Cal. App. 3d 961, 229 Cal. Rptr. 360 (Ct. App. 1986)

Bouvia v. *Super. Ct. of Los Angeles County,* 179 Cal. App. 3d 1127, 225 Cal. Rptr. 297 (Ct. App. 1986)

Bouvia v. *Los Angeles County,* 195 Cal. App. 3d 1075, 241 Cal. Rptr. 239 (Ct. App. 1987)

Conservatorship of Morrison v. *Abramovice,* 253 Cal. Rptr. 530 (Ct. App. 1988)

Conservatorship of Drabick, 200 Cal. App. 3d 185, 245 Cal. Rptr. 840, cert. denied, 109 S. Ct. 399 (1988)

McMahon v. *Lopez,* 199 Cal. App. 3d 832, 245 Cal. Rptr. 172 (Ct. App. 1988)

Westhart v. *Mule,* 213 Cal. App. 3d 454, 261 Cal. Rptr. 640 (1989)

Donaldson v. *Van de Kamp,* 2 Cal. App. 4th 1614, 4 Cal. Rptr. 2d 59 (Ct. App. 1992)

Colorado
Lovato v. *Dist. Ct. in & for Tenth Judicial Dist.,* 198 Colo. 419, 601 P.2d 1072 (1979)

Department of Institutions, *Grand Junction Regional Center* v. *Carothers,* 821 P.2d 891 (Colo. Ct. App. 1991)

---

*This chart of cases was compiled by the National Center for State Courts (NCSC, 1992, p. 171) and is current through May 1992. Cases involving religious objections to medical treatment and refusals of prisoners to accept food are not included.

Connecticut

Foody v. *Manchester Memorial Hospital,* 40 Conn. Supp. 127, 482 A.2d 713 (Super. Ct. 1984)

McConnell v. *Beverly Enterprises, Inc.* 209 Conn. 692, 553 A.2d 596 (1989)

Delaware

Severens v. *Wilmington Medical Center,* 425 A.2d 156 (Del. Ch. Ct. 1980), cert. granted for questions, 421 A.2d 1334 (Del. 1980)

In re Shumosic, C.M. No. 5515 (Del. Ch. Sept. 27, 1988), reviewed in 13 MPDLR 215

Florida

Satz v. *Perlmutter,* 362 So.2d 160 (Fla. Dist. Ct. App. 1978)

In re Guardianship of Barry, 445 So.2d 365 (Fla. Dist. Ct. App. 1984)

John F. Kennedy Memorial Hosp. v. *Bludworth,* 452 So.2d 921 (Fla. 1984)

Corbett v. *D'Alessandro,* 487 So.2d 368 (Fla. Dist. Ct. App. 1986)

In re Guardianship of Browning, 568 So.2d 4 (Fla. 1990)

Georgia

Kirby v. *Spivey,* 167 Ga. App. 751, 307 S.E.2d 538 (1983)

In re L.H.R., 253 Ga. 439, 321 S.E.2d 716 (1984)

State of Georgia v. *McAfee,* 259 Ga. 579, 385 S.E.2d 651 (1989)

In re Doe, No. D-93064 (Ga. Super. Ct. Oct. 17, 1991), reprinted in 7(4) Issues L. & Med. 521

Illinois

In re Estate of Longeway, 133 Ill.2d 33, 549 N.E.2d 292 (1989)

In re Estate of Sidney Greenspan, 137 Ill.2d 1, 558 N.E.2d 1194 (1990)

Indiana

Payne v. *Marion General Hospital,* 549 N.E.2d 1043 (1990)

In re Lawrence, 579 N.E.2d 32 (Ind. 1991)

Iowa

Morgan v. *Olds,* 417 N.W.2d 232 (Iowa Ct. App. 1987)

Louisiana

In re P.V.W., 424 So.2d 1015 (La. 1982)

Maine

In re Gardner, 534 A.2d 947 (Me. 1987)

In re Swan, 569 A.2d 1202 (1990)

Maryland

In re Riddlemoser, 564 A.2d 812 (1989)

Massachusetts

Superintendent of Belchertown State School v. *Saikewicz,* 373 Mass. 728, 370 N.E.2d 417 (1977)

Custody of a Minor, 379 N.E.2d 1053 (Mass. 1978)

In re Dinnerstein, 6 Mass. App. Ct. 466, 380 N.E.2d 134 (1978)

Lane v. *Candura,* 376 N.E.2d 1232 (Mass. App. Ct. 1978)

In re Spring, 380 Mass. 629, 405 N.E.2d 115 (1980)

Commissioner of Correction v. *Myers*, 379 Mass. 255, 399 N.E.2d 452 (1979)
Custody of a Minor, 385 Mass. 697, 434 N.E.2d 601 (1982)
In re Hier, 18 Mass. App. Ct. 200, 464 N.E.2d 959 (1984)
Brophy v. *New England Sinai Hosp.*, 398 Mass. 417, 497 N.E.2d 626 (1986)
Care and Protection of Beth, 412 Mass. 188, 587 N.E.2d 1377 (1992)
Guardianship of Doe, 411 Mass. 512, 583 N.E.2d 1263 (1992)

Minnesota
In re Torres, 357 N.W.2d 332 (Minn. 1984)
In re Conservatorship of Wanglie, No. PX-91-283 (Minn. Dist. Ct. June 28, 1991), reviewed in 16(1) MPDLR 46

Missouri
In re Busalacchi, 1991 Mo. App. LEXIS 315 (1991)

Nevada
McKay v. *Bergstedt*, 801 P.2d 617 (Nev. 1990)

New Jersey
In re Quinlan, 70 N.J. 10, 355 A.2d 647 (1976), cert. denied sub nom., Garger v. New Jersey, 429 U.S. 922, 97 S. Ct. 319, 50 L. Ed. 2d 289 (1976)
In re Schiller, 148 N.J. Super. 168, 372 A.2d 360 (Super. Ct. Ch. Div. 1977)
In re Quackenbush, 156 N.J. Super. 282, 383 A.2d 785 (Morris County Ct. 1978)
In re Conroy, 98 N.J. 321, 486 A.2d 1209 (1985)
Iafelice v. *Luchs*, 206 N.J. 103, 501 A.2d 1040 (Super. Ct. Law Div. 1985)
Warthen v. *Toms River Community Hosp.*, 199 N.J. Super. 18, 488 A.2d 229 (Super. Ct. App. Div. 1985)
In re Clark, 210 N.J. Super. 548, 510 A.2d 136 (Super. Ct. Ch. Div. 1986)
In re Requena, 213 N.J. Super. 475, 517 A.2d 886 (Super. Ct. Ch. Div. 1986), aff'd, 213 N.J. Super. 443, 517 A.2d 869 (Super. Ct. App. Div. 1986)
Strachan v. *John F. Kennedy Memorial Hosp.*, 209 N.J. Super. 300, 507 A.2d 718 (Super. Ct. App. Div. 1986)
In re Visbeck, 210 N.J. Super. 527, 510 A.2d 125 (Super. Ct. Ch. Div. 1986)
McVey v. *Englewood Hosp. Assoc.*, 216 N.J. Super. 502, 524 A.2d 450 (Super. Ct. App. Div. 1987)
In re Farrell, 108 N.J. 335, 529 A.2d 404 (1987)
In re Peter, 108 N.J. 365, 529 A.2d. 404 (1987)
In re Clark (II), 151 A.2d 276, 212 N.J. Super. 408, aff'd, 524 A.2d 448, 216 N.J. Super. 497 (1987)
In re Moorhouse, 250 N.J. Super. 307, 593 A.2d 1256 (App. Div. 1991)

New York
In re Eichner, 73 A.D.2d 431, 426 N.Y.S.2d 517 (1980)
In re Jones, 433 N.Y.S.2d 984 (Sup. Ct. 1980)
In re Storar, 52 N.Y.2d 363, 420 N.E.2d 64, 438 N.Y.S.2d 266, cert. denied, 454 U.S. 858, 102 S. Ct. 309, 70 L. Ed.2d 153 (1981)
In re Lydia E. Hall Hosp. (Hall I), 116 Misc.2d 477, 455 N.Y.S.2d 706 (Sup. Ct. 1982)

In re Lydia E. Hall Hosp. (Hall II), 117 Misc.2d 1024, 459 N.Y.S.2d 682 (Sup. Ct. 1982)

A.B. v. *C.*, 124 Misc.2d 672, 477 N.Y.S.2d 281 (Sup. Ct. 1984)

Saunders v. *State*, 129 Misc.2d 45, 492 N.Y.S.2d 510 (Sup. Ct. 1985)

In re O'Brien, 135 Misc.2d 1076, 517 N.Y.S.2d 346 (Sup. Ct. 1986)

Vogel v. *Forman*, 134 Misc.2d 395, 512 N.Y.S.2d (Sup. Ct. 1986)

Delio v. *Westchester County Medical Center*, 129 A.D.2d 1, 516 N.Y.S.2d 677 (1987)

In re Beth Israel Medical Center, 136 Misc.2d 931, 519 N.Y.S.2d 511 (Sup. Ct. 1987)

Workman's Circle Home v. *Fink*, 135 Misc.2d 270, 514 N.Y.S.2d 893 (Sup. Ct. 1987)

Hayner v. *Child's Nursing Home*, RJI No. 0188-015609 (N.Y. Sup. Ct. 1988), reviewed in 13 MPDLR 353

In re O'Connor, 72 N.Y.2d 517, 531 N.E.2d 607, 534 N.Y.S.2d 886 (Ct. App. 1988, amended 1989)

Alvarado v. *New York City Health and Hospitals Corp.*, 547 N.Y.S.2d 190 (1989)

Elbaum v. *Grace Plaza of Great Neck, Inc.*, 148 A.2d 244, 544 N.Y.S.2d 840 (1989)

Gannon v. *Albany Memorial Hospital*, No. 0189-017460 (N.Y. Sup. Ct., Apr. 3, 1989), reviewed in 13 MPDLR 440

In re Hallahan, No. 16338 (N.Y. Sup. Ct., Aug. 28, 1989), reviewed in 14 MPDLR 32

In re Klein, 145 A.D.2d 145, 543 N.Y.S.2d 397 (1989)

In re Application of Kruczlnicki, IAS No. 56/189-0077 (N.Y. Sup. Ct. 1989), reviewed in 13 MPDLR 353

Wickel v. *Spellman*, 552 N.Y.S.2d 437 (1990)

Ohio

Leach v. *Akron General Medical Center*, 68 Ohio Misc. 1, 426 N.E.2d 809 [22 Ohio Op. 3d 49] (Ct. C.P. 1980)

Estate of Leach v. *Shapiro* (Leach II), 12 Ohio App.3d 393, 469 N.E.2d 1047 (1984)

Couture v. *Couture*, 48 Ohio App.3d 208, 549 N.E.2d 571 (1989)

In re Guardianship of Crum, 61 Ohio Misc. 2d 596, 580 N.E.2d 876 (1991)

Pennsylvania

In re Jane Doe, 16 Phila. 229 (1987)

Milton S. Hershey Medical Center v. *Pennsylvania Department of Public Welfare*, 565 A.2d 210 (1989)

Tennessee

Dockery v. *Dockery*, 559 S.W.2d 952 (Tenn. Ct. App. 1977)

State Dept. of Human Resources v. *Northern*, 563 S.W.2d 197 (1978)

Doe v. *Wilson*, No. 90-364-II (Tenn. Ch. Ct. Feb 16, 1991), reviewed in 14 MPDLR 404

Washington

In re Welfare of Bowman, 94 Wash.2d 407, 617 P.2d 731 (1980)

In re Welfare of Colyer, 99 Wash.2d 114, 660 P.2d 738 (1983)

Dinino v. *State ex rel. Gorton*, 102 Wash.2d 327, 684 P.2d 1297 (1984)

In re Guardianship of Ingram, 102 Wash.2d 827, 689 P.2d 1363 (1984)

In re Guardianship of Hamlin, 102 Wash.2d 810, 689 P.2d 1372 (1984)

In re Guardianship of Grant, 109 Wash.2d 545, 747 P.2d 445 (1987)

Famam v. *Crista Ministries*, 116 Wash.2d 659, 807 P.2d 830 (1991)
State v. *Yates*, 64 Wash. App. 345, 824 P.2d 519 (1992)

Wisconsin
In re Guardianship of L.W. (Lenz v. L.E. Phillips Career Development Center), 482 N.W.2d 60 (Wisc. 1992)

District of Columbia
In re A.C., 573 A.2d 1235 (1990)

Federal Cases
Union Pacific Railroad v. *Botsford*, 141 U.S. 250, 251 (1891)
Schloendorff v. *Society of New York Hospital*, 211 N.Y. 125, 105 N.E. 92 (1914)
Griswold v. *Connecticut*, 381 U.S. 479 (1965)
Roe v. *Wade*, 410 U.S. 113 (1973)
Youngberg v. *Romero*, 457 U.S. 307, 321 (1982)
Tune v. *Walter Reed Army Medical Hosp.*, 602 F. Supp. 1452 (D. D.C. 1985)
Ross Hilltop Rehab. Hospital, 676 F. Supp. 1528 (1987)
Gray v. *Romeo*, 697 F. Supp. 580 (D. R.I. 1988)
Sanchez v. *Fairview Developmental Center*, No. CV 88-0129 FFF (Tx) (C.D.Cal. March 30, 1988), reviewed in 13 MPDLR 214
Gray v. *Romeo II*, 709 F. Supp. 325 (Dist. R.I. 1989)
Cruzan v. *Director, Missouri Department of Health*, 110 S. Ct. 2841 (1990)
Planned Parenthood of Southeastern Pennsylvania v. *Casey*, 112 S. Ct. 2791 (1992)

Statutory-Law Citations

State Acts
Alabama Natural Death Act [1981], Ala. Code secs. 22-8A-1 to 10 (1990).
Alaska Rights of the Terminally Ill [1986], Alaska Stat. secs. 18.12.010 to 12.100 (1991).
Alaska Statutory Form Power of Attorney Act [1988], Alaska Stat. secs. 13.26.332 to 26.353 (1985 & Supp. 1992).
Arizona Medical Treatment Decision Act [1985], Ariz. Rev. Stat. Ann. secs. 36-3201 to 3210 (West 1986).
Arizona Powers of Attorney Act [1974], Ariz. Rev. Stat. Ann. secs. 14-5501 to 5502 (West 1975).
Arkansas Rights of the Terminally Ill or Permanently Unconscious Act [1987], Ark. Code Ann. secs. 20-17-201 to 17-218 (1991).
California Natural Death Act [1976], Cal. Health and Safety Code secs. 7185 to 7195 (West 1970 & Supp. 1989).
California Durable Power of Attorney for Health Care Act [1984, 1985, 1988, 1990], Cal. Civ. Code secs. 2430 to 2445 (West 1974 & Supp. 1993).
Colorado Medical Treatment Decision Act [1985, 1989], Colo. Rev. Stat. Ann. secs. 15-18-101 to 113 (West 1989 & Supp. 1992).
Colorado Powers of Attorney Act [1973], Colo. Rev. Stat. Ann. secs. 15-14-501 to 502 (West 1989).

Connecticut Removal of Life Support Systems Act [1985], Conn. Gen. Stat. Ann. secs. 19a-570 to 575 (West 1986 & Supp. 1992).

Connecticut Statutory Short Form Power of Attorney Act [1965], Conn. Gen. Stat. Ann. secs. 1-42 to 56 (West 1988 & Supp. 1993).

Delaware Death with Dignity Act [1982, 1983], Del. Code Ann. tit. 16, secs. 2501 to 2509 (1983).

District of Columbia Uniform Determination of Death Act of 1981 [1982], D.C. Code Ann. secs. 6-2421 to 2430 (1981 & Supp. 1989).

District of Columbia Health-Care Decisions Act of 1988 [1989], D.C. Code Ann. secs. 21-2201 to 2213 (1981 & Supp. 1989).

Florida Life-Prolonging Procedure Act [1984, 1985, 1990], Fla. Stat. Ann. secs. 765.01 to .15 (1986).

Florida Durable Power of Attorney Act [1974, 1977, 1983, 1988, 1990], Fla. Stat. Ann. secs. 709.08 (1988 & Supp. 1993).

Florida Health Care Advance Directives [1992], Fla. Stat. Ann. secs. 765.101 to .401 (1986 & Supp. 1993).

Georgia Living Wills Act [1984, 1986, 1987, 1989], Ga. Code Ann. secs. 31-32-1 to 12 (1991 & Supp. 1992).

Georgia Durable Power of Attorney for Health Care Act [1990], Ga. Code secs. 31-36-1 to 13 (1991 & Supp. 1992).

Hawaii Medical Treatment Decisions [1986], Haw. Rev. Stat. secs. 327D-1 to 27 (1986 & Supp. 1992).

Idaho Natural Death Act [1977, 1986, 1988], Idaho Code secs. 39-4501 to 4509 (1985 & Supp. 1991).

Illinois Living Will Act [1984, 1988], Ill. Ann. Stat. ch. 110½, paras. 701 to 708 (Smith-Hurd 1978 & Supp. 1992).

Iowa Life-Sustaining Procedures Act [1985], Iowa Code Ann. secs. 144A.1 to .11 (West 1989).

Kansas Natural Death Act [1979], Kan. Stat. Ann. secs. 65-28,101 to 28,109 (1992).

Kentucky Living Will Act [1990], Ky. Rev. Stat. secs. 311.622 to .644 (1990 & Supp. 1992).

Louisiana Declarations Concerning Life-Sustaining Procedures Act [1984, 1985, 1990], La. Rev. Stat. Ann. secs. 40:1299.58.1 to .58.10 (West 1992).

Maine Uniform Rights of the Terminally Ill Act [1985, 1989, 1991], Me. Rev. Stat. Ann. tit. 18-A, secs. 5-701 to 714 (West 1981 & Supp. 1991).

Maryland Life-Sustaining Procedures Act [1985, 1986, 1987], Md. Code Ann., Health-Gen. secs. 5-601 to 614 (1990 & Supp. 1992).

Maryland Durable Power of Attorney Act [1957, 1974], Md. Code Ann., Est. & Trusts secs. 13-601 to 603 (1991).

Massachusetts Health Care Proxies Act [1990], Mass. Gen. Laws Ann. ch. 201D secs. 1 to 17 (1990 & Supp. 1992).

Michigan Power of Attorney for Health Care Act [1990], Mich. Comp. Laws, secs. 700.496 (1980 & Supp. 1992).

Minnesota Living Will Act [1989, 1991, 1992], Minn. Stat. Ann. secs. 145B.01 to .17 (1989 & Supp. 1993).

Mississippi Withdrawal of Life-Saving Mechanisms Act [1984], Miss. Code Ann. secs. 41-41-101 to 121 (1981 & Supp. 1992).

Mississippi Durable Power of Attorney for Health Care Act [1990], Miss. Code Ann. secs. 41-41-151 to 183 (1981 & Supp. 1992).

Missouri Life Support Declarations Act [1985], Mo. Ann. Stat. secs. 459.010 to .055 (Vernon 1992).

Montana Rights of the Terminally Ill Act [1985, 1989, 1991], Mont. Code Ann. secs. 50-9-101 to 206 (1991).

Nevada Withholding or Withdrawal of Life-Sustaining Treatment Act [1977, 1985, 1987, 1991], Nev. Rev. Stat. Ann. secs. 449.535 to .690 (Michie 1991).

New Hampshire Living Wills Act [1985, 1992], N.H. Rev. Stat. Ann. secs. 137-H:1 to H:16 (1990 & Supp. 1992).

New Jersey Advance Directives for Health Care Act [1992], N.J. Stat. Ann. secs. 26:2H-53 to 78 (West 1987 & Supp. 1992).

New Jersey Powers of Attorney Unaffected by Disability of Principal According to its Act [1972], N.J. Stat. Ann. sec. 46:2B-8 (West 1989).

New Mexico Right to Die Act [1977, 1984], N.M. Stat. Ann. secs. 24-7-1 to 7-11 (Michie 1991).

New York Health Care Agents and Proxies Act [1991], N.Y. Pub. Health Law secs. 2980 to 2994 (McKinney 1985 & Supp. 1992).

North Carolina Right to Natural Death Act [1977, 1979, 1981, 1983, 1991], N.C. Gen. Stat. secs. 90-320 to 322 (1990 & Supp. 1992).

North Dakota Uniform Rights of the Terminally Ill Act [1989, 1991], N.D. Cent. Code secs. 23-06.4-01 to .4-14 (1991).

Ohio Durable Power for Health Care Act [1989, 1991], Ohio Rev. Code Ann. secs. 1337.11 to .17 (Anderson 1979 & Supp. 1991).

Oklahoma Rights of the Terminally Ill or Persistently Unconscious Act [1985, 1987, 1990, 1992], Okla. Stat. Ann. tit. 63, secs. 3101.1 to .16 (West 1984 & Supp. 1993).

Oregon Rights with Respect to Terminal Illness Act [1977, 1983], Or. Rev. Stat. secs. 127.605 to .650 (1990).

Pennsylvania Abortion Control Act [1993], Pa. Stat. Ann. tit. 18, sec. 3201 et sec.

Pennsylvania Advance Directive for Health Care Act [1991], Pa. Stat. Ann. tit. 20, secs. 5401 to 5416 (1975 & Supp. 1992).

Pennsylvania Power of Attorney Act [1982], Pa. Stat. Ann. tit. 20, secs. 5601 to 5616 (1975 & Supp. 1992).

Rhode Island Rights of the Terminally Ill Act [1991, 1993], R.I. Gen. Laws secs. 23-4.11-1 to .11-14 (1989 & Supp. 1992).

South Carolina Death with Dignity Act [1986, 1988], S.C. Code Ann. secs. 44-77-10 to 77-160 (Law. Co-op. 1985 & Supp. 1992).

South Dakota Living Will Act [1991], S.D. Codified Laws Ann. secs. 34-12D-1 to 12D-22 (1991).

Tennessee Right to Natural Death Act [1985, 1989, 1991, 1992], Tenn. Code Ann. secs. 32-11-101 to 112 (1984 & Supp. 1992).

Texas Natural Death Act [1977, 1979, 1983, 1985, 1989, 1990, 1991], Tex. Health & Safety Code Ann. secs. 672.001 to .021 (West 1992).

Utah Personal Choice and Living Will Act [1985, 1991], Utah Code Ann. secs. 75-2-1101 to 1118 (1978 & Supp. 1992).

Vermont Terminal Care Document Act [1982], Vt. Stat. Ann. tit. 18, secs. 5251 to 5262 (1987); tit. 13, sec. 1801 (1974).

Virginia Health Care Decisions Act [1983, 1984, 1988, 1989, 1991, 1992], Va. Code Ann. secs. 54.1-2981 to 2993 (Michie 1991 & Supp. 1992).

Washington Natural Death Act [1979], Wash. Rev. Code Ann. secs. 70.122.010 to .905 (West 1992).

West Virginia Natural Death Act [1984, 1991], W. Va. Code secs. 16-30-1 to 13 (1991 & Supp. 1992).

Wisconsin Natural Death Act [1984, 1986, 1988, 1991, 1992], Wis. Stat. Ann. secs. 154.01 to .15 (West 1989 & Supp. 1992).

Wyoming Living Will Act [1984, 1985, 1987, 1991, 1992], Wyo. Stat. secs. 35-22-101 to 109 (1988 & Supp. 1992).

Other Related Acts

Patient Self-Determination Act (PSDA): The Omnibus Budget Reconciliation Act of 1990, Pub. L. secs. 4206, 4751 (OBRA), 42 U.S.C. sec. 1395cc(f)(1) & 42 U.S.C. sec. 1396a(a) (Supp 1991)

Uniform Rights of the Terminally Ill Act, 9B U.L.A. 609 (1987 & Supp. 1992)

About the Book and Authors

RIGHT-TO-DIE ISSUES are no longer confined to the back corridors of hospitals or the front pages of newspapers that trumpet news of Dr. Kevorkian's latest assisted suicide. A perverse combination of high-tech medicine, consumerism, demographic trends, and economic realities is forcing increasing numbers of Americans and their families to deal with end-of-life decisions—decisions that were the exclusive purview of physicians in years past. As living wills proliferate and baby boomers age, the debate is bound to intensify, forcing our public policy system to face—and attempt to resolve—the cultural, legal, and emotional dilemmas embedded in this political and medical minefield.

Deathright offers the first comprehensive survey of right-to-die issues, potential policy resolutions, judicial decisions, and legislative activity throughout the fifty states. Covering everything from pet cemeteries to holistic hospices, the denial of death to death watches, and near-death experiences to the living death of persistent vegetative states, James Hoefler and Brian Kamoie provide a balanced and readable account of the current right-to-die landscape.

With a minimum of technical jargon and an emphasis on facts, figures, and engaging case studies—including the stories of Karen Ann Quinlan, Nancy Cruzan, and Jack Kevorkian—the authors clearly demonstrate the emerging challenges raised by our constitutionally protected and statutorily regulated deathright. Appropriate for health-care professionals, public policy students, medical ethicists, and anyone who will confront questions about assisted suicide, euthanasia, informed consent, or medical self-determination, *Deathright* is a book for our time.

James M. Hoefler is assistant professor of political science and coordinator of the Policy Studies Program at Dickinson College. **Brian E. Kamoie,** research assistant to Professor Hoefler, graduated from Dickinson College in 1993 and is currently a student at the George Washington University School of Law.

Index